Respiratory Nursing at a Glance

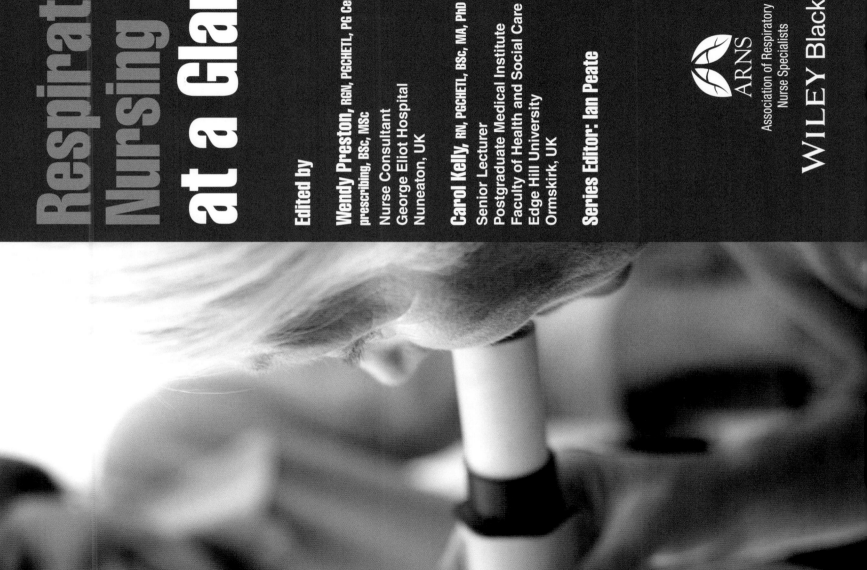

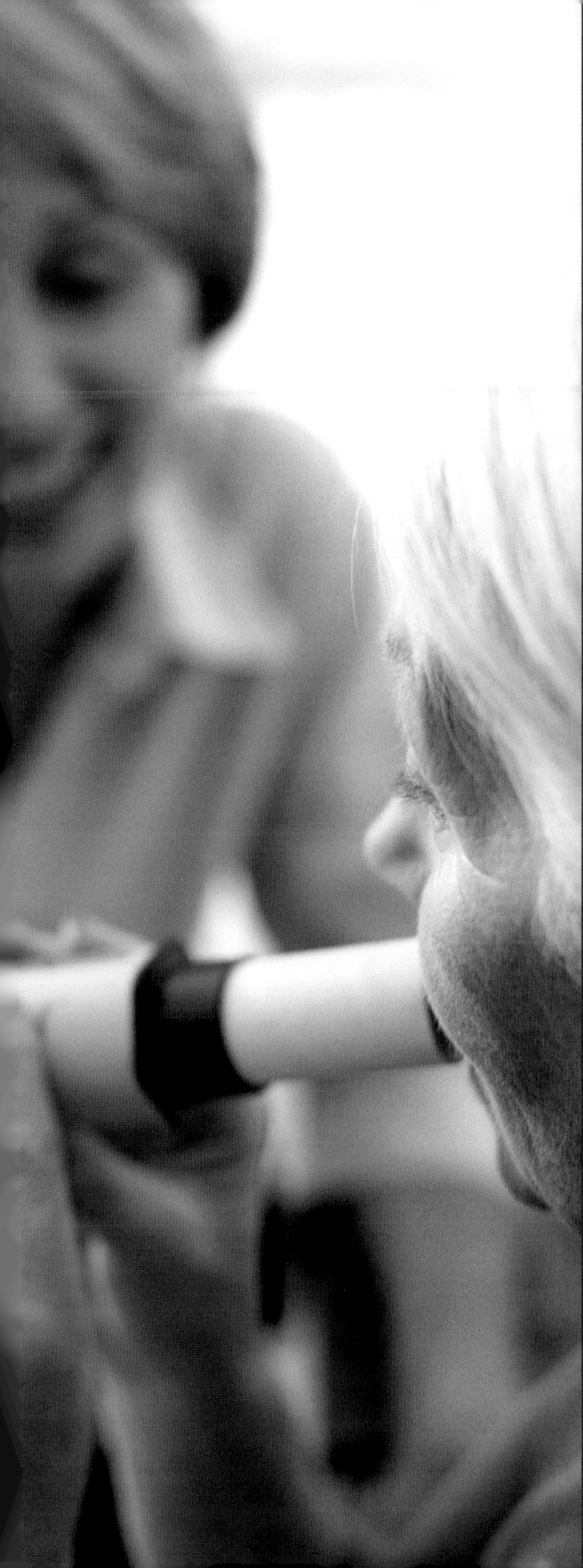

Respiratory Nursing at a Glance

Edited by

Wendy Preston, RGN, PGCHETL, PG Cert in Non-medical prescribing, BSc, MSc
Nurse Consultant
George Eliot Hospital
Nuneaton, UK

Carol Kelly, RN, PGCHETL, BSc, MA, PhD
Senior Lecturer
Postgraduate Medical Institute
Faculty of Health and Social Care
Edge Hill University
Ormskirk, UK

Series Editor: Ian Peate

ARNS
Association of Respiratory Nurse Specialists

WILEY Blackwell

This edition first published 2017 © 2017 by John Wiley and Sons, Ltd
Registered office: John Wiley & Sons, Ltd, The Atrium, Southern Gate, Chichester, West Sussex, PO19 8SQ, UK

Editorial offices: 9600 Garsington Road, Oxford, OX4 2DQ, UK
The Atrium, Southern Gate, Chichester, West Sussex, PO19 8SQ, UK
111 River Street, Hoboken, NJ 07030-5774, USA

For details of our global editorial offices, for customer services and for information about how to apply for permission to reuse the copyright material in this book please see our website at www.wiley.com/wiley-blackwell

Library of Congress Cataloging-in-Publication Data

Names: Preston, Wendy, editor. | Kelly, Carol (Carol Ann), editor.
Title: Respiratory nursing at a glance / edited by Wendy Preston, Carol Kelly.
Other titles: At a glance series (Oxford, England)
Description: Chichester, West Sussex ; Hoboken, NJ : John Wiley & Sons Inc., 2017. | Series: At a glance series | Includes bibliographical references and index.
Identifiers: LCCN 2016007514 | ISBN 9781119048305 (pbk.) | ISBN 9781119048299 (Adobe PDF) | ISBN 9781119048275 (epub)
Subjects: | MESH: Respiratory Tract Diseases—nursing | Handbooks
Classification: LCC RC735.5 | NLM WY 49 | DDC 616.2/004231—dc23
LC record available at http://lccn.loc.gov/2016007514

A catalogue record for this book is available from the British Library.

Wiley also publishes its books in a variety of electronic formats. Some content that appears in print may not be available in electronic books.

Cover image: © Getty/IAN HOOTON/SPL

Set in 9.5/11.5pt Minion Pro by Aptara
Printed and bound in Singapore by Markono Print Media Pte Ltd

1 2017

Contents

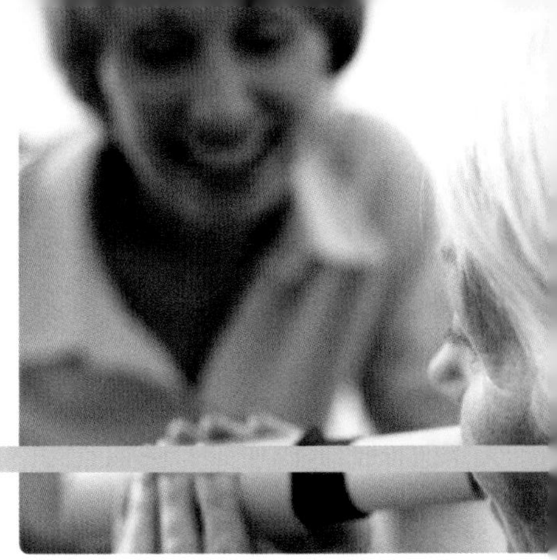

Contributors

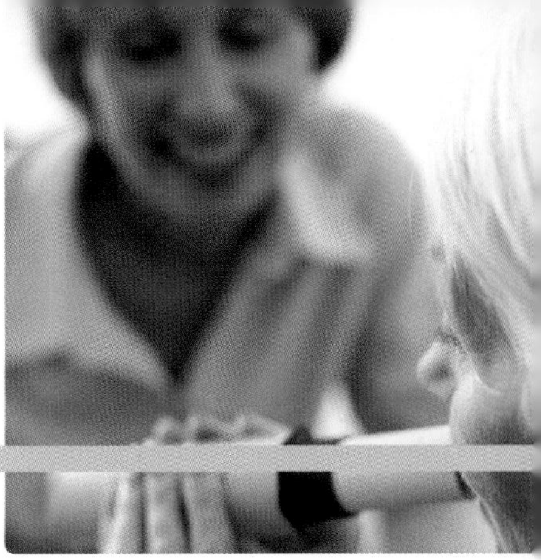

Joe Annandale, Chapters 52, 60
Katy Beckford, Chapter 11
Andrew Booth, Chapter 44
Joanne Bousanquet, Chapter 6
Michaela Bowden, Chapters 12, 45
Dave Burns, Chapters 13, 49
Julie Cannon, Chapter 32
Caroline Cowperthwaite, Chapter 30
Jo Coyle, Chapter 12
Alexander Christie, Chapter 11
Nicola Cross, Chapter 51
Jennifer Daniels, Chapter 30
Annette Duck, Chapters 55, 61
Jan Dunne, Chapter 30
Paula Dyce, Chapter 30
Jenny Fleming, Chapter 57
Elizabeth Gillam, Chapter 53
Beverly Govin, Chapter 30
Karen Heslop-Marshall, Chapters 56, 58
Matthew Hodson, Chapters 22, 25
Tracy Kates, Chapter 27
Carol Kelly, Chapters 7, 17, 57
Lynn Keogan, Chapters 59, 62
Dave Lynes, Chapter 40
Victoria Malone, Chapter 30
Mike McKevitt, Chapter 42
Shauna McKibbon, Chapters 8, 9
Tom Moreton, Chapters 26, 36, 37, 38
Sarah Murphy, Chapter 35
Sandra Olive, Chapters 19, 46, 47
Lorraine Ozerovitch, Chapter 31
Minesh Parbat, Chapter 48
Ella Pereira, Chapter 40
Wendy Preston, Chapters 2, 3, 4, 10, 29, 36, 38, 48, 54
Sam Prigmore, Chapter 5
Jaclyn Proctor, Chapter 16
Heather Randle, Chapter 3
Elaine Reid, Chapter 53
Jo Riley, Chapters 21, 43
Ann-Marie Russell, Chapters 23, 33, 34
Jane Scullion, Chapter 14
Rebecca Sherrington, Chapter 1
Clare Sumner, Chapter 30
Heidi Swift, Chapters 20, 50
Lisa Taylor, Chapter 24
Emma Vincent, Chapter 2
Liz Walker, Chapter 28
Lindsay Welch, Chapter 18
Carol White, Chapter 15
Steven Wibberley, Chapter 42
Jane Young, Chapters 39, 41

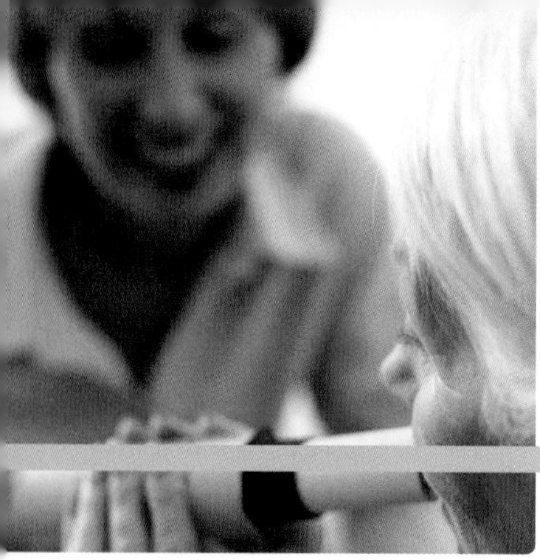

Preface

Respiratory nursing covers a diverse range of respiratory diseases including acute, chronic and acute on chronic presentations. Nurses caring for these patients need a variety of skills and approaches to provide holistic management in both the short and the long term. An insight into normal and abnormal anatomy and physiology is required but this needs to be related to the symptoms that the patient presents with; awareness of assessment, investigation, holistic treatment and care required for quality patient management are necessary in today's health care arena.

This book aims to provide a summary of topics related to respiratory nursing in an easy to read format with illustrations and diagrams to aid clarity. It is designed to provide a quick reference guide to common respiratory conditions, presentations and treatment options that require nursing care. Additionally, a focus on respiratory health will enable the nurse to promote preventative measures in both health and disease in order to prevent, minimise or control respiratory disease.

The book has been organised into parts, each containing chapters that focus on individual aspects of respiratory care. You may choose to read the book as a whole in order to gain an overview of respiratory nursing issues, or you may use it as a reference book which will guide you to further reading for each topic.

Respiratory Nursing at a Glance is aimed at nurses, health care professionals and students (nursing, medical and professions allied to medicine) at all levels providing an overview of relevant topics. As part of an established series it will be large enough to provide informative illustrations while being concise enough to provide quick reading and an overview of topics. The focus of nursing care adds depth by including holistic care from birth to death covering subjects like childhood development of the respiratory system, communication and end-of-life care. This book spans both acute and chronic spectra of respiratory disease and in doing so provides a comprehensive overview of the various disease trajectories followed by the majority of patients.

Wendy Preston
Carol Kelly

About ARNS

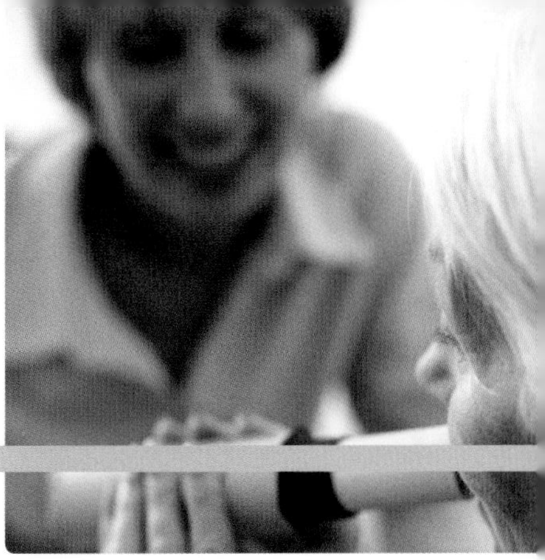

This book has been developed in collaboration with the Association of Respiratory Nurse Specialists (ARNS), which was created in 1997 by respiratory nurses and is still the only nursing-led organisation within the respiratory specialty field in the UK. ARNS has approximately 1500 members who are represented by an executive committee consisting of a broad range of expert respiratory nurses from a variety of backgrounds: nurse consultants, researchers, academics and nurse specialists working within primary, secondary and tertiary care.

ARNS collaborates with other respiratory care organisations, as well as government and NHS initiatives in order to influence policy and developments for respiratory services, such as the National Insititute for Health and Care Excellence (NICE) and British Thoracic Society (BTS) Guidelines.

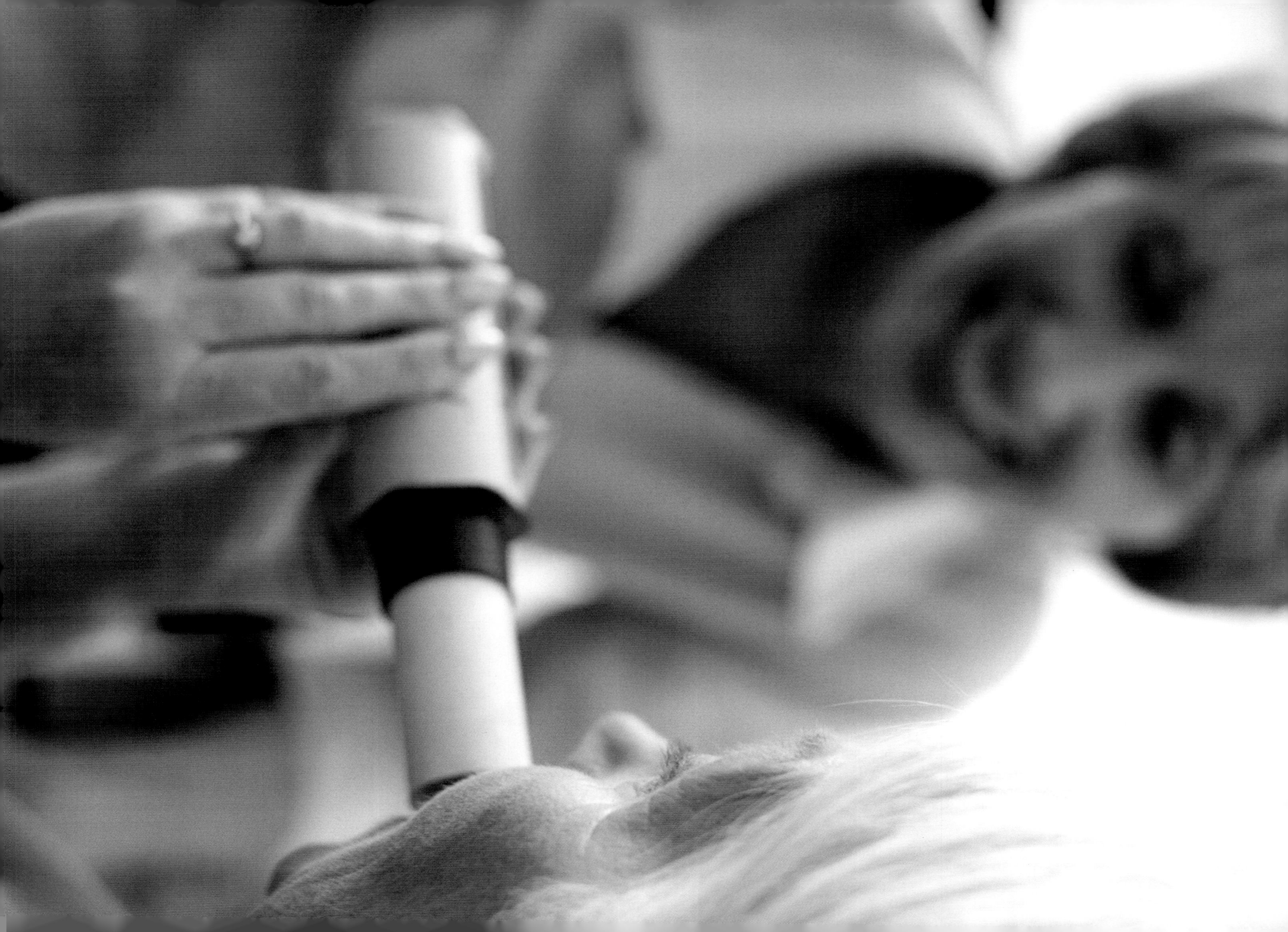

The context of respiratory nursing

Part 1

Chapters

Overview

Part 1 sets out to orientate the reader to the context of respiratory nursing, from its historical roots, through the various present day working environments where respiratory patients are cared for, and offers a vision for the future. It is hoped this will demonstrate the diversity and wide-reaching influence of respiratory nursing.

1 The origins of respiratory nursing

Box 1.1 Criteria for the nurse specialist
Source: Adapted from Giles M, et al. (2014) *BMC Nursing*, 13: 30.

- Practitioner involved in direct care
- Teacher of patients, relatives, staff and students
- Consultant for other nurses and other professions
- Researcher in relation to area of specialisation
- Change agent
- Manager

Figure 1.1 TB Ward, National Jewish Hospital
Source: https://commons.wikimedia.org/wiki/File:National_Jewish_Hospital2.jpg. CC0-1.0 public domain.

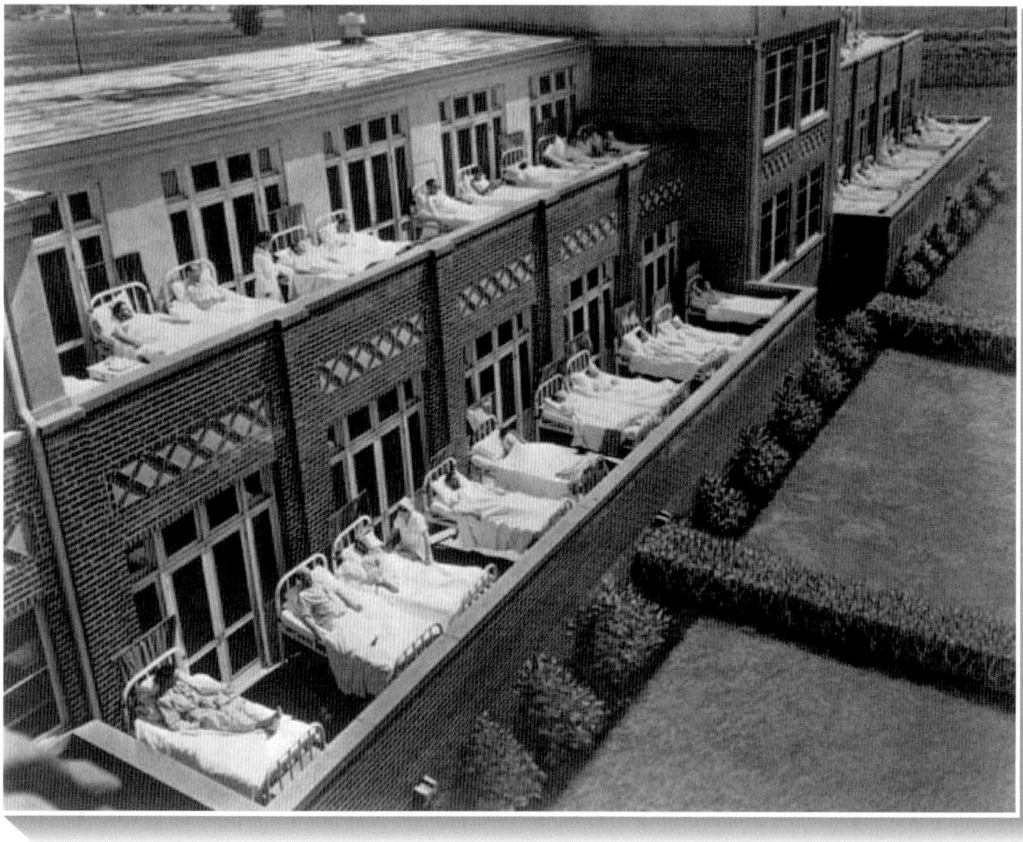

The concept of specialist nursing

Before the influence of Florence Nightingale and the advent of modern nursing, the concept of nursing specialties was unknown. Nurses were expected to provide nursing care no matter what illness afflicted their patients. Patients in hospital were not segregated according to diseases until the early years of the twentieth century, when they were placed in specific areas according to their medical diagnosis. Following scientific and medical advances made during and after the Second World War, this knowledge gave the impetus to emerging medical specialties (Donahue, as cited in MacKinnon, 2002).

While nurses have been working within specialisms for over a century, Castledine (2004) argues that the first development of the clinical nurse specialist emerged in the UK in the mid 1970s. He argued that while the numbers of specialist nurses were increasing in the early 1980s, there was lack of guidance on the criteria for such posts and the first generation of nurse specialists developed lacking direction or control. It was this lack of evaluation or audit that later led to problems in identifying the necessary characteristics of the clinical nurse specialist (Castledine, 2004).

What is a specialist nurse?

The second generation of clinical nurse specialists evolved in the 1990s in response to the publication of the Scope of Professional Practice (UKCC, 1992) and in reaction to the reduction in junior doctors' hours and shortages of medical staff. However, it was not until the publication of the PREP (post Registration, Education and Practice) report (UKCC, 1994) that specialist nursing practice was defined as 'Exercise higher levels of judgement and discretion in clinical care. Demonstrate higher levels of clinical decision making, monitor and improve standards of care through supervision of practice, clinical nursing audit, developing and leading practice, contributing to research, teaching and supporting professional colleagues' (UKCC, 1994).

Although there were more specialist nurses, particularly respiratory nurse specialists, in post by the mid 1990s, within the nursing press it was argued that very few fulfilled the criteria set out in the literature (Christmann, 1965; Peplan, 1965; Oda, 1977) and summarised by Girard (1987) (Box 1.1).

The respiratory nurse specialist

The roots of respiratory nursing can be traced to the care and management of patients with tuberculosis (TB) and included roles such as the TB family visitor (similar to today's health visitor) and the ward nurse who attended patients on the old TB wards (Figure 1.1).

Since the 1980s, as advances in medicine and changes in the delivery of health care continued, this resulted in an increasing number of respiratory nurse specialists working in a wide range of respiratory settings, for example working within TB clinics, sleep apnoea services, asthma and chronic obstructive pulmonary disease (COPD) nurse led clinics, ventilation services, pulmonary rehabilitation programmes and running nurse-led community based centres for people with respiratory disease. As the number of nurses working in respiratory care settings has increased, the improvements in knowledge and evidence of the psychosocial issues related to respiratory care, respiratory management and technologies have made a significant difference to the understanding of the needs of patients living with a respiratory condition.

Since the 1990s, the role of the nurse consultant has evolved including within respiratory care. There are a number of such posts currently established across the UK, although those roles vary and titles are inconsistent nationwide. These inconsistencies and variability in nurse consultant roles still needs to be addressed across all specialities (Giles et al. 2014).

Todays respiratory nurses

It should not be forgotten that there are many other nurses, in hospital and community settings, as well as other professionals and providers who contribute to the specialist care of the person with a respiratory condition. Frequent changes in political climate, organisational changes, rising costs, pressures on health services and rapid advance of medicine and technology over the last 20 years have inevitably led to the creation of new and more effective ways for improving health care (BTS, 2014). With the predicted demands in numbers of the population with respiratory conditions in the UK, and the evidence of increasing morbidity, change is needed if the care of people with respiratory conditions in the UK is to improve.

While it is recognised that new roles will be developed (BTS, 2014), and specialist nurses roles will continue to evolve, health care providers should recognise the contributions to respiratory care made by nurse specialists over the past 20 years. There is a need to be cautious about replacing any roles before we have a clear idea of the pros or cons of specialist nurses. Modern respiratory nursing requires skill in leadership, management and providing compassionate nursing care and also recognising the cultural, physical, psychosocial and spiritual framework in which people with respiratory diseases live.

Summary

The development of advanced or specialist nursing has been long and complex, but while this process has led to innovations and developments within nursing, it could be argued that it has also led to confusion about what specialist nursing comprises. Specialist nursing is one of the most scrutinised and researched concepts, but there is still a long way to go. Specialist nursing can be described as a role, specialist or generalist in nature, or a level of practice, and as scoping areas of clinical, managerial, educational and research skill. Far more research is needed on the role and its effectiveness within clinical practice.

Further reading

British Thoracic Society (BTS). (2014) The role of the respiratory specialist in the integrated care team: A report from the British Thoracic Society. https://www.brit-thoracic.org.uk/document-library/delivery-of-respiratory-care/integrated-care/role-of-the-respiratory-specialist-in-the-integrated-care-team-june-2014/ (accessed 20 February 2016).

2 Working in secondary care

The delivery of effective, competent and safe respiratory care is a priority for specialist nurses working within hospitals. Engaging patients in their own health care is now recognised as a major component in enhancing a service that is not only patient-centred, but also of high quality. As much respiratory care is of chronic disease, it has to be organised in a way that is integrated with other resources so that contradictions and overlaps are avoided. This signposting and sharing of resources promotes the most effective and efficient combination of health professionals needed to deliver the complex care needs of this group of patients.

The role of the respiratory nurse

The role of the respiratory nurse in secondary care is vital in coordinating a care plan that is holistic, dignified and of a compassionate nature. Holistic patient care requires a multi-disciplinary team (MDT) approach involving health care professionals from a range of health and social settings and from a variety of organisations (e.g. in the UK from the NHS and local authority). The MDT includes physiotherapists, occupational therapists, psychologists and pharmacists. All have a key role in holistic care and input which may be for a short period (e.g. to give an opinion or specific therapy) or long term as part of a care plan (e.g. care provider).

What is involved?

Secondary care predominantly addresses diagnostics in the patient with complex needs and the acute and palliative changes that occur in chronic respiratory conditions, such as asthma, chronic obstructive pulmonary disease (COPD), interstitial lung disease, bronchiectasis and cystic fibrosis. In addition, the management of infections such as pneumonia, influenza and tuberculosis are common. The respiratory nurse provides care around exacerbation management, smoking cessation, disease education, energy conservation, rehabilitation, chest clearance and palliation. The role has been identified as a key component in providing support for the patient and their carer. In recent decades the number of different types of respiratory nurses employed by the NHS has increased and become more specialised. Roles are varied, with some covering respiratory disease in general with perhaps an area of speciality, while others are very specialised and focus on patients with a particular diagnosis, for example interstitial lung disease.

Advancing practice

Different grades of nurses have evolved, with training now available to advance practice for health assessment, diagnostics and independent prescribing. Respiratory nurses can be caseworkers for their patients to allow coordination and continuity of care. The role is enhanced in many ways:

1 Problem solver
2 Advocacy
3 Educator
4 Leader
5 Signposting
6 Surrogate for resources
7 Researcher
8 Prescriber.

In turn, this specialist role can have a positive effect on NHS resources through improved nurse metrics and patient satisfaction, reduced admissions and readmissions and improved self-management strategies. However, with financial pressures putting these roles under threat, specialist nurses need to ensure they have evidence to prove they enhance services, and that they are cost effective. Audit, metrics and acquiring commissioned tariffs are crucial for long-term sustainability.

Secondary care provision varies significantly. For example, in the UK, services run across into or from primary care to provide integration and some trusts also manage GP practices. Ambulatory care provides acute care without hospital admission and is discussed further in Chapter 4.

Changing contracts, raised patient expectation and pay stagnation continue to affect morale in the current NHS. However, respiratory nursing remains a challenging and rewarding specialism which allows practitioners to assess, provide and evaluate evidence-based care on the 'front line'.

National Early Warning Score

The national Early Warning Score (EWS) is utilised in the secondary care environment to help identify patients who are clinically unstable and to prompt early escalation in their clinical management. Many hospitals use a EWS score routinely. For patients with chronic respiratory diseases their baseline score may be high because of increased respiratory rates and low oxygen saturations and in this case a modified score can be used. It is important that a comprehensive history includes the patient's baseline function and observations (e.g. oxygen saturation levels). Most systems can be adjusted to take this into account to avoid inappropriate escalation.

Further reading

Royal College of Physicians (2015) National Early Warning Score (EWS). https://www.rcplondon.ac.uk/projects/outputs/national-early-warning-score-news (accessed 20 February 2016).

3 Working in primary care

The majority of care takes place in the primary care setting, approximately 90% of care interactions in the UK. As well as general practice, primary care also covers a full range of community care such as district nursing, pharmacists and dentists.

The primary care setting is becoming more diverse to meet the needs of a growing and ageing population. This can bring opportunities for nurses and an increased range of roles and advancing practice across a 24-hour period:

- Practice nurse and advanced nurse practitioner
- Out-of-hours GP service
- Walk-in and urgent care
- District nursing
- Community matron
- Long-term condition teams
- Intermediate care (Chapter 4)
- Respiratory community services
- Smoking cessation services
- Palliative care teams (Chapter 4).

Practice nursing

Practice nursing is a vast branch of nursing ranging significantly in scope and competence level. For many patients with a respiratory condition the practice nurse will be their key contact and coordinate care, often for entire families. They carry out annual reviews for long-term conditions such as asthma and chronic obstructive pulmonary disease (COPD). Many are qualified independent prescribers who diagnose, initiate treatment and titrate to optimise symptom control, and then develop and agree self-management plans with patients (Chapter 39).

A holistic approach is required to treat the patient not the disease, as many patients have co-morbidities (e.g. diabetes and heart disease). Practice nurses are often generalists and need to be multi-skilled with competency based qualifications, for example assessing and interpreting spirometry (Chapter 21).

Scope of practice and level varies significantly depending on variables such as the size of the practice. A large multi-GP practice may have several practice nurses who have a sub-speciality (e.g. lead the COPD or asthma clinic). Their role is also pivotal in public health and making every contact count. Many are qualified stop smoking advisers (Chapters 6 and 10). There are some strategies used in primary care to promote best practice and evidence-based care. The Quality and Outcomes Framework (QOF) sets out key elements of care that are monitored to improve outcomes for patients.

The World Health Organization identified that there is a need to identify all patients nearing the end of their life, not just those with cancer. Sixty-five per cent of deaths are non-cancer related, which includes respiratory causes, and these should receive equitable care (WHO 2015). General practice is in a prime position to meet the gold standards framework in end of life care (Chapter 61).

When general practice surgeries are closed, different systems are in place to provide out-of-hours service. This provides many opportunities for nurses at a variety of levels: from telephone triage nurses who assess patients, prioritise care and signpost to other services and self-care to advanced nurses who work on the same rota as GPs to assess, diagnose and treat patients in clinic environments and on home visits. A significant proportion of the workload is respiratory disease, infections and exacerbations. Communication with patients' own GPs is important as long-term conditions can often be suspected and further investigation required.

Walk-in centres and urgent care

Walk-in centres and urgent care are similar services that can be part of the out-of-hours service. Triage is again a key role and many services are nurse led. Joined up care is essential and can influence long-term management. For example, for an asthmatic patient who has frequent exacerbations and requires repeat prescriptions for an inhaler, their practice nurse needs to be aware of this in order to prompt a review of the management plan with the patient.

Community care

Community care is organised in many ways, depending on country and region. People with long-term conditions such as respiratory diseases often need their treatment coordinating by a case manager or a community matron. These are very experienced nurses who have health assessment and prescribing skills with a key role in admission avoidance.

Traditional roles such as district nurses continue to deliver the majority of care at home to people with long-term conditions, often in conjunction with community matrons and/or case managers. It is essential that nurses in these roles receive training in respiratory disease management and are able to access the wider multi-disciplinary team.

Further reading

The Primary Care Respiratory Society UK. www.pcrs-uk.org (accessed 20 February 2016).

4 Ambulatory, intermediate and tertiary care

Care is delivered in a wide range of settings and is not exclusive to primary and secondary care. This chapter discusses the ambulatory care setting, intermediate (community) and tertiary care.

Ambulatory care

Traditionally, the care of many patients with emergency conditions has focused on inpatient hospital management but recently there has been increasing evidence that care can be safely and effectively managed out of hospital. Many acute medical conditions including respiratory disease can be effectively managed in this manner, with greater patient satisfaction. Effective ambulatory care provision is about providing same-day emergency care and avoiding admitting patients to hospital unless absolutely necessary.

The NHS as a whole is under pressure, with a shortage of acute beds. The ambulatory model used by different specialties has demonstrated a reduction in admissions and saved a considerable number of bed days. The Directory of Ambulatory Emergency Care for Adults lists pathways that can be transformed to either partial or full ambulatory care.

Ambulatory care teams work with a range of specialties to develop algorithms and pathway protocols, targeting those that GPs refer on a regular basis and seek alternatives to admission. There are some emergency department pathways that could be treated with ambulatory care thus avoiding admission. Examples of respiratory pathways:

- Respiratory infections (community-acquired pneumonia and lower respiratory tract infection)
- Pulmonary embolism
- Pneumothorax
- Pleural effusion
- Chronic obstructive pulmonary disease (COPD).

Feedback from patients and carers on ambulatory treatment has been very positive. GPs have given positive feedback to the service and on average 40% of referrals, during the service's opening times, have resulted in admission avoidance.

Ambulatory care complements services such as virtual ward and community matrons to facilitate acute review in timely manner when a patient's condition deteriorates, thus avoiding admission and disturbance of care provision. When the acute stage is resolving, care can then be transferred back to these community services or to intermediate care.

Intermediate care

Intermediate care services are provided to patients to help them avoid going into hospital unnecessarily or to help them be as independent as possible after discharge from hospital. These services are generally time-limited, until the person has regained independence or medical stability, and are provided in people's own homes, in community hospitals or sometimes within local nursing homes. They should be multi-disciplinary and include clinical assessment, therapy (e.g. chest physiotherapist) and rehabilitation.

Intermediate care is necessary to ensure that older people with complex needs are seen by the right service for their needs at the right time, preventing admissions to acute hospitals or reducing length of stay. It also helps to ensure that life-changing decisions are not made prematurely about long-term care needs.

Palliative care is an essential element of many respiratory pathways and is often required in conjunction with respiratory and generic teams. Palliative care teams are structured in various ways, discussed in more detail in Chapter 61. Patients with respiratory disease should have equal access to services and specialist advice. It should be remembered that most palliative care is given by community teams such as district nurses and education should be provided.

Tertiary care

Tertiary care is specialised consultative health care, often on an inpatient basis and on referral from a primary or secondary health professional. It usually takes place in a facility that has personnel and facilities for advanced medical investigation and treatment, such as a tertiary referral hospital. Some people with complex respiratory disease or rare conditions require referral to tertiary care.

Often, care will be shared between tertiary care and either secondary or primary care (or both). This is to facilitate the expert input for patient care while reducing the amount of times patients need to travel or be away from their relatives and carers.

Further reading

NHS Institution for Innovation and Improvement (2012) *Directory of Ambulatory Emergency Care for Adults,* 3rd edn. www.institute.nhs.uk/ambulatory_emergency_care/public_view_of_ambulatory_emergency_care/directory.html (accessed 20 February 2016).

NHS Choices (2015) Your care after discharge from hospital. www.nhs.uk/conditions/social-care-and-support-guide/pages/hospital-discharge-care.aspx (accessed 20 February 2016).

5 The future of respiratory nursing

Respiratory nurses

The need for nurses to develop expertise in caring for patients with respiratory conditions has grown steadily over the last half a century. Traditional nursing roles have been expanded, with advanced skills including physical assessment, performing diagnostic tests and non-medical prescribing. More patients with respiratory disease have benefited from the additional contribution of a holistic approach to their management, delivered by nurses. The origins of respiratory nursing lie in disease control and public health, in caring for people with tuberculosis, but as a speciality it has grown in popularity as it enables nurses to develop expertise and advanced skills and provide care in all health care settings.

Provision of health care

Current health polices (NHS 2014) focus on the need to tackle the root causes of ill health, providing individuals with more control of their care, addressing the care needs of an ageing population and the opportunity to develop and deliver new models of care, to expand and strengthen primary and out of hospital care. This has resulted in a shift in care from being hospital based to providing care closer to home. This means there is the need for specialists to be located in hospital, the community and primary care settings. This approach to care can be achieved through integrated models of care, and provides an opportunity for nurses with respiratory experience and expertise to care for people with respiratory illnesses in a range of venues, at different stages of their disease trajectories (i.e. chronic disease management or acute care).

The respiratory population

The burden of respiratory disease continues to grow, despite the advances in respiratory medicine (Chapter 9). Smoking-related respiratory disease continues to be a major public health problem and nurses' roles in smoking cessation will continue to be important (Chapter 10).

The number of premature babies surviving is increasing, many of whom will have required ventilator support. Some children require long-term ventilation, and therefore need on-going support and education. With the advances in treatment options, for example, lung transplantation, prophylactic antibiotic therapy has increased the survival rate of some inherited diseases, such as cystic fibrosis, chronic lung diseases such as chronic obstructive pulmonary disease (COPD) and interstitial lung disease.

As people are living longer, many will have respiratory disease along with other long-term conditions, which will be managed in general practice or by community-based teams. It is inevitable that many will develop an acute respiratory problem (e.g. community-acquired pneumonia), which can result in an admission to hospital for appropriate treatment and intervention.

It is therefore clear that the number of people with respiratory-related illnesses will be significant and therefore there will be the need for nurses with respiratory experience and skills to care for and support them.

Respiratory nursing in the future

The fundamentals of nursing care will be applicable to people with respiratory conditions to assist in the management of the multitude of symptoms that they may experience. All nurses should be able to check inhaler technique as many of the respiratory medications are delivered via an inhaled route, provide symptom control and slow down disease progression. Many frequently prescribed interventions are costly and therefore a value-based approach to care should be adopted.

Acute-based care

Non-invasive ventilation has significantly improved the survival rate for respiratory patients admitted with acute hypercapnic respiratory failure, in particular patients with COPD. These patients need to be cared for by staff who have experience in managing patients requiring ventilation (Chapter 52).

Advances in treatment include new drugs for some respiratory conditions such as monoclonal antibodies for severe asthma and novel treatments for idiopathic pulmonary fibrosis. These require careful assessment and monitoring, as well as administration, which could be provided by respiratory nurses. Working as part of a multi-disciplinary team, there are numerous opportunities to expand nursing roles, to provide timely diagnosis and treatment of respiratory conditions. Examples include nurses performing bronchoscopies, nurse-led pleural services and tracheostomy management.

Community-based care

For many respiratory diseases there is no cure, and the mainstay of treatment is symptom management, early identification of exacerbations and prompt intervention. This involves supporting and empowering patients to manage their conditions and ensuring regular reviews of symptoms and disease progression. For this to be effective, nurses will need to have the appropriate knowledge and expertise.

Interventions previously delivered in a hospital setting have been successfully integrated into the community setting. Support, education and review of patients with complex needs, such as patients with neuromuscular conditions requiring ventilatory support, and their carers, is essential to enable them to stay at home, and such care lends itself to nurses with respiratory expertise.

As there is no cure for many respiratory diseases, the ability to support and care for patients and their carers at the advanced and terminal stages of their illness is vital, and therefore application of specialist knowledge and expertise in both respiratory and palliative care is required.

Further reading

NHS England, Care Quality Commission, Health Education England, Monitor, NHS Trust Development Authority, Public Health England (2014) *NHS Five Years Forward*. www.england.nhs.uk/ourwork/futurenhs/ (accessed 21 February 2016).

6 Respiratory public health

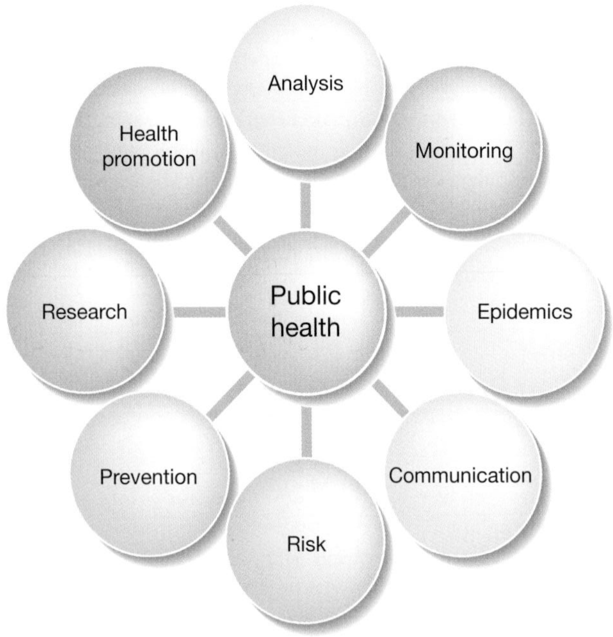
Public health
Analysis
Monitoring
Epidemics
Communication
Risk
Prevention
Research
Health promotion

Figure 6.1 Facets of public health

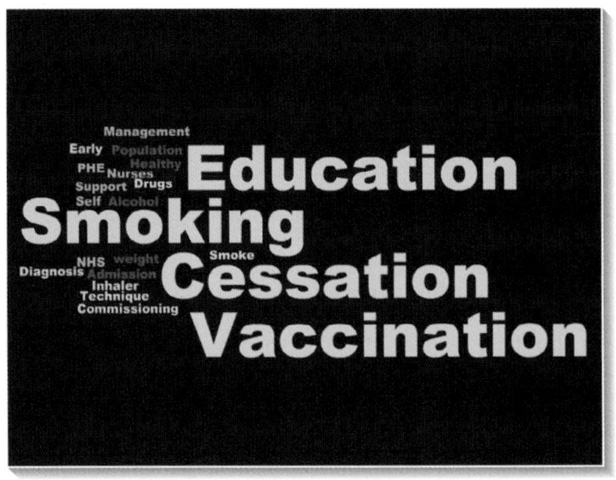
Management
Early
Population
PHE
Healthy
Nurses
Support
Drugs
Self
Alcohol
Education
Smoking
NHS
weight
Smoke
Diagnosis
Admission
Inhaler
Technique
Commissioning
Cessation
Vaccination

Figure 6.2 Public health interventions

The impact of lung diseases remains as great today as it was at the turn of the century and is likely to remain so for several decades. Each year in the European Union, one in eight of all deaths is caused by respiratory diseases and lung conditions cause at least 6 million hospital admissions (ERS, 2013). In the UK, the number of people affected by asthma is amongst the highest in the world and the UK has one of the highest asthma mortality rates in Europe (RCP, 2014).

From a public health perspective, the challenges nurses face in terms of population health and well-being are huge; however, every single nurse and midwife can act to make every contact count and become a health promoting practitioner. Nurses are in key positions to support patients at population, community and individual levels, to make decisions and choices that are positive for their health (Figure 6.1).

Population level

- An evaluation of screening for chronic obstructive pulmonary disease (COPD), against the National Screening Committee criteria, recommended against population screening as there was insufficient evidence of its effectiveness. However, they also stated that cost-effective evidence does exist for case-finding symptomatic individuals and this should continue.
- Nurses, midwives and allied health professionals (AHPs) have a role in raising awareness of health issues and influencing policies that affect health (www.arns.co.uk).
- Charity groups have a key role in respiratory public health (Chapter 29).
- The Cold Weather Plan for England sets out a series of clear actions triggered by a Met Office alert system. These actions are to be taken by the NHS, social care and other public agencies – professionals working with vulnerable people as well as by individuals and local communities themselves – designed to minimise the effects of severe cold weather on health.
- Provide the right care in the right place at the right time – agreeing locally a pathway of care – including timing and location of initial assessment and delivery of care (hospital, GP surgery, community care, or in their own home).
- Ensure structured hospital admissions – ensuring patients are seen by a respiratory specialist on admission to hospital and receive key interventions promptly, such as non-invasive ventilation for patients with COPD,and self-management plans.
- Support post-discharge – ensuring people who have been admitted to hospital with an exacerbation of COPD or an asthma attack are given support to prevent readmissions.

Commissioning

Admission to hospital is a major adverse outcome for people with COPD and is not always necessary. Because spend on COPD admissions is so high, action to prevent admissions could save substantial amounts of money as well as improving outcomes for people with COPD.

Local clinical commissioning groups that have achieved lower emergency admission rates have done so by:

- Smoking cessation services and health promotion, often in partnership with local and education authorities
- Reviewing admissions to identify frequent exacerbators
- Early discharge schemes and hospital at home services commissioned to support evidence-based admission avoidance
- Preventive care should include clear action plans, optimisation of therapy and support for self-management and home provision of standby medication
- Referral for pulmonary rehabilitation, a treatment that has been shown to reduce admissions, improve exercise capacity and improve health-related quality of life
- Prompt support for people when they develop new or worsening symptoms, with access to specialist-led care in the community.

Interventions at an individual level

See Figure 6.2.

Early diagnosis

It is important that all patients with respiratory diseases are diagnosed as early as possible so that treatment can be used to try to slow down deterioration.

Smoking

It has been well established that stopping smoking will slow the rate of deterioration of lung function and prevent flare ups. Health care professionals are advised to follow NICE guidance when providing advice and support for smoking cessation (Chapter 10).

Education

All patients with asthma should receive a written personalised action plan. These are provided as part of structured education, and can improve outcomes such as self-efficacy, knowledge and confidence. For people with asthma who have had a recent acute exacerbation resulting in admission to hospital, written personalised action plans can reduce readmission rates (Chapter 41).

Inhaler technique

Training and assessment need to take place before any new inhaler treatment is started, to ensure that changes to treatment do not fail because of poor technique (Chapter 44).

Self-management

There is good evidence that prompt therapy in exacerbations results in less lung damage, faster recovery and fewer admissions (and subsequent readmissions) to hospital. A self-management plan is essential and discussed in detail in Chapter 39.

Vaccinations

Pneumococcal vaccination and an annual influenza vaccination should be offered to all patients with chronic respiratory disease (Chapter 25).

Further reading

A Framework for Personalised Care and Population Health for Nurses, Midwives, Health Visitors and Allied Health Professionals Caring for populations across the life course (2014) https://www.gov.uk/government/uploads/system/uploads/attachment_data/file/377450/Framework_for_personalised_care_and_population_health_for_nurses.pdf (accessed 21 February 2016)

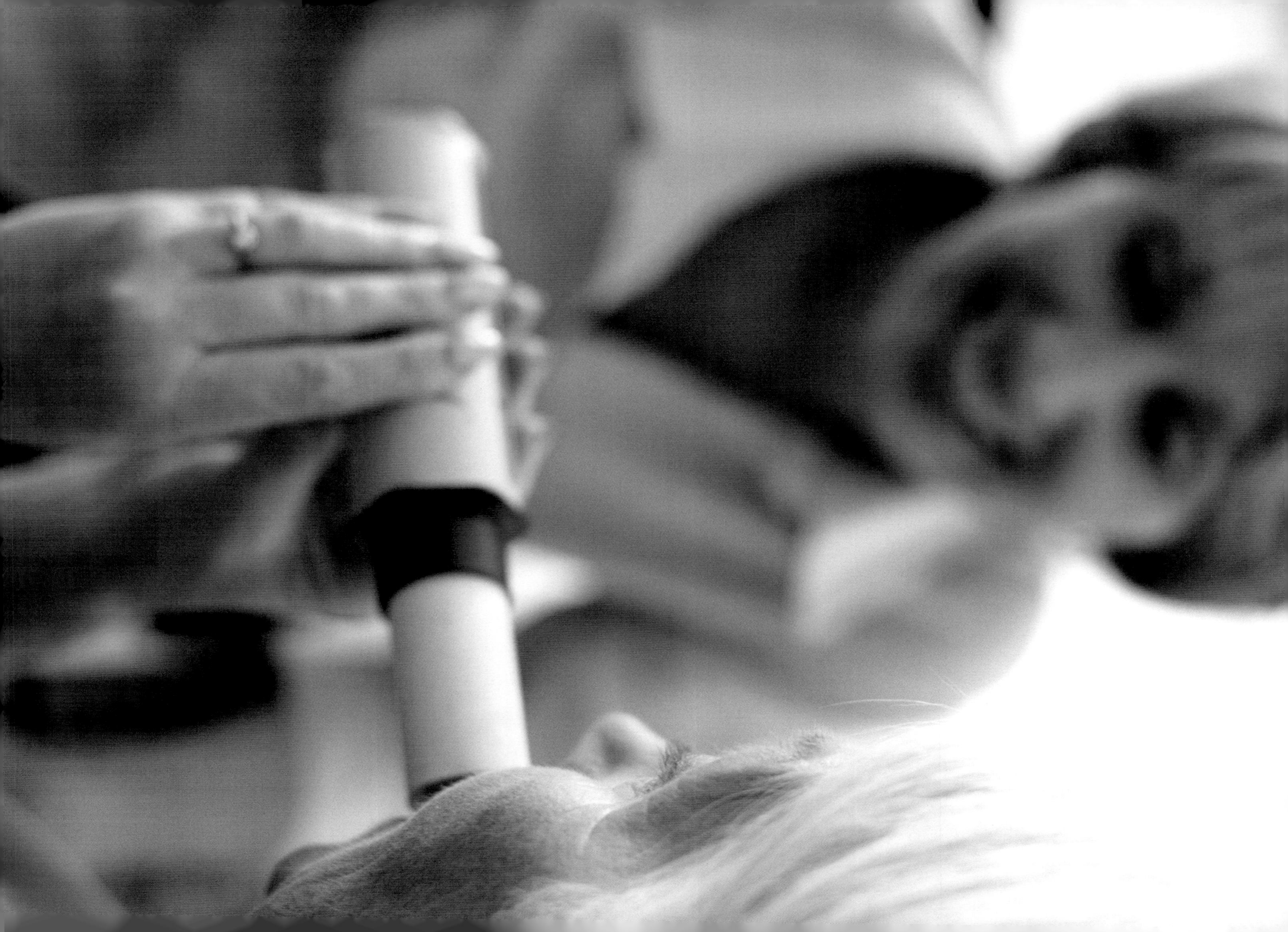

Respiratory health

Part 2

Chapters

Overview

Part 2 sets out the various influences on the health and well-being of respiratory patients, and highlights how nurses can influence this. The range of approaches is diverse and encompasses respiratory health, both with and without respiratory disease.

7 The respiratory system

Figure 7.1 Major structures of the upper and lower respiratory tract
Source: Peate I, Nair M. (eds.) (2011) Fundamentals of Anatomy and Physiology for Student Nurses. Reproduced with permission of John Wiley & Sons Ltd.

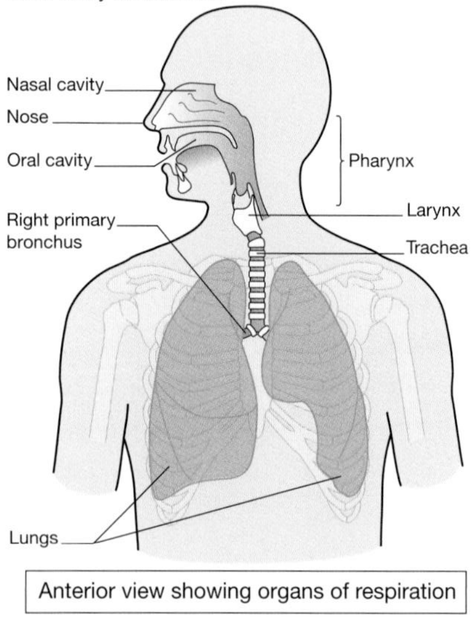

Nasal cavity
Nose
Oral cavity
Pharynx
Larynx
Right primary bronchus
Trachea
Lungs
Anterior view showing organs of respiration

Figure 7.2 The muscles involved in ventilation
Source: Peate I, Nair M. (eds.) (2011) Fundamentals of Anatomy and Physiology for Student Nurses. Reproduced with permission of John Wiley & Sons Ltd.

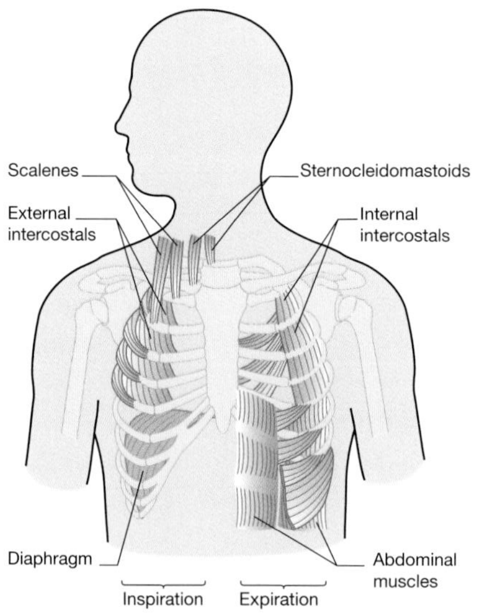

Scalenes
Sternocleidomastoids
External intercostals
Internal intercostals
Diaphragm
Abdominal muscles
Inspiration
Expiration

Figure 7.3 External respiration
Source: Peate I, Nair M. (eds.) (2011) Fundamentals of Anatomy and Physiology for Student Nurses. Reproduced with permission of John Wiley & Sons Ltd.

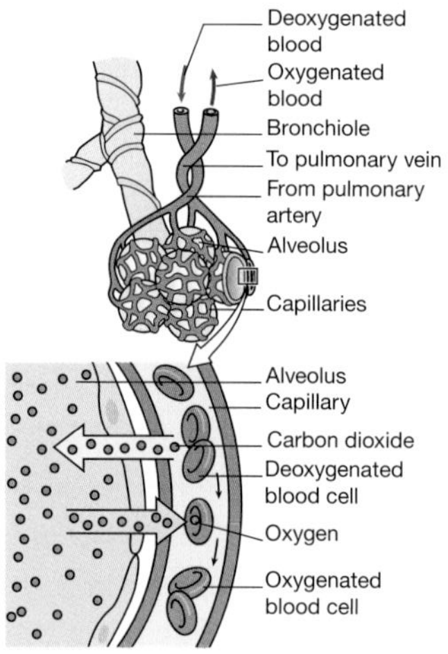

Deoxygenated blood
Oxygenated blood
Bronchiole
To pulmonary vein
From pulmonary artery
Alveolus
Capillaries
Alveolus
Capillary
Carbon dioxide
Deoxygenated blood cell
Oxygen
Oxygenated blood cell

Figure 7.4 Diagramatic representation of the major lung volumes and capacities
Source: Peate I, Nair M. (eds.) (2011) Fundamentals of Anatomy and Physiology for Student Nurses. Reproduced with permission of John Wiley & Sons Ltd.

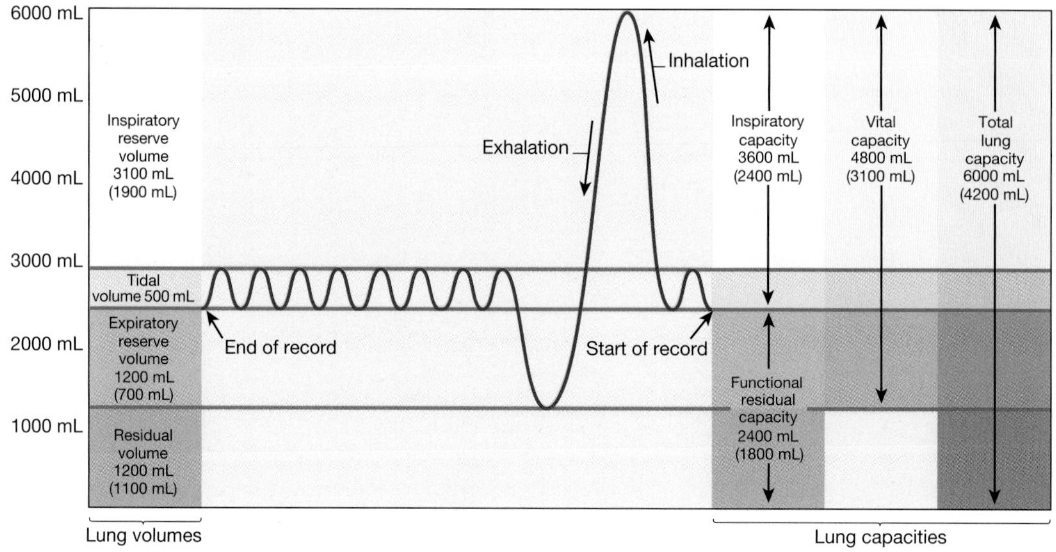

6000 mL
5000 mL
4000 mL
3000 mL
2000 mL
1000 mL
Inspiratory reserve volume 3100 mL (1900 mL)
Tidal volume 500 mL
Expiratory reserve volume 1200 mL (700 mL)
Residual volume 1200 mL (1100 mL)
End of record
Exhalation
Inhalation
Start of record
Inspiratory capacity 3600 mL (2400 mL)
Functional residual capacity 2400 mL (1800 mL)
Vital capacity 4800 mL (3100 mL)
Total lung capacity 6000 mL (4200 mL)
Lung volumes
Lung capacities

Figure 7.5 The oxyhaemoglobin dissociation curve

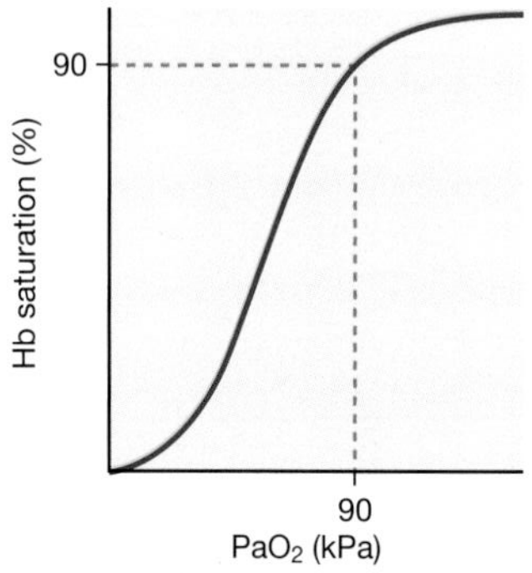

90
Hb saturation (%)
90
PaO2 (kPa)

Figure 7.6 The carriage of carbon dioxide in the blood

CO_2	+	H_2O	⇔	H_2CO_3	⇔	H^+	+	HCO_3^-
Carbon dioxide		Water		Carbonic acid		Hydrogen ions		Carbon dioxide

The respiratory system is one of the major systems of the body and primarily consists of two lungs (Figure 7.1). Its main function is to facilitate gas exchange through ventilation (the process of breathing) and respiration. Respiration can be expressed in two ways: internal respiration and external respiration. External respiration refers to exchange of gases at alveolar/capillary level, whereby oxygen enters the blood and carbon dioxide leaves to be excreted through exhalation. Internal respiration refers to metabolism at cell level were oxygen is combined with carbohydrates to produce energy; carbon dioxide is a waste product of this metabolic process.

The mechanics of breathing

Pulmonary ventilation describes the process more commonly known as breathing. In order for air to pass in and out of the lungs a change in pressure needs to occur. Before inspiration, intrapulmonary pressure – the pressure within the lungs – is the same as atmospheric pressure. During inspiration the thorax, through contraction of the diaphragm and intercostals muscles (Figure 7.2), expands and intrapulmonary pressure falls below atmospheric pressure. Because intrapulmonary pressure is now less than atmospheric pressure air will naturally enter the lungs until the pressure difference no longer exists. Expiration is the opposite: the diaphragm and intercostals muscles relax, intrapulmonary pressure increases and air is forced out of the lungs.

The work of breathing

During inspiration respiratory muscles overcome various factors that hinder thoracic expansion, including elastic recoil, resistance to airflow through narrow airways, and surface tension forces at liquid–air interface. The energy required by the respiratory muscles to overcome these hindering forces is referred to as work of breathing. Lung compliance (elasticity of the lungs), ensuring the expenditure of minimum energy, is aided by the production of a detergent-like substance called surfactant by type 2 cells within the alveloi, which reduces the surface tension occurring when the alveoli meet capillary blood flow.

Work of breathing is also required to overcome airway resistance. As air flows through the bronchial tree resistance to airflow occurs as the gas molecules begin to collide with one another in the increasingly narrow airways. Many lung diseases can affect lung compliance and airway resistance and therefore increase the work of breathing. Any increase in airway resistance and lung compliance will inevitably increase the work of breathing.

Respiration

The process of external respiration involves the movement of gases across the alveolar–capillary membrane, this movement of gases occurs through the process of diffusion. Gases diffuse along their partial pressure gradient: that is, gases move from areas of high pressure to areas of low pressure (Figure 7.3).

Transport of gases

Both oxygen and carbon dioxide are transported from the lungs to body tissues in blood plasma and haemoglobin, found within erythrocytes (red blood cells).

The major source of transport for oxygen therapy is haemoglobin (Hb), contained in red blood cells; 97% of oxygen is carried by the Hb and 3% dissolved in the plasma. Because there is a fixed amount of Hb circulating in the blood, the amount of oxygen carried is often referred to in terms of saturation of Hb.

There is a defined relationship between the partial pressure of oxygen and the percentage of saturated haemoglobin, represented by the oxyhaemoglobin dissociation curve. Importantly, this curve is not linear but sigmoid in shape: a unique property that influences saturation and desaturation (Figure 7.5) and therefore facilitates uptake and release of oxygen.

Acid–base balance

Another important function of the respiratory system is the maintenance of acid–base balance. The majority of carbon dioxide is transported as bicarbonate ions (HCO_{3-}). As carbon dioxide enters the red blood cell it combines with water to form carbonic acid (H_2CO_3). Carbonic acid then quickly dissociates into hydrogen ions (H^+) and bicarbonate ions (HCO_{3-}) (Figure 7.6). Arterial blood pH is mainly influenced by the levels of H^+; the more H^+ ions the more acidic the blood. If blood pH falls out of its optimum range of 7.35–7.45 an acid–base imbalance can occur. The respiratory system can help to maintain acid–base balance by controlling the expulsion and retention of carbon dioxide.

Volumes and capacities

Lung volumes and capacities measure or estimate the amount of air passing in and out of the lungs. Each individual has a total lung capacity (TLC), the total amount of air the lungs can contain. TLC is dependent upon age, sex and height; it can be subdivided into a range of potential or actual volumes of air. For example, the amount of air that passes in and out of the lungs during one breath is called the tidal volume (VT). After a normal, quiet breath there is still room for a deeper inspiration that could fill the lungs (IRV). Likewise, after a normal, quiet breath, there remains the potential for a larger exhalation, expiratory reserve volume (ERV). Tidal volume, inspiratory reserve volume and expiratory reserve volume can all be measured. However, because a small volume of air always remains in the lungs, total lung capacity can only be estimated, even after a maximal exhalation. This small volume of remaining air is called residual volume (RV) (Figure 7.4).

The control of breathing

The rate and depth of breathing are controlled by the respiratory centres, which are found in the brainstem. Within the medulla oblongata there are specialised chemoreceptors, which continually analyse carbon dioxide levels within cerebrospinal fluid (CSF). As levels of carbon dioxide rise messages are sent to the diaphragm and intercostal muscles instructing them to contract. Another set of chemoreceptors found in the aorta and carotid arteries analyse levels of oxygen as well as carbon dioxide. If oxygen falls or carbon dioxide rises, messages are sent to the respiratory centres stimulating further contraction. Breathing is refined by other areas in the brain to prevent the lungs from becoming overinflated.

Further reading

Wheeldon A. (2011) The respiratory system. In: Peate I, Nair M (eds) *Fundamentals of Anatomy and Physiology for Student Nurses*. Oxford: Wiley-Blackwell.

8 Preventing respiratory disease

Figure 8.1 Percentage of hospital admissions in selected European Union countries, by respiratory condition. CF, cystic fibrosis; ILD, interstitial lung disease; LRI, lower respiratory infection.
Source: The European Lung White Book Respiratory Health and Disease in Europe, 2nd edn. © 2013 European Respiratory Society, Sheffield, UK. Reproduced with permission of the European Respiratory Society.

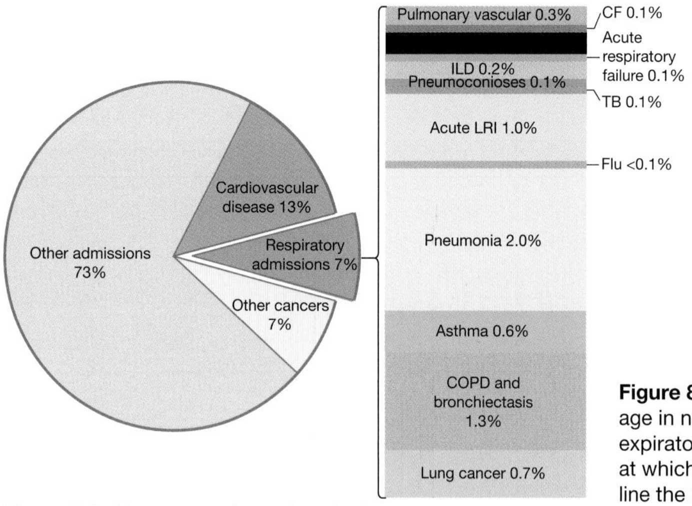

Other admissions 73%
Cardiovascular disease 13%
Respiratory admissions 7%
Other cancers 7%
Pulmonary vascular 0.3%
CF 0.1%
Acute respiratory failure 0.1%
ILD 0.2%
Pneumoconioses 0.1%
TB 0.1%
Acute LRI 1.0%
Flu <0.1%
Pneumonia 2.0%
Asthma 0.6%
COPD and bronchiectasis 1.3%
Lung cancer 0.7%

Figure 8.2 Frequency of cough and wheeze is highest in Swiss adults living close to the highway
Source: Hazenkamp-von Arx ME, et al. (2011) *Environ Health*. 10: 13.

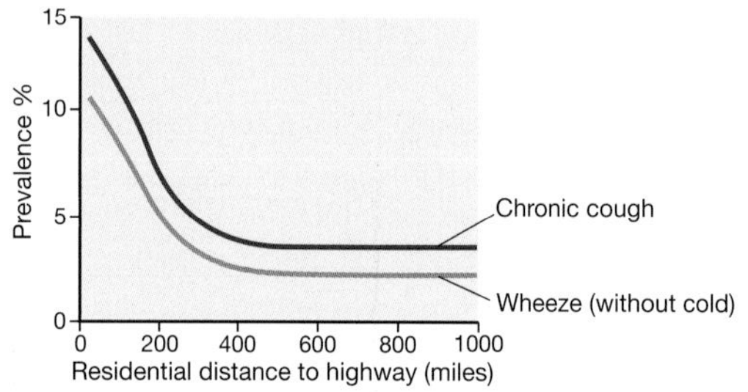

Prevalence %
15
10
5
0
0
200
400
600
800
1000
Residential distance to highway (miles)
Chronic cough
Wheeze (without cold)

Figure 8.3 The dangers of second-hand smoke exposure

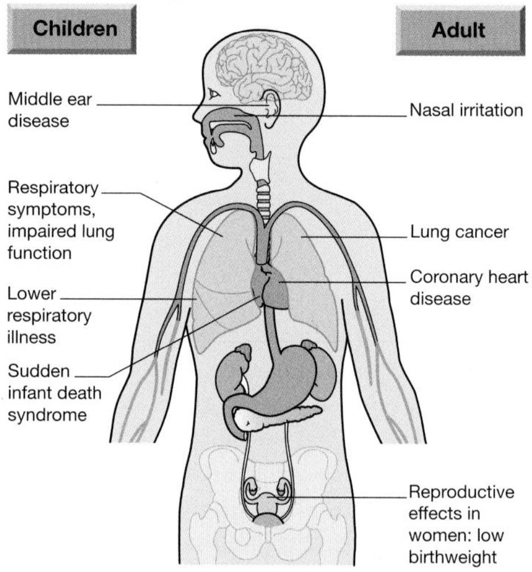

Children
Adult
Middle ear disease
Respiratory symptoms, impaired lung function
Lower respiratory illness
Sudden infant death syndrome
Nasal irritation
Lung cancer
Coronary heart disease
Reproductive effects in women: low birthweight

Figure 8.4 Schematic diagram of the decline in lung function with age in non-smokers, smokers and those who quit. FEV_1, forced expiratory volume in 1 s. The horizontal pink line indicates the level at which symptoms are likely to be disabling and the broken black line the level at which death is likely. Note that stopping smoking slows the rate of decline of lung function
Source: The European Lung White Book Respiratory Health and Disease in Europe, 2nd edn. © 2013 European Respiratory Society, Sheffield, UK. Reproduced with permission of the European Respiratory Society.

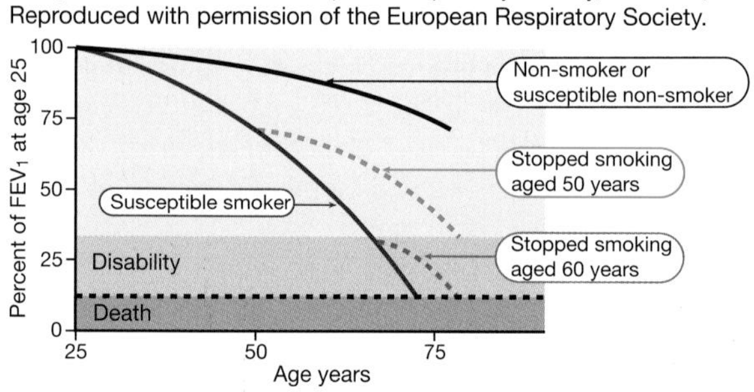

Percent of FEV1 at age 25
100
75
50
25
0
25
50
75
Age years
Non-smoker or susceptible non-smoker
Stopped smoking aged 50 years
Susceptible smoker
Stopped smoking aged 60 years
Disability
Death

Box 8.1 Clinical approach: components of a thorough occupational exposure history
Source: The European Lung White Book Respiratory Health and Disease in Europe, 2nd edn. © 2013 European Respiratory Society, Sheffield, UK. Reproduced with permission of the European Respiratory Society

- **Job type and activities:** employer, what products the company produces, job title, years worked, description of job tasks or activities, description of all equipment and materials the patient used, description of process changes and dates they occured, any temporal association between symptoms and days worked.
- **Exposure estimate:** visible dust or mist in the air and estimated visibility, dust on surfaces, visible dust in sputum (or nasal discharge) at the end of work shift, hours worked per day and days per week, open or closed work process system, presence and description of engineering controls on work processes (for instance, wet process, local exhaust ventilation), personal protective equipment used (type, training, testing for fit and comfort and storage locations), sick co-workers.
- **Bystander exposures at work:** job activities and materials used at surrounding workstations, timing of worksite cleaning (during or after shift), individual performing cleanup and process used (wet versus dry).
- **Bystander exposure at home:** spouse's job, whether spouse wears work clothes at home and who cleans them, surrounding industries.
- **Other:** hobbies, pets, problems with home heating or air-conditioning, humidifier and hot tub use, water damage in the home.

Table 8.1 The main respiratory health effects of common indoor pollutants. ETS, environmental tobacco smoke; PM, particulate matter; VOC, volatile organic compound
Source: The European Lung White Book Respiratory Health and Disease in Europe, 2nd edn. © 2013 European Respiratory Society, Sheffield, UK. Reproduced with permission of the European Respiratory Society.

Pollutants	Health effects
Combustion products and ETS (CO, CO_2, NO, SO_2, PM, wood/coal smoke)	• Respiratory symptoms • Lung function reduction • Bronchial hyperresponsiveness • Asthma • COPD
VOCs (alkanes, formaldehyde, esters, ketones)	• Upper/lower respiratory tract irritation • Asthma
Biological organisms (fungal spores, bacteria, viruses)	• Respiratory infections
Allergens (pollens, moulds, mites, cockroaches, insects, dander, feathers)	• Sensitisation (specific/total IgE) • Respiratory allergic diseases • Hypersensitivity pneumonitis • Chronic cough
Random	• Lung cancer

Chronic respiratory disease

In Europe, approximately 7% of all hospital admissions are due to lung disease (Figure 8.1) with almost half of respiratory admissions potentially preventable (ERS, 2013).

Genetic susceptibility

The most common chronic respiratory diseases – asthma and COPD – as well as emphysema, pulmonary fibrosis, sarcoidosis, respiratory infections, pneumonia, tuberculosis and lung cancer, are complex diseases that result from interaction among many genetic risk factors and multiple environmental exposures. As altering the former is currently impracticable, attention should be directed to the management of important environmental factors, such as physical inactivity, air pollution, smoking and diet.

Primary prevention

Primary prevention of chronic respiratory diseases requires the reduction or avoidance of personal exposure to common risk factors, to be started during pregnancy and childhood.

Early life events

Major early-life risk factors for respiratory disease include abnormal antenatal lung growth, low birth weight, prematurity and broncho-pulmonary dysplasia, passive smoke exposure and viral infections. Tobacco smoke exposure, during pregnancy and after birth, can have respiratory repercussions throughout childhood, and is a risk factor for asthma and infectious illness.

Diet and nutrition

Aspects of diet are risk factors for several respiratory diseases, with normal weight and overweight people having lower respiratory mortality than underweight people. Clinical recommendations include a balanced diet with a lot of fruit, vegetables and fish, reducing salt intake, restricting the amount of trans- and omega-6 fatty acids in the diet, maintaining an ideal weight, with a body mass index (BMI) of 21–30 and undertaking moderate exercise (Chapters 11 and 12).

Outdoor environment

Air pollution is not a lifestyle choice but a ubiquitous involuntary environmental exposure, which can affect 100% of the population from the womb to death. Short-term respiratory effects include daily mortality, daily respiratory exacerbations with long-term consequences on mortality and life expectancy. Research has shown that proximity to green space reduced respiratory disease prevalence; people with lower education levels living close to green space had lower annual prevalence rates of COPD than those living further away (Marmot, 2010) (Figure 8.2).

Occupational risk factors

Occupational agents, such as the inhalation of specific particles, gases, fumes or smoke, are responsible for about 15% (in men) and 5% (in women) of all respiratory cancers, 17% of all adult asthma cases, 15–20% of COPD and 10% of interstitial lung disease. Workplace interventions include reduced exposure to asbestos and latex in hospitals. However, it is difficult to measure the effects of such interventions because of the long latency of occupational respiratory diseases. A thorough clinical assessment (Box 8.1) is essential in the prevention, detection and management of occupational risk factors (Chapter 32).

Passive smoking

Passive smoking is the exposure to second- or third-hand smoke by breathing ambient air containing toxic substances resulting from the combustion of tobacco products after birth; or the exposure *in utero* to maternal blood contaminated with the combustion of tobacco smoking products.

Environmental tobacco smoke or passive smoke is classed as a human carcinogen by the World Health Organization and there are no safe levels of exposure (Figure 8.3).

Tobacco smoking

At least one in four adults across Europe smoke, exceeding 40% in some countries (ERS, 2013). Smoking is a cause of childhood asthma and a risk factor for the development of asthma in adults. It is associated with increased risk of mortality, asthma attacks and exacerbations, greater severity, more difficulty in controlling asthma and deteriorating lung function (Figure 8.4). Smoking predisposes to infection and is a serious complicating factor for tuberculosis (Chapter 10).

Indoor environment

Indoor air pollution results from human activity such as tobacco smoking, burning fuel for heat or cooking, the use of cleaning materials and solvents or due to natural pollutants such as allergens, dampness and mould. There is strong evidence of increased risk of acute lower respiratory infections in childhood (at least 2 million deaths annually in children under 5 years of age; ERS, 2013). There is also evidence of an association with the risk of developing COPD, mostly for women, and with the risk of tuberculosis and asthma (Table 8.1).

Secondary and tertiary prevention

This involves collaboration among health care systems and (non) governmental organisations to achieve changes in policy, which are essential if one intends to reduce the population's exposure to disease determinants and pollution risks. However, there are a number of mechanisms for health care professionals to assist in the prevention of respiratory disease.

Health education

The population must be fully informed about what constitutes a healthy lifestyle, such as healthy nutritional habits, regular exercise and avoidance of tobacco, airway irritants and allergens.

Personalised approach

Health care professionals should take into account any circumstances that may affect the outcomes of care or disease prevention. For example, the causes of asthma are not well understood but as 90% of asthma deaths have preventable features, patients should be aware of triggers for symptoms to maintain asthma control and prevent deterioration (DH, 2011).

Behaviour change

Successful prevention, treatment and burden of the disease can be reduced by ensuring people take action to avoid the causes or exacerbating factors of respiratory disease, such as cigarette smoke, diet and workplace dusts and gases.

Further reading

World Health Organization. (2016) *Chronic Respiratory Diseases Prevention and Control.* http://www.afro.who.int/en/clusters-a-programmes/dpc/non-communicable-diseases-managementndm/programme-components/chronic-respiratory-diseases.html (accessed 23 March 2016).

9 Epidemiology and contributing factors

Table 9.1 Female and male age-standardised mortality rates (ASMRs), for three major categories of cause of death, 2001 and 2011: England and Wales
Source: Office of National Statistics.

Year	Rate per million					
	Cause of death (broad disease group)					
	Circulatory diseases (female)	Circulatory diseases (male)	Cancer (female)	Cancer (male)	Respiratory diseases (female)	Respiratory diseases (male)
2001	1986	3221	1647	2348	648	975
2011	1110	1803	1478	2023	573	798

Table 9.2 Standardised mortality ratios for selected diseases of the respiratory system by social class. England and Wales, men aged 20-64, 1991/93

Social class	All causes	TB	Cancer of bronchus, trachea & lung	Pneumonia	COPD	Bronchitis and emphysema
		(10–18, 137)	162	480–486	496	490–492
I–professional	66	32	45	58	21	44
II–mangerial/	72	47	61	69	42	43
IIIN–skilled (non-mangerial)	100	75	87	106	78	81
IIIM–skilled (manual)	117	94	138	93	131	125
IV–partly skilled	116	141	132	108	146	137
V–unskilled	189	285	206	197	298	268
England and Wales	100	100	100	100	100	100
Ratio unskilled: Pra	2.8	8.9	4.6	3.4	14.2	6.1
Number of deaths	175,847	252	16,082	2916	3095	1331

Figure 9.1 The 10 most common causes of death in 2012
Source: WHO World Health Statistics 2014. Reproduced with permission of WHO.

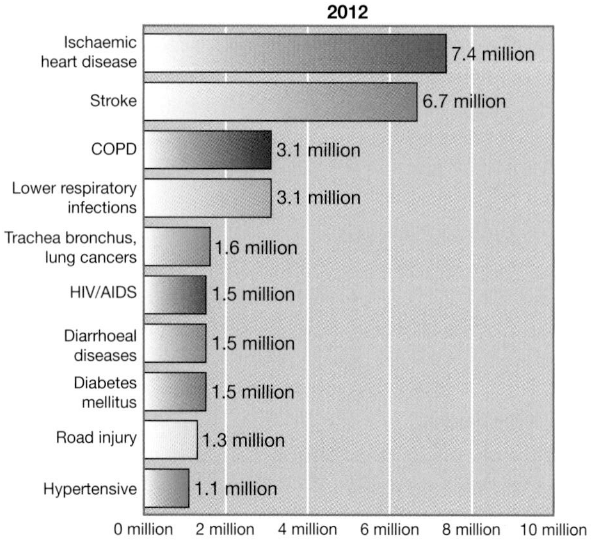
2012
Ischaemic heart disease
7.4 million
Stroke
6.7 million
COPD
3.1 million
Lower respiratory infections
3.1 million
Trachea bronchus, lung cancers
1.6 million
HIV/AIDS
1.5 million
Diarrhoeal diseases
1.5 million
Diabetes mellitus
1.5 million
Road injury
1.3 million
Hypertensive
1.1 million
0 million
2 million
4 million
6 million
8 million
10 million

Table 9.3 Current annual mortality from work-related respiratory diseases in Britain, 2012

Disease	Annual deaths 2012
Mesothelioma	2535
Asbestos-related lung cancer	More than 2000
Laryngeal cancer due to asbestos	Approx. 3
Lung cancer due to other agents	Approx. 2800
COPD	Approx. 4000
Pneumoconiosis: Coal worker's Pneumoconiosis: Asbestosis: Silicosis:	 140 464 11
Farmer's lung and other allergic alveolitis	10
Byssinosis	1
Total	Approx. 12,000

Figure 9.2 The burden of asthma, COPD, lung cancer and tuberculosis, around 2010, in the 28 countries of the European Union
Source: The European Lung White Book Respiratory Health and Disease in Europe, 2nd edn. © 2013 European Respiratory Society, Sheffield, UK. Reproduced with permission of the European Respiratory Society.

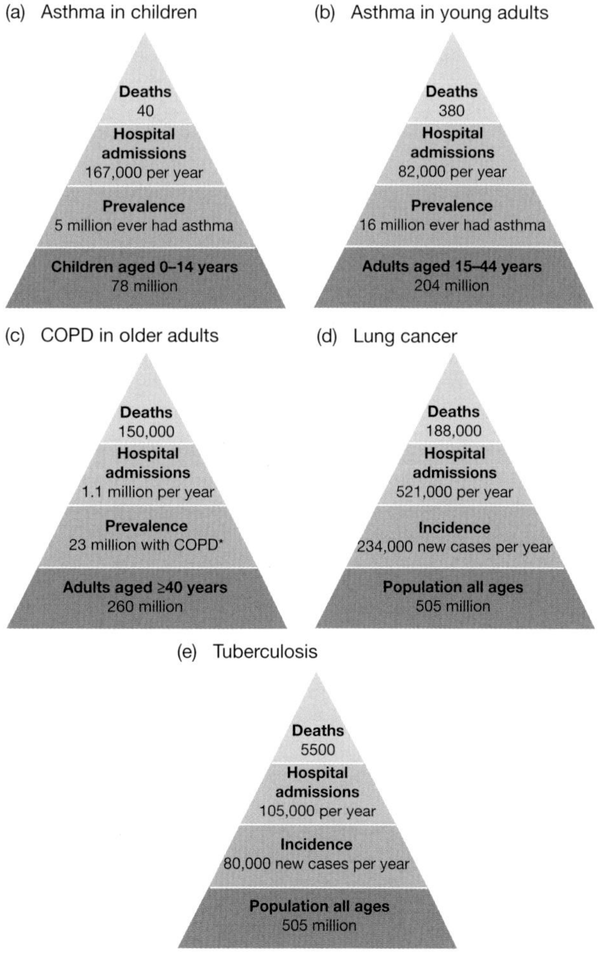
(a) Asthma in children
Deaths
40
Hospital admissions
167,000 per year
Prevalence
5 million ever had asthma
Children aged 0–14 years
78 million
(b) Asthma in young adults
Deaths
380
Hospital admissions
82,000 per year
Prevalence
16 million ever had asthma
Adults aged 15–44 years
204 million
(c) COPD in older adults
Deaths
150,000
Hospital admissions
1.1 million per year
Prevalence
23 million with COPD*
Adults aged ≥40 years
260 million
(d) Lung cancer
Deaths
188,000
Hospital admissions
521,000 per year
Incidence
234,000 new cases per year
Population all ages
505 million
(e) Tuberculosis
Deaths
5500
Hospital admissions
105,000 per year
Incidence
80,000 new cases per year
Population all ages
505 million

Respiratory diseases are among the leading causes of death worldwide (Figure 9.1) and accounted for 9.5 million deaths worldwide during 2012, one-sixth of the global total (WHO, 2014). Figure 9.2 summarises the prevalence of asthma, chronic obstructive pulmonary disease (COPD), lung cancer and tuberculosis in Europe (2010). In the UK, respiratory diseases accounted for 14% of all deaths in 2011 (ONS, 2011). However, in England and Wales the male mortality rate for respiratory diseases decreased by 18% between 2001 and 2011, while the rate for females fell by 12% (ONS, 2010). Such improvements are a result of legislative measures and tobacco control strategies to reduce exposure to second-hand smoke, restrictions on marketing of foods high in sugar, fat and salt, national frameworks to drive up standards of treatment and care and advances in stem cell research and regenerative medicine.

Contributing factors

Age

In 2009, mortality rates for diseases of the respiratory system were highest among those aged 90 years and over; 266.6 per million males and 180.9 per million females, respectively (ONS, 2010) while the most commonly reported long-term illnesses in children and babies are conditions of the respiratory system.

Sex

In 2009, males accounted for 59% of deaths from diseases of the respiratory system, a rate 60% lower than in 1971, while among females the mortality rate was 39% lower, falling from 909 per million in 1971 to 552 per million in 2009. Table 9.1 shows the male–female mortality rate across the three broad disease groups from 2001 to 2011 (ONS, 2011).

Ethnicity

Self-reported rates of respiratory disease also vary by ethnic group, with rates highest in black Caribbean men and lowest in Chinese respondents and in Indian and Bangladeshi women (BTS, 2006).

For asthma, non-UK-born people have been shown to have a reduced risk of new or first consultation than people of the same ethnic group born in the UK (Netuveli et al., 2005). This suggests that changes in environmental exposures (e.g. pollutants and allergens) and conditions (e.g. housing and diet) or changes in lifestyle (e.g. Westernised diet) and behaviour (e.g. smoking) upon migration and settlement can alter susceptibility to respiratory disease, especially in early life.

There are ethnic disparities in the UK, with black and minority men in deprived urban areas at higher risk of COPD because of the interplay between ethnic identity, socio-economic status and living environment. These factors result in incidence and mortality rates from respiratory disease being higher in disadvantaged groups and areas.

Social class

In the UK, social inequality causes a higher proportion of deaths in respiratory disease than any other disease area, with 44% of all deaths from respiratory disease associated with social class inequalities compared with 28% of deaths from ischaemic heart disease (BTS, 2006). Men aged 20–64 employed in unskilled manual occupations are around 14 times more likely to die from COPD, and 9 times more likely to die from tuberculosis, than men employed in professional roles, while the standardised mortality ratio for respiratory diseases shows a threefold difference across all social classes (Table 9.2). Deprived populations have the highest prevalence and the highest under-diagnosis of COPD, with the gap in life expectancy between the areas with the worst health and deprivation and the average – around an 8% gap for men and 12% gap for women (DH, 2011).

Occupation

There are currently approximately 12,000 deaths each year from occupational respiratory diseases, about two-thirds of which are due to asbestos-related diseases or COPD (Table 9.3) (HSE, 2014). Because of the long latency period following exposure, current deaths reflect the effect of past working conditions. In 2013/14, 28,000 people who worked in the last year and 127,000 who had ever worked currently have breathing or lung problems they thought were caused or made worse by work, with an estimated 10,000 new cases of breathing or lung problems caused or made worse by work each year (HSE, 2014).

Smoking

Smoking is one of the main risk factor for respiratory diseases including COPD, as well as for cardiovascular diseases, cancers of several organs and many other pathological conditions (Chapter 10).

Co-morbidities

It is estimated that two-thirds of the patients with COPD have at least one co-morbidity (Raherison and Girodet, 2009). COPD and mental health impact on each other in two ways: first, people with mental health problems smoke much more than the rest of the population, consuming 42% of all cigarettes smoked in England (McManus et al., 2010) and, secondly, people who are diagnosed with COPD are prone to mental health problems such as depression and anxiety because of their diagnosis (DH, 2011). In the UK, 40% of people with COPD also have heart disease, and significant numbers have depression and/or anxiety disorder.

Those with asthma are more likely to have other allergic conditions, including hay fever and allergic rhinitis. The most frequently reported asthma co-morbid conditions include rhinitis, sinusitis, gastroesophageal reflux disease, obstructive sleep apnoea, hormonal disorders and psychopathologies. These conditions can share a common pathophysiological mechanism with asthma, can influence asthma control, its phenotype and response to treatment; and be more prevalent in asthmatic patients but without obvious influence on this disease (Boulet and Boulay, 2011).

Further reading

European Respiratory Society European Lung white book: The burden of lung disease. (ERS) (2013) http://www.european-lung.org/assets/files/publications/lung_health_in_europe_facts_and_figures_web.pdf

10 Smoking and smoking cessation

Figure 10.1 Just a few of the 4000 chemicals legally allowed in cigarettes

- Cadmium (batteries)
- Stearic acid (candle wax)
- Hexamine (barbecue lighter)
- Toluene (industrial solvent)
- Nicotine (insecticide)
- Ammonia (toilet cleaner)
- Methanol (rocket fuel)
- Paint
- Carbon monoxide
- Arsenic (poison)
- Methane (sewer gas)
- Acetic acid (vinegar)
- Butane (lighter fluid)

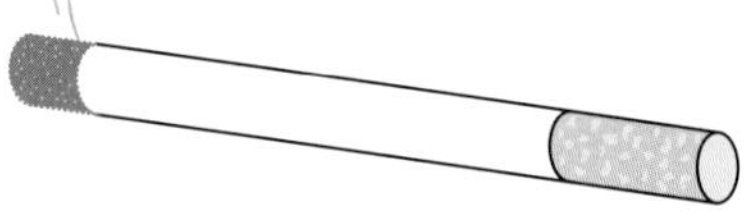

Figure 10.2 Effect of smoking on all organs

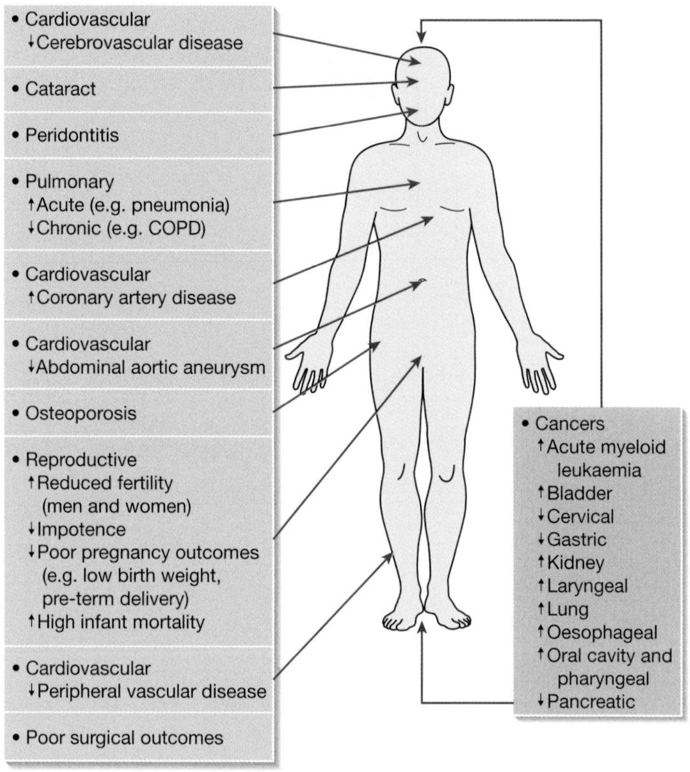
• Cardiovascular
↓Cerebrovascular disease
• Cataract
• Peridontitis
• Pulmonary
↑Acute (e.g. pneumonia)
↓Chronic (e.g. COPD)
• Cardiovascular
↑Coronary artery disease
• Cardiovascular
↓Abdominal aortic aneurysm
• Osteoporosis
• Reproductive
↑Reduced fertility (men and women)
↓Impotence
↓Poor pregnancy outcomes (e.g. low birth weight, pre-term delivery)
↑High infant mortality
• Cardiovascular
↓Peripheral vascular disease
• Poor surgical outcomes
• Cancers
↑Acute myeloid leukaemia
↑Bladder
↓Cervical
↓Gastric
↑Kidney
↑Laryngeal
↑Lung
↑Oesophageal
↑Oral cavity and pharyngeal
↓Pancreatic

Figure 10.3 Cost-effectiveness analysis of smoking cessation when compared with other elements of a COPD treatment plan. A cost/ QALY of £30,000 or less is classed as cost-effective and should be recommended according to NICE.
Source: Reproduced with permission of London Respiratory Network.

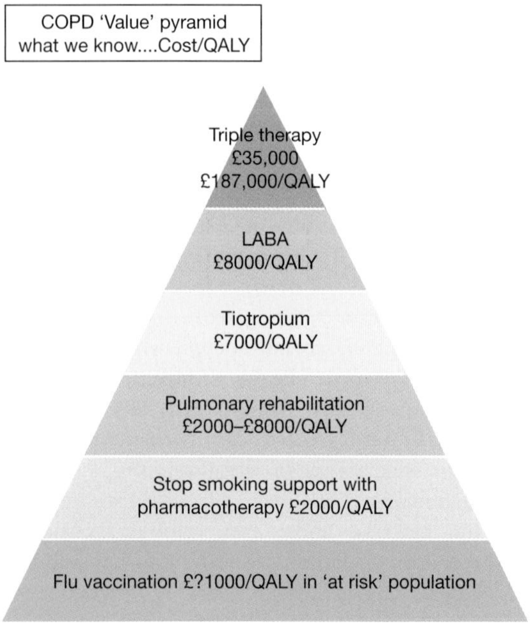
COPD 'Value' pyramid
what we know....Cost/QALY
Triple therapy
£35,000
£187,000/QALY
LABA
£8000/QALY
Tiotropium
£7000/QALY
Pulmonary rehabilitation
£2000–£8000/QALY
Stop smoking support with pharmacotherapy £2000/QALY
Flu vaccination £?1000/QALY in 'at risk' population

Figure 10.5 The cycle of change

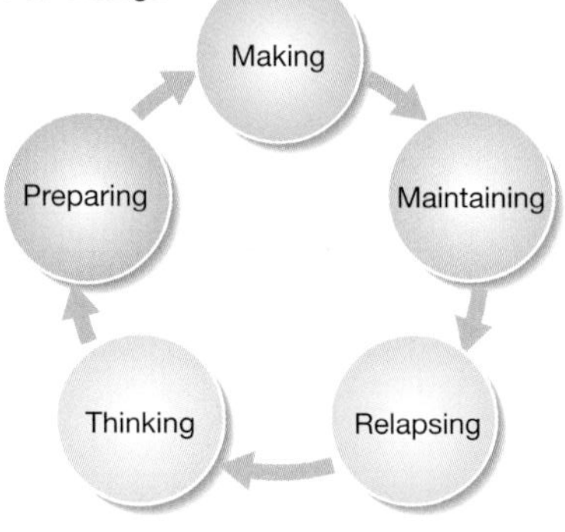
Making
Maintaining
Relapsing
Thinking
Preparing

Figure 10.4 Forced Expiratory Volume (FEV_1) and the decline with age in various groups. The stage of likely disability and death is also indicated

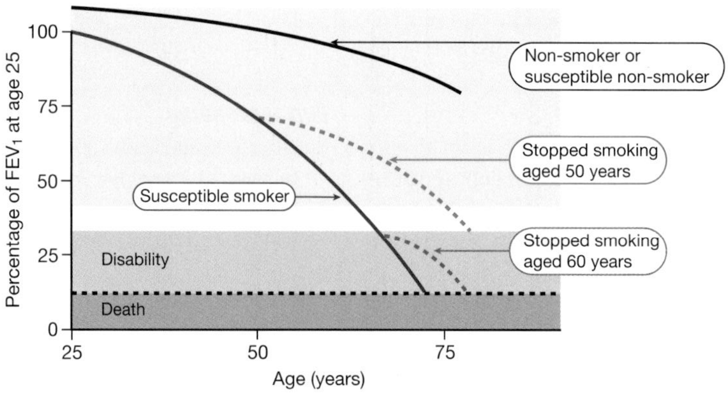
Non-smoker or
susceptible non-smoker
Stopped smoking
aged 50 years
Susceptible smoker
Stopped smoking
aged 60 years
Disability
Death
Percentage of FEV1 at age 25
100
75
50
25
0
25
50
75
Age (years)

Tobacco

Tobacco, for recreational use, dates back to the sixteenth century in England. It is smoked to obtain the drug nicotine, principally to relieve symptoms of nicotine withdrawal. Nicotine is an agonist that releases dopamine which gives the 'feel good' effect but it has a very short half-life meaning this effect is short and another dose is required. Although nicotine itself has few serious adverse effects on health, the smoker exposes themselves to serious harm from the 4000 chemicals (Figure 10.1), many of which are carcinogenic, including tar, oxidant gases and carbon monoxide.

Respiratory health burden of tobacco smoking and prevalence

The side effects of smoking only became noticeable in the 1920s. Many of these adverse effects and life-limiting illnesses are caused by these chemicals (Figure 10.1). The widespread effects of tobacco smoking can be seen in Figure 10.2. In addition to well-known smoking- related conditions such as chronic obstructive pulmonary disease (COPD) and lung cancer, it is worth noting that smokers with asthma have more severe symptoms and are less responsive to corticosteroid treatment. Second-hand exposure to other people's tobacco smoke is also a cause of ill health. Smoking in pregnancy can also cause harm as well as risks to children's future health.

Smoking cessation

Smoking cessation should be seen as a treatment and in a current smoker it is one of the most cost-effective options in chronic disease management (Figure 10.3). This is especially important in COPD as it is the only intervention that will slow disease progression (Figure 10.4).

The body starts to recover in as little as 20 minutes when a person quits smoking.

- After 20 minutes blood pressure and pulse start returning to normal
- After 24 hours carbon monoxide is eliminated from the body and the lungs start to clear out smoking debris
- After 48 hours ability to taste and smell improves
- After 3–9 months lung function improves up to 10%
- After 5 years the risk of heart attack falls to about half that of a smoker
- After 10 years the risk of lung cancer is halved and the risk of heart ischaemia falls to that of someone who has never smoked.

Smoking is a relapsing addiction and many people have 6–7 attempts before quitting long term (Figure 10.5). Receiving behavioural support, for example from a NHS Stop Smoking Service, will quadruple chance of success (NICE, 2008). It is also recommended that therapy is combined with nicotine replacement therapy and/or medication.

Nicotine replacement therapy replaces to some extent the nicotine a person would have received from smoking. The dose depends on the amount of cigarettes smoked, intensity and pattern of habit. NICE (2008) recommends a long- acting product (e.g. a patch) and a short-acting product of which there are many varieties; these provide a dose of nicotine to help cravings. Most are absorbed sublingually (e.g. gum, spray or inhalator). The dose is usually titrated down over a 12-week period.

Varenicline is a partial antagonist that prevents nicotine reaching receptors, it also releases dopamine to help with cravings. The dose is titrated meaning the person smokes for 8–14 days before quitting. The course of oral tablets is usually 12 weeks.

Bupropion is an older drug not now commonly used. Its primary use was as an antidepressant and it was found the oral tablets had the beneficial side effect of assisting smoking cessation. A course usually lasts 8–12 weeks.

Other drugs

Tobacco is also smoked in conjunction with other drugs such as heroin, cannabis and shisha. The risk of lung disease is enhanced when smoking these drugs, possibly as a result of unfiltered smoke, the heat of the smoke and the increased depth of inhalation to optimise the effect of the drug.

Electronic cigarettes and vaping

Electronic nicotine delivery devices (ENDDs) are electronic devices that mimic real cigarettes and release vapour. There are hundreds of different types of devices and is a growing trend for 'switchers' who want a safer way of consuming nicotine or by those attempting to quit. More research is needed especially into the effects on tobacco cessation and the safety of inhalation of the flavours used. Regulation commenced in the UK in 2016.

Further reading

Action on Smoking and Health http://www.ash.org.uk/ (accessed 22 February 2016).

11 Exercise and pulmonary rehabilitation

Figure 11.1 The cycle of inactivity

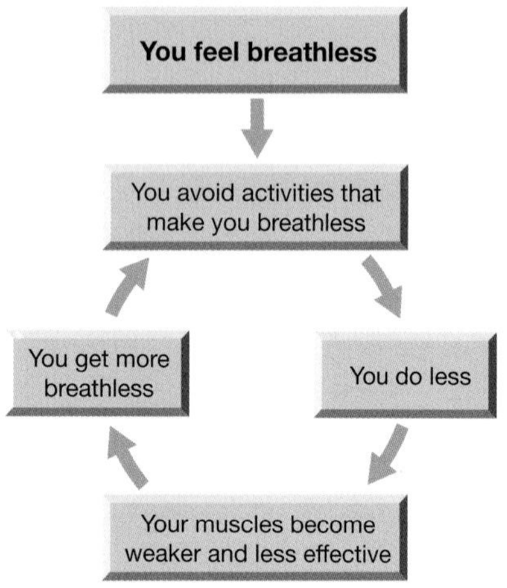
You feel breathless
You avoid activities that make you breathless
You do less
Your muscles become weaker and less effective
You get more breathless

Box 11.1 Benefits of exercise

1 Reduces body fat	11 Maintains mobility
2 Increases lifespan	12 Improves memory
3 Oxygenates body	13 Improves coordination
4 Strengthens muscles	14 Strengthens bones
5 Manages chronic pain	15 Improves complexion
6 Wards off viruses	16 Detoxifies body
7 Reduces diabetes risk	17 Decreases stress
8 Strengthens heart	18 Boosts immune system
9 Clears arteries	19 Lowers blood pressure
10 Boosts mood	20 Reduces cancer risk

Figure 11.2 Cost-effectiveness analysis of PR compared with other COPD treatments.
Source: Reproduced with permission of London Respiratory Network.

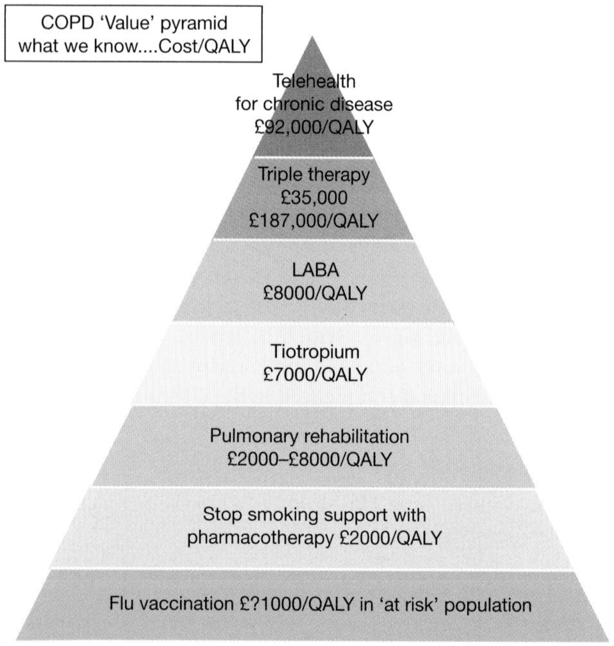
COPD 'Value' pyramid
what we know....Cost/QALY
Telehealth
for chronic disease
£92,000/QALY
Triple therapy
£35,000
£187,000/QALY
LABA
£8000/QALY
Tiotropium
£7000/QALY
Pulmonary rehabilitation
£2000–£8000/QALY
Stop smoking support with
pharmacotherapy £2000/QALY
Flu vaccination £?1000/QALY in 'at risk' population

Figure 11.3 Key components of PR.
Source: Bernard S, et al. (2014) *Rev Port Pneumol* 20: 92–100. Reproduced with permission of Elsevier.

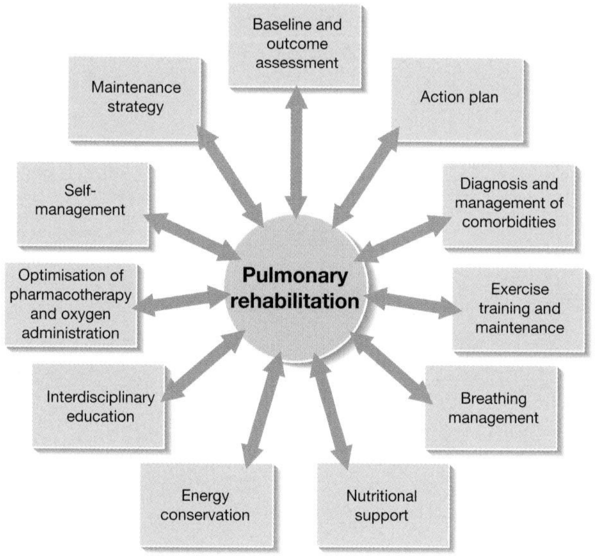
Pulmonary rehabilitation
Baseline and outcome assessment
Action plan
Diagnosis and management of comorbidities
Exercise training and maintenance
Breathing management
Nutritional support
Energy conservation
Interdisciplinary education
Optimisation of pharmacotherapy and oxygen administration
Self-management
Maintenance strategy

Exercise

Fitness is a part of everyday life. It enables us to get up, get washed and dressed and go out and live our lives. Unfortunately, if you have a respiratory condition such as chronic obstructive pulmonary disease (COPD) where breathlessness is a symptom, it can be difficult to be active. There is a sense of fear of getting breathless so activities are avoided. However, if activities are avoided and less activity is undertaken, the muscles become weaker and less effective, thus leading to an increased experience of dyspnoea. The person then becomes deconditioned and starts to avoid more activities and becomes even weaker and more breathless on less activity. This is known as the cycle of inactivity (Figure 11.1). Exercise helps to break this cycle and increases the strength and capacity for work of the muscles. For our muscles to maintain strength we need to exercise them on a regular basis and it is imperative that this is reinforced to the breathless person. Exercise should be encouraged no matter how little the individual is able to do. Chair-based exercises are a good start; these can then be progressed once muscle strength improves.

Benefits of exercise

There are many benefits to exercise (Box 11.1):

- Reduced sensation of breathlessness – getting breathless can be frightening but exercising in a safe environment and experiencing breathlessness can reduce the sensation of it
- Stronger, more efficient muscles – improved oxygen uptake to the muscles reduces ventilator demand
- Improved balance and coordination
- Reduced anxiety and depression
- Increased confidence and motivation
- Regulation of appetite
- Improved sense of well-being
- Reduced progression of osteoporosis
- Improved sleep
- Reduction of high blood pressure to healthy levels
- Improved flexibility and suppleness
- Assists secretion clearance from the airways
- Improved posture
- Reduction in cholesterol levels.

Pulmonary rehabilitation

NICE (2010) defined pulmonary rehabilitation (PR) as 'a multidisciplinary programme of care for patients with chronic respiratory impairment that is individually tailored and designed to optimise each patient's physical and social performance and autonomy'. It is an exercise and education programme where patients come twice a week for a minimum of 6 weeks (BTS, 2013) and is very cost effective (Figure 11.2). The exercises should include both muscle strengthening using weights, such as bicep curls, and aerobic exercises, such as walking or steps.

Even though it is a group programme providing peer support, the exercises should be tailored and progressed to each patient's ability and requirements. PR is run in a number of locations such as hospitals, community centres, church halls, and the types of exercises and equipment vary across different services based on location and resources. The programme is run at a ratio of up to 16 patients to 2 clinicians. Programmes are run as either a cohort or a rolling programme.

- Cohort: patients all start and finish at the same time; they are progressing together and receive education in a logical order. However, when people drop out or miss sessions the spaces cannot be filled.
- Rolling programme: patients are starting and finishing at different points. If a session is missed it can be made up or if someone drops out their space can be filled. The new starters can get support and encouragement from those who have already commenced on the programme. A rolling programme also provides flexibility to allow those who have recently exacerbated to participate.

Which programme your local service delivers will depend on availability of staff and venues.

PR education

NICE (2010) and BTS (2013) encourage a multi-disciplinary approach to PR and as well as the physical training and should incorporate 'disease education, nutritional, psychological and behavioural intervention' (Figure 11.3).

The education element can vary from service to service but should generally include the following:

- Disease education
- Breathing control
- Medication
- Chest clearance
- Energy conservation and pacing
- Diet and nutrition
- Self-management
- Goal planning
- Continuing exercising after PR
- Psychological support.

Other topics that could be covered:

- End of life
- Social services support
- Acute/secondary care advice
- Non-invasive ventilation.

The talks are delivered by physiotherapists, nurses, psychologists, occupational therapists, social workers, chest physicians and palliative care nurses, depending on availability of personnel and expertise.

Inclusion and exclusion criteria

Inclusion criteria:

- Confirmed respiratory diagnosis
- Medical Research Council (MRC) scale 3 and above (Figure 15.3)
- Stable blood pressure.

Exclusion criteria:

- Unstable cardiac disease
- Lung cancer
- Unable to mobilise
- Unmotivated
- Cognitive impairment
- Recent cardiac or abdominal surgery.

PR assessment

Prior to being accepted onto the programme an initial assessment will need to be completed. This includes a walking test which is normally an incremental shuttle walk test (bleep test) or a 6 minute walk test. This provides a baseline of exercise tolerance and provides an outcome measure to use at the end of the programme. It also includes a psychological assessment and exploration of symptoms using quality of life tools.

If you have any further questions and about PR then contact your local respiratory team.

Further reading

British Thoracic Society (BTS) (2013) Guideline on pulmonary rehabilitation in adults: British Thoracic Society Pulmonary Rehabilitation Guideline. *Thorax* 68(Suppl 2): 1–30.

12 Nutrition and hydration

Table 12.1 Consequences of malnutrition

Body system	Effect
Muscle	Inactivity increases risk of pressure ulcers blood clots and falls. Reduced ability to cough, heart failure and increased risk of chest infection
Kidneys	Inability to regulate salts and fluids which can leave over/under hydration
Immunity	Reduced ability to fight infection
Brain	Apathy, depression, introversion and self-neglect. Impaired regulation of temperature leading to hypothermia
Reproduction	Decreases fertility, if present in pregnancy can cause the baby to be predisposed to diabetes, strokes and heart disease in later life

Table 12.3 Indications for enteral feeding

Indication	Some examples
Swallowing difficulties (dysphagia)	Cerebral vascular accident Motor neurone disease Multiple sclerosis Brain tumours Burns
Upper GI obstruction	Oesophageal cancer (not indicated for PEG insertion due to risk of seeding the cancer in the stoma) Stricture Tumours
Increased nutritional requirements	Liver disease Cystic fibrosis Crohn's disease Renal disease COPD Malnutrition
Psychological requirements	Anorexia nervosa
Unconscious patients	The ventilated patient Head trauma

Figure 12.2 Delivery method of total parenteral nutrition (TPN) –either through a central line of peripherally as a PICC line

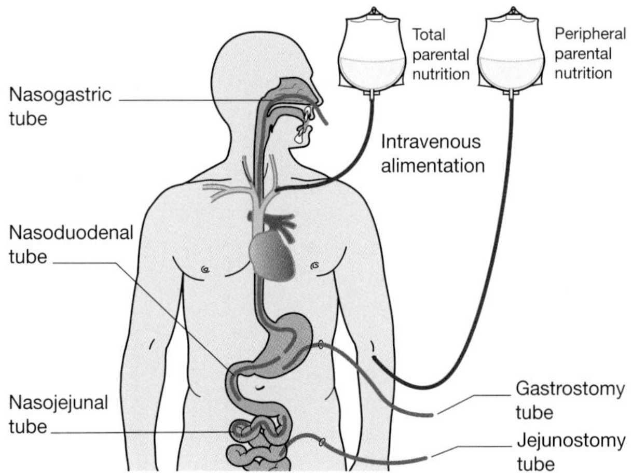
Total parental nutrition
Peripheral parental nutrition
Nasogastric tube
Intravenous alimentation
Nasoduodenal tube
Nasojejunal tube
Gastrostomy tube
Jejunostomy tube

Table 12.2 Consequences of micronutrient deficiencies

Micro-nutrient	Effect of deficiency
Iron	Iron deficiency anaemia
Zinc	Skin rashes, reduced ability to fight infection
Vitamin B12	Anaemia, nerve complications
Vitamin D	Rickets in children, osteomalacia in adults, tirednesss
Vitamin C	Scurvy
Vitamin A	Night blindness

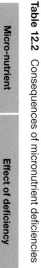

Figure 12.1 Nasal feeding tubes for gastric and jejunal feeding

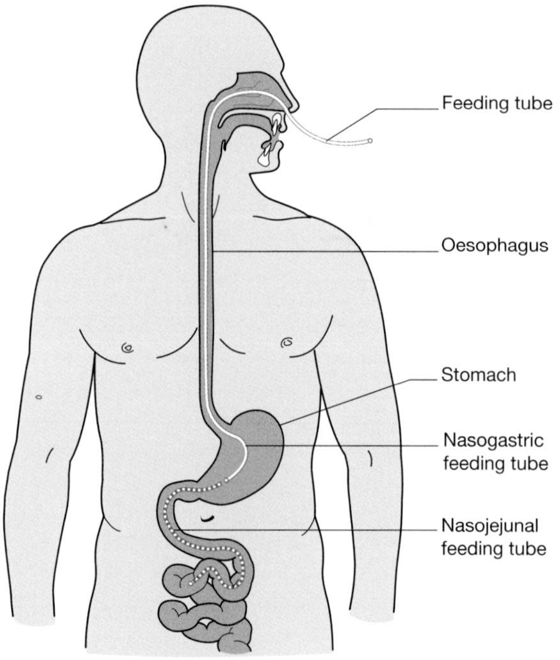
Feeding tube
Oesophagus
Stomach
Nasogastric feeding tube
Nasojejunal feeding tube

Figure 12.3 Gastrostomy tube held in place using a balloon

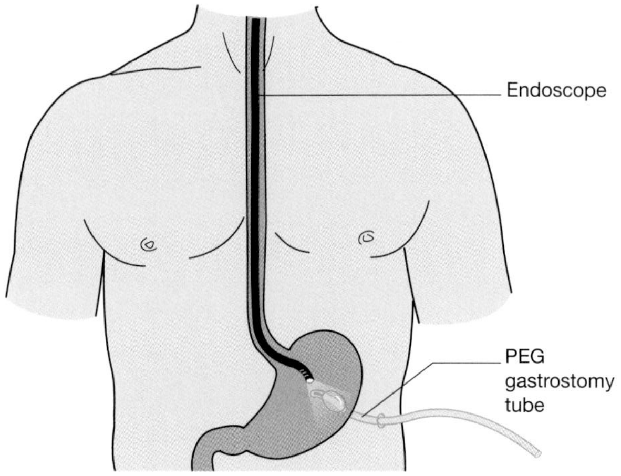
Endoscope
PEG gastrostomy tube

Good nutrition and hydration are fundamental for health, wound healing, to maintain well-being and prevent malnutrition. Dehydration and malnutrition can cause ill health and poor recovery (Table 12.1). Steer et al. (2010) found patients with chronic obstructive pulmonary disease with a body mass index (BMI) <18.5 kg/m^2 who were hospitalised for an infective exacerbation were 2.5 times more likely to die during admission than those with a higher BMI. Malnutrition is common in respiratory disease associated with reduced nutritional intake and increased calorific demand so maintaining good nutrition and hydration are essential for improving treatment outcomes for patients.

It is important to ensure patients are offered a variety of food and drinks as this is part of basic care alongside pain relief and assisting with activities of daily living. Health care professionals should also ensure appropriate support is available for those patients who need supplementation of nutrition and hydration.

Malnutrition and screening

Screening for malnutrition and the potential to be at risk of malnutrition should be carried out by health care providers across all health care settings. A validated screening tool such as the Malnutrition Universal Screening Tool (MUST) can be used to identify these patients. The MUST uses three areas to enable the health care provider to calculate a score which will instruct on the best course of action. The tool uses a BMI, percentage of weight loss over 3 months and an acute illness indicator to identify a total score.

If patients have fluid imbalance such as oedema or ascites, interpretation of an accurate BMI can be difficult and weight loss underestimated, so use of mid upper arm circumference (MUAC) measurement can be used and weight recorded when fluid balance has been achieved.

Nutrition and hydration support

Nutrition and hydration support should be considered if a patient has a low BMI >18.5 kg/m^2, if they have unintentional weight loss of >10% in the last 3–6 months, or of a BMI of >20 kg/m^2 and unintentional weight loss >5% in the last 3–6 months. Patients who feel breathless can have difficulty eating and drinking enough to achieve adequate intake of protein and micronutrients. The problem is multi-factorial including physical issues of breathlessness, dry or sore mouth from medications, difficulty preparing meals because of fatigue and social isolation removing the pleasure element of eating. All these elements need to be addressed: such as planning activity of eating, small frequent meals that are easy to chew, oral care and promoting the pleasure of eating.

Forms of nutritional support include oral supplementation such as high calorie diets, prescribed supplements and the fortification of foods.

It is always best to encourage patients to eat orally, if deemed safe to do so, prior to the consideration of enteral tube feeding (ETF). If patients have an adequate accessible gastrointestinal tract and sustainable absorption, then ETF is the safest way to feed a person either orally, or in the form of tube feeding such as a nasogastric tube (NGT) (Table 12.3). ETF can be used for short or long-term feeding support, depending on the patient's medical condition (Table 12.3; Figure 12.1).

When making a decision that a patient may need ETF, generally it is best practice to discuss with the patient reasons for using tube feeding and involve them in this treatment plan. It can sometimes be useful to include family members of the patient to help them make a decision; however, it is essentially the patient's choice, if they have capacity.

When considering long-term tube feeding such as percutaneous endoscopic gastrostomy (PEG) or radiological inserted gastrostomy (RIG), it is good practice to provide a multi-disciplinary approach in making this decision as well as using a holistic approach. Topics to be considered are whether the risks of the procedure outweigh the benefits, complications such as post procedure chest infection, bleeding, mortality, stoma infection and more serious complications such as peritonitis, small bowel and colonic injury all need to be considered. If placed in endoscopy, the patient needs to be medically fit enough for the gastroscopy (Figure 12.3). Complications associated with endoscopy and sedation include cardiopulmonary compromise, respiratory depression, hypoxia, aspiration and possibly myocardial infarction and haemorrhage.

Parenteral nutrition

Total parenteral nutrition (TPN) is a way of supplying all the nutritional needs of the body by bypassing the digestive system and administering nutrient-rich solution directly into a central vein generally via central venous catheter or peripherally inserted central line (PICC) (Figure 12.2). TPN is used when individuals cannot or should not obtain their nutrition through eating. TPN is used when the intestines are obstructed, when the small intestine is not absorbing nutrients properly or a gastrointestinal fistula is present. Risks associated with TPN include line infection, sepsis, deranged liver function bloods, variable blood glucose levels and thrombosis and pneumothorax from line insertion.

Further reading

NICE (2014) Nutritional support for adults: oral nutrition support, enteral tube feeding and parenteral nutrition. https://www.nice.org.uk/guidance/cg32 (accessed 22 February 2016).

13 The upper airways

Figure 13.1 Naso-bronchial reflexes
Source: Bergeron C, Hamid Q. (2005) *Allergy, Asthma & Clinical Immunology* 1: 81–87.

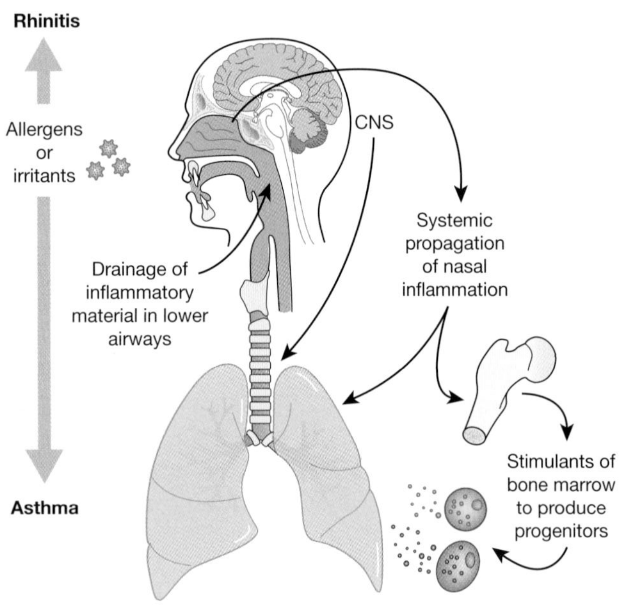
Rhinitis
Allergens
or
irritants
CNS
Drainage of
inflammatory
material in lower
airways
Systemic
propagation
of nasal
inflammation
Stimulants of
bone marrow
to produce
progenitors
Asthma

Figure 13.2 The inflammatory process

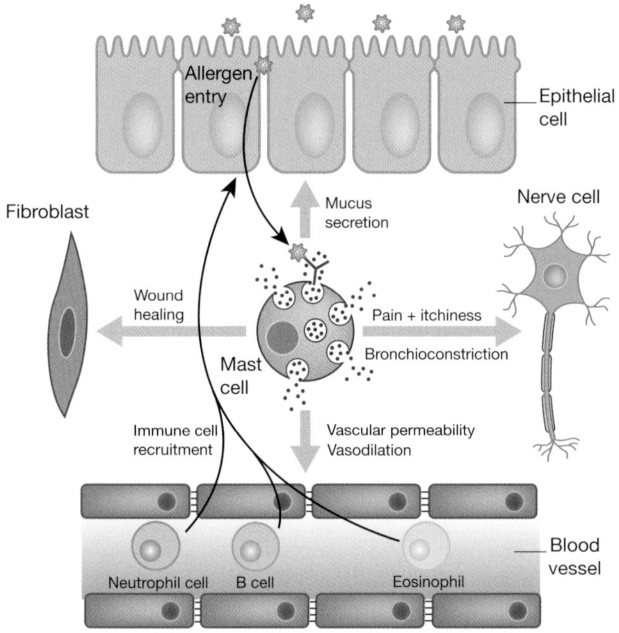
Allergen
entry
Epithelial
cell
Fibroblast
Mucus
secretion
Nerve cell
Wound
healing
Pain + itchiness
Bronchioconstriction
Mast
cell
Immune cell
recruitment
Vascular permeability
Vasodilation
Neutrophil cell
B cell
Eosinophil
Blood
vessel

Figure 13.3 Nasal cavity: allergic rhinitis

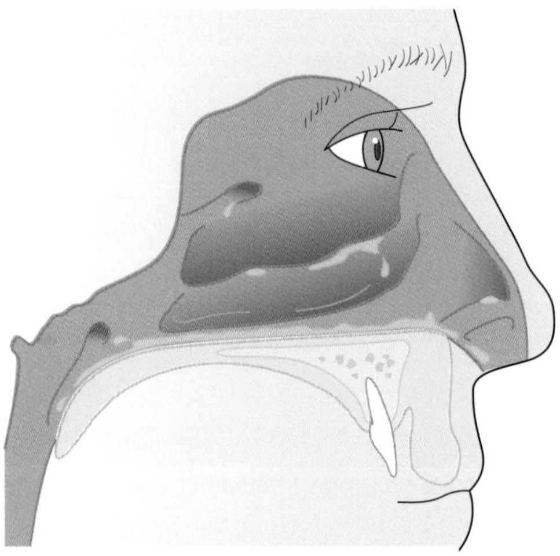

Figure 13.4 Correct administration of nose drops

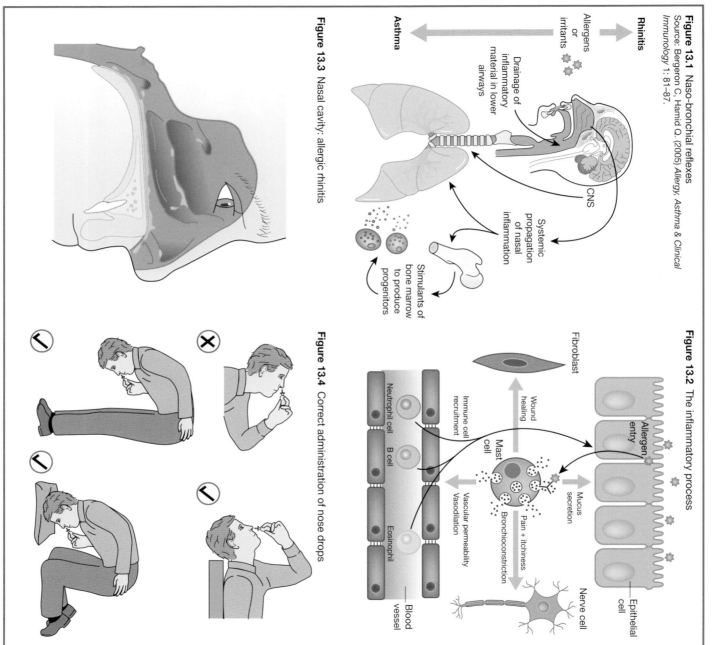

Asthma, allergic rhinitis (AR) and atopic dermatitis are the three most common manifestations of allergy. Various studies have demonstrated links between these conditions, and their development in individuals has been termed 'the atopic march', reviewed by Bantz et al. (2014).

In terms of pathophysiology, asthma and AR share many similarities: the inflammatory process is the same, characterised by mast cell degranulation, early and late phase responses, and eosinophils being key players in both conditions (Figure 13.1 and Figure 13.2). AR can cause considerable morbidity. It can be classified in a number of ways, conventionally being thought of as seasonal allergic rhinitis (SAR) or perennial allergic rhinitis (PAR). In addition, it can be thought of as mild, or moderate/severe.

Epidemiological studies vary in findings, but approximately 70% of people with asthma have some degree of AR, while approximately 40% of people with AR have some form of lower airways involvement, which can manifest as asthma. These findings underpin the notion of 'united airways', with the recommendation that where allergic inflammation exists at one end of the airway (e.g. asthma), the other end of the airway should also be assessed in some way for allergic inflammation (e.g. AR) (Figure 13.3). The importance of this was demonstrated by Baser et al. (2007). Eighty nine patients with AR but no diagnoses of asthma were screened for asthma using symptom questionnaires and lung function testing. Following screening and appropriate trials of treatment, approximately 25% of the group were confirmed as having a new diagnosis of asthma.

Many patients who have AR may not consult a health care professional for advice, relying instead on over-the-counter medications which may not always be the correct choice for their level of disease. Where AR and asthma coexist, poorly controlled AR has been shown to impact negatively upon asthma control, leading some authorities to suggest that optimising AR management can lead to improved asthma control. This is debateable to some extent and randomised controlled trials (e.g. Dahl et al., 2005) studying the impact of AR treatment on asthma control have concluded that where the two conditions coexist they should both be treated optimally, regardless of the presence of the other condition.

There are a number of guidelines for the management of AR, such as those published by the British Society for Allergy and Clinical Immunology (BSACI, 2008). Most guidelines are uniform in their advice. Common strategies – once the diagnosis has been confirmed – include:

- Allergen avoidance (there is limited evidence for this, however, and it can difficult to implement in many cases)
- Immunotherapy (desensitisation) – highly specialised, and can be very effective but requires expert selection of patients and administration of therapy
- Pharmacotherapy: therapies include antihistamines (systemic and topical), topical corticosteroids (seen as the gold standard treatment), cromones (useful in certain situations) and leukotriene receptor antagonists (LTRAs)
- Nasal douches have been shown to have benefits in some trials.

Practical advice for systemic antihistamine use

- Try to start these before AR symptoms develop (for seasonal AR BSACI advise 2 weeks' pre-treatment)
- Use second generation antihistamines (e.g. cetirizine, loratidine) as these are much less sedating than first generation preparations
- If a particular drug does not work, or becomes less effective, swapping to another preparation usually helps
- Shop around – generic antihistamines can be substantially cheaper than brand names but are equally effective
- Antihistamines are very effective in controlling itchiness, runny nose, sneezing and eye symptoms; however, they are not so effective when nasal congestion is a problem and topical corticosteroids should be considered in this situation.

Practical advice for topical corticosteroid use

- Newer drug preparations (fluticasone, mometasone) have extremely low bioavailability and so pose much less risk of systemic side effects than older versions which should be used with caution where use will be long term.
- It is essential to ensure device technique is correct. Patients should be advised to clean the nose thoroughly, point the nozzle of the device towards the side of the nose and avoid vigorous inhalation as this will simply take the drug away from the nose where it is needed to the back of the throat (patients reporting unpleasant taste is a good indicator that poor control results from poor technique) (Figure 13.4).

Nasal decongestants are available over-the-counter. They can be very effective at reducing congestion. However, they should only be used in the short term (i.e. 2–3 days, with an absolute maximum of 10 days; beyond this there is the risk of rhinitis medicamentosa, a form of rebound rhinitis where congestion recurs more severely and is less responsive to treatment).

AR and asthma together

Some evidence suggests treating AR can improve asthma control, but this is debatable. Where asthma control is suboptimal, the essential actions are to check inhaler technique and adherence with inhaled corticosteroids, as there are common causes of poor control. Current smoking can also cause problems as this reduces corticosteroid efficacy (Chaudhuri et al., 2003). If treatment and adherence have been optimised and AR is present, it should certainly be treated effectively regardless of other considerations, and any of the options for managing AR outlined can be considered. One further consideration where AR and asthma coexist is the use of an LTRA. These are an option in step 3 of UK asthma management guidelines, and are licensed for seasonal AR and asthma, and many clinicians report excellent results in some patients at least. One advantage of these drugs is that they are presented in tablet or capsule form, which is preferable for patients in terms of ease of use.

Further reading

British Society for Allergy and Clinical Immunology (2008) Rhinosinusitis and nasal polyposis. http://www.bsaci.org/guidelines/rhinosinusitis-nasal-polyposis (accessed 22 February 2016).

14 Respiratory disease and sexuality

Figure 14.1 Sexual positions

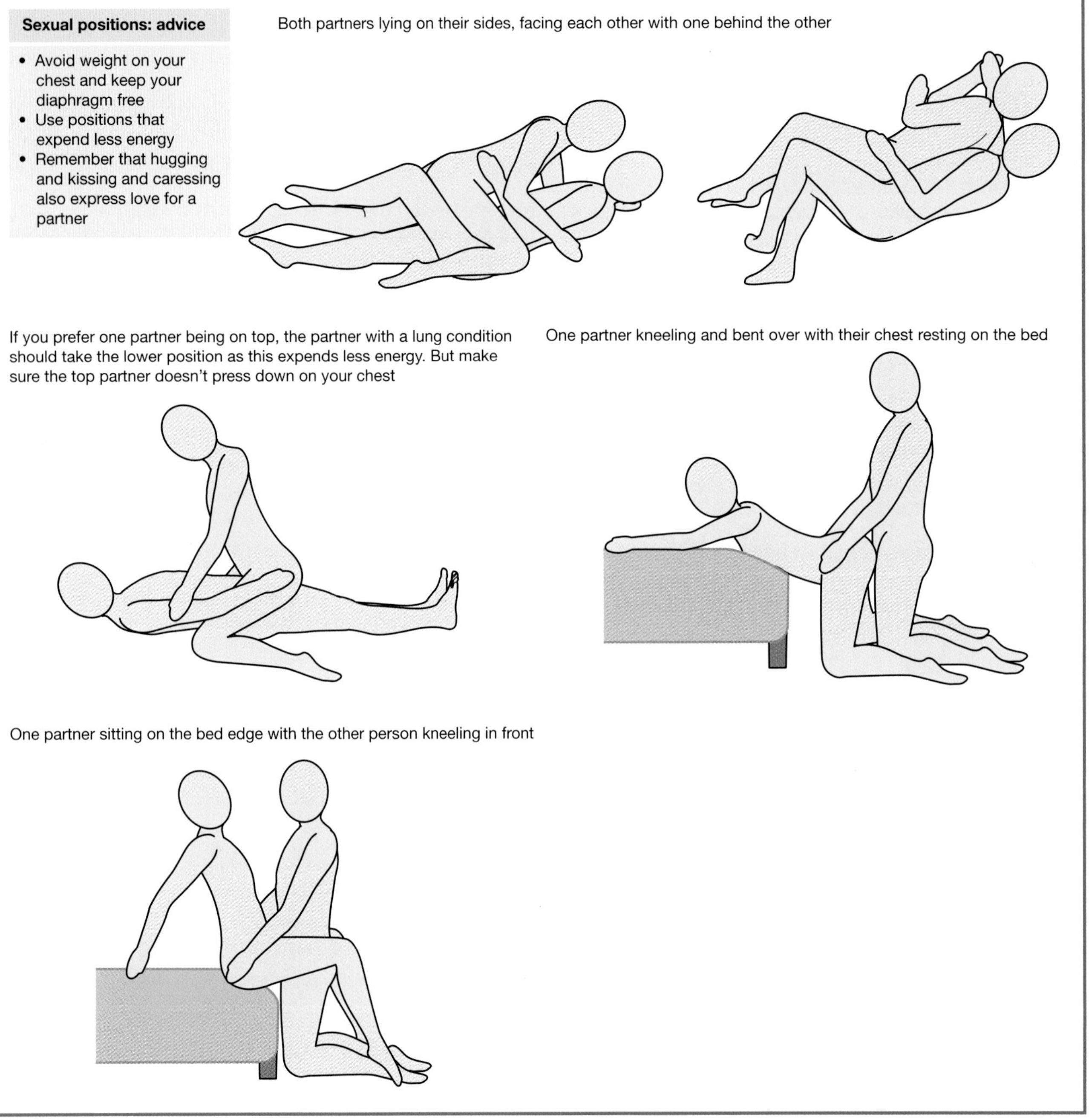
Sexual positions: advice
• Avoid weight on your chest and keep your diaphragm free
• Use positions that expend less energy
• Remember that hugging and kissing and caressing also express love for a partner
Both partners lying on their sides, facing each other with one behind the other
If you prefer one partner being on top, the partner with a lung condition should take the lower position as this expends less energy. But make sure the top partner doesn't press down on your chest
One partner kneeling and bent over with their chest resting on the bed
One partner sitting on the bed edge with the other person kneeling in front

What is it all about?

People with any chronic illness, including a respiratory disorder, have a range of physical, psychological, social and emotional needs in the same way as people without a chronic illness. Somewhere in the rehabilitative process of the patient with lung disease, after medical and physical needs have been addressed, other issues can arise.

Sex is a biological term, depicting our gender, and to be human is to be a sexual being. Sex, who we are and our sexuality means our physical responses are an essential part of our lives. Sexuality involves emotions, our understanding of ourselves and our interactions with others.

Sex and respiratory disease

Sexual problems and breathlessness are often how people adapt to their disease, rather than the disease itself. The most important message we can give to our patients is that an increased breathing rate during sex is normal and harmless, and that the breathlessness this can cause is not dangerous.

Breathless patients can enjoy their love life but often fear intimacy because of breathlessness. A British Lung Foundation (BLF) survey in 2003, Breathing Fears, surveyed 1388 people with COPD and found that because of their breathlessness they felt that they had missed out on:

- 2.89 million kisses
- 3.15 million hugs
- 3.82 million chances to make love.

How to raise the issue?

Not everyone is comfortable with discussing sexual issues with patients and it is important to be aware of your own limitations. If the subject comes up and you do not want to handle it then acknowledge the problem and provide further information as to where to obtain help. It is important to know how far to go and when to to ask for help. Sensitivity is important.

Is it all about breathlessness?

Patients may worry about increased breathlessness during sexual activity; however, although breathing rates can alter, the physical stress of sexual intercourse is limited and comparable to climbing one or two flights of stairs. Regardless of the activity, helping patients to accept that they will experience some breathlessness is essential.

It can also be useful to review the patient's medication; many can affect libido and sexual functioning as can co-morbid conditions such as diabetes and cardiovascular disease. And it may not be all about breathlessness; it might be a relationship difficulty, which can be trickier to deal with.

The nurse's role

The nurse's role is to support and encourage those who are struggling with their feelings. It is important to be prepared and this means having some educational material available and not being embarrassed when the issue is raised. Be responsive and acknowledge the problem and, where possible, be useful. Always use comfortable terminology. Not all patients will wish to discuss what to many is a very personal part of their lives but those who do will need practical advice such as energy conservation, using bronchodilators prior to sexual activity, using oxygen if prescribed and practical advice on positions that need less effort (Figure 14.1).

Be a good listener and acknowledge the problem even if you do not feel able to offer practical advice. By helping patients to cope with the impact of the disease process on their lives, including their sexual lives, focuses on the impact of chronic lung disease and the symptoms it causes in patients.

Further reading

British Lung Foundation (BLF) Leaflets available at www.blf.org.uk/publications (accessed 22 February 2106).

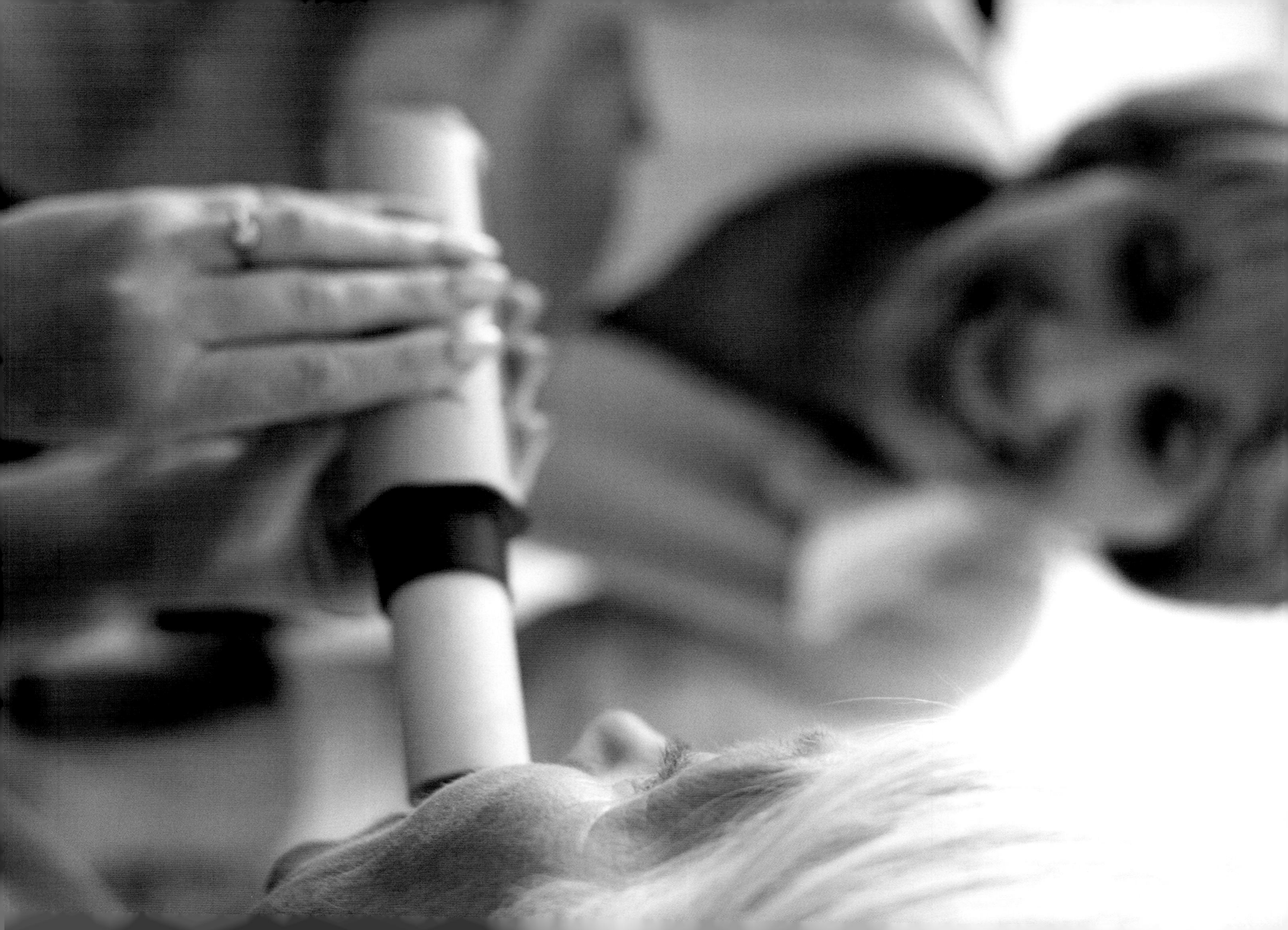

Assessment and diagnosis of respiratory disease

Part 3

Chapters

Overview

Assessment and diagnosis is an essential part of any nursing intervention. With the advancement of practice, many nurses now have skills that enable them to undertake a comprehensive assessment and be involved in diagnostics. Part 3 provides an overview of approaches and procedures involving the assessment and diagnosis of various presentations related to patients with respiratory conditions.

15 Respiratory history taking

Figure 15.1 Misunderstanding and confusion

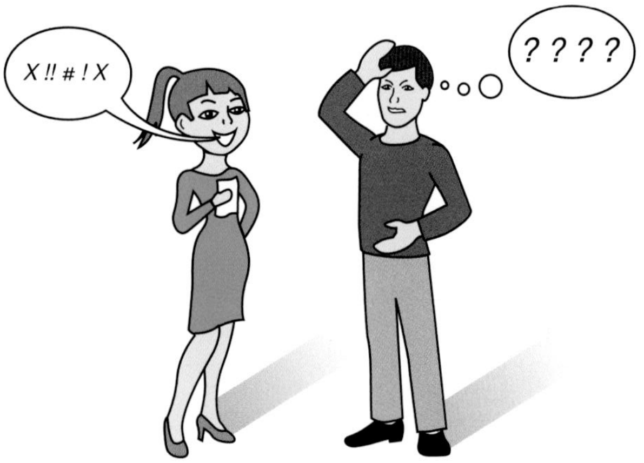
X !! # ! X
? ? ? ?

Figure 15.2 Document the consultation as the patient says it

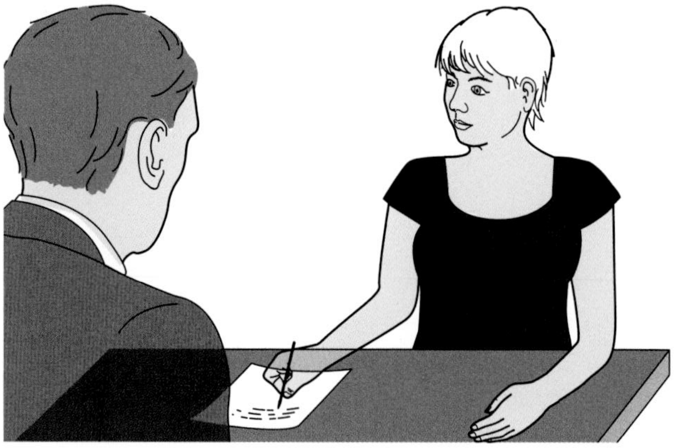

Table 15.1 Example of the hospital clerking model

The hospital clerking model	
HPC	History of present complaint
PMH	Past medical history
DRUGS	Medication
FH	Family history
SH	Social history
DQ	Direct questions
EXAM	Examination
Inv	Investigation
D	Diagnosis

Table 15.2 Example of a BORG visual analogue dyspnoea scale

1	Not breathless at all
2	Very, very slight
3	Very slight
4	Slight
5	Moderate
6	Severe
7	
8	Very severe
9	
10	Very, very severe

Table 15.3 MRC dyspnoea scale, which can be useful but does not consider other co-morbidities such as arthritis or heart failure

Grade	Impact
1	Not troubled by breathlessness except on vigorous exercise
2	Short of breath when hurrying or walking up inclines
3	Walks slower than people of the same age on the level because of breathlessness or has to stop for breath when walking at ownpace
4	Stops for breath after 100 metres or after a few minutes on the level
5	Too breathless to leave the house or breathless when dressing or undressing

Why take a history?

Respiratory history taking is an essential part of a patient's assessment. Often it is from good clinical history taking that a diagnosis is made. This communication forms part of a therapeutic relationship from which the development of trust begins or is built upon. An effective consultation is a two-way process which is fundamentally reliant on good communication skills – both verbal and non-verbal. This is a clear opportunity for clinicians to enable patients to express the reasons why they have presented themselves. These reasons include reaching their tolerance limits of anxiety, problems living with presenting symptoms, prevention of symptoms or for administration reasons (form filling). Poor communication can lead to conflicting messages, misunderstanding, dissatisfaction, all of which may lead to complaints or litigation (Figure 15.1). Top tips for good communication: make sure you speak clearly, avoid medical jargon and emotive words and listen to your patient.

Which consultation model?

Consultation models offer a systematic approach to obtaining the information required in order to formulate an opinion, share information and agree goals and clarify consent especially in relation to third parties. The type of consultation model used, however, is dictated by the severity of the illness, the patient and access to their background history, time and environment. There are several models available; Table 15.1 is an example of the hospital clerking model. The clinical situation can dictate use of open-ended or reflective questioning such as 'Do you have a cough?' (closed question) or 'Can you tell me a bit more about your cough?' (open ended) then a clarifying question from the clinician that demonstrates listening such as 'OK, can you remember when your cough first started?' Clarify the meaning of terms like 'allergy', be non-judgemental and objective. Consider, culture, personal space and physical contact. Be mindful that you are dealing with feelings, such as anger and frustration, and this must be acknowledged.

Gathering information

Information should be gathered in a systematic way, starting with the patient's presenting complaint in their own words and recorded in this exact way (Figure 15.2). The history of that complaint should be explored using your knowledge and skills to direct questioning and clarify points on the way. For example, a 63-year-old male smoker would imply with his age that he is a long-term smoker and increases the probability for certain diagnoses related to this. Another example: a patient presents with persistent cough and haemoptysis and weight loss for 2 months, increases the likelihood of lung cancer rather than chronic obstructive pulmonary disease (COPD). If the same man was complaining of chest pain, has he pulled a muscle coughing or is this cardiac in nature? The main signs and symptoms of a respiratory disease according to Bourke (2015) are dyspnoea, wheeze, cough, sputum, haemoptysis, and chest pain and for all of these, onset, duration, variability, contributing and relieving factors should be analysed. Tools for measuring subjective experiences of a symptom, such as dyspnoea, can be useful (Chapter 17). Wheeze is associated with airway narrowing and again onset, variability either diurnal or associated with certain days/environments can determine possible causes (e.g. occupational). A cough is a reflex action meant to clear the airways, but can be caused by an irritant or drug induced and is described a dry or productive. Sputum colour, taste, presence of blood, viscosity, amount and ease of clearance can aid differential diagnosis. Chest pain on inspiration or cough is described as pleuritic pain; however, explore the site, any radiation to other areas and type of pain (i.e. tightness, soreness or crushing).

It is important to take a full history including medical and surgical complaints, medications, lifestyle choices, social and psychological history, occupational and family history, childhood diseases, immunisation and recent travel. This information creates an overall picture of the patient to aid decision making, diagnosis and plan care.

Past medical history

This extracts past medical conditions that may be contributing to the presenting complaint (e.g. breathlessness can be caused by a number of conditions). Medication history including immunisations leads on from this as the appropriateness of drugs, compliance, optimisation, side effects and allergies could also be a contributing factor. Lifestyle choices such as smoking history, recreational drug use and alcohol intake can be more prevalent in certain diseases. Social history leads to enquiry on what support network is available in the home, if the patient is vulnerable, any identified possible links to poor living standards, pets and possible risks and the level of independence they manage to achieve, and enquiry into any recent foreign travel. This links to family history to explore any possible familial disease or inherited diseases. Childhood diseases and exposure to illnesses (travel) such as tuberculosis can lead to delayed problems so this should also be considered.

Some diseases such as COPD are more highly associated with anxiety and depression (Chapter 23) so recording psychological problems and any issues regarding capacity and consent need to be explored. Some occupations pose a direct health risk for certain diseases, such as asbestos exposure and sarcoidosis. Data should include length of time in each job and if there were any health problems when they retired if applicable and known exposure to any toxins, dust and chemicals. This list is not exhaustive so information gathered should be used to further direct the consultation and complement the respiratory examination.

Further reading

Douglas G, Nicol F, Robertson C. (eds.) (2013) *Macleod 's Clinical Examination*, 13th edn. Churchill Livingstone.

16 Respiratory clinical examination

Table 16.1 Respiratory inspection, palpation, percussion and auscultation (IPPA)

	Pneumonia	Pneumothorax	Plural effusion	COPD
History/ inspection	Cough, sputum production, fever	Dyspnoea, chest pain, Hx of trauma. ↑VP* in tension	Dyspnoea, mild non-productive cough, chest pain	Chronic smoking repeated respiratory infections, dyspnoea, cough
Palpation	• ↑Tactile fremitus • ↓Chest expansion – unilateral	• ↓Tactile fremitus • Tracheal deviation if tension (away from affected side) • ↓Chest expansion unilateral	• ↓Tactile fremitus • Tracheal deviation (away from affected side) if >1000 mL	• ↓Chest expansion bilaterally
Percussion	Dull	Hyper-resonant	Stony dull	Hyper-resonant
Auscultation	• Bronchial breathing • Added sounds: crackles and wheeze • ↑Vocal resonance (whispering pectoriloquy)	• ↓Vesicular breath sounds • Added sounds	• ↓Vesicular breath sounds • Crackles at the upper edge of the effusion • Pleural friction rub • Muffled vocal resonance	• ↓Vesicular breath sounds • Added sound: wheeze, crackles

*VP, venous pressure

Figure 16.1 Clubbing/Schamroth's sign DPD, distal phalangeal depth: IPD, interphalangeal depth. DPD : IPD is the phalangeal depth ratio, the DPD being smaller than the IPD in the normal finger, but the DPD is greater than the IPD in finger clubbing

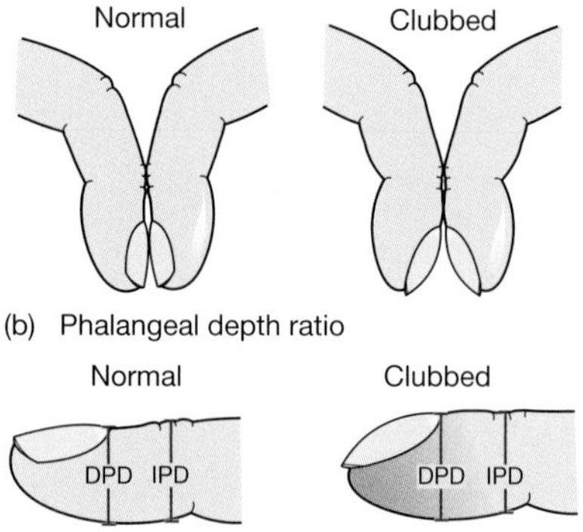
(a) Schamroth's sign
Normal
Clubbed
(b) Phalangeal depth ratio
Normal
Clubbed
DPD IPD
DPD IPD

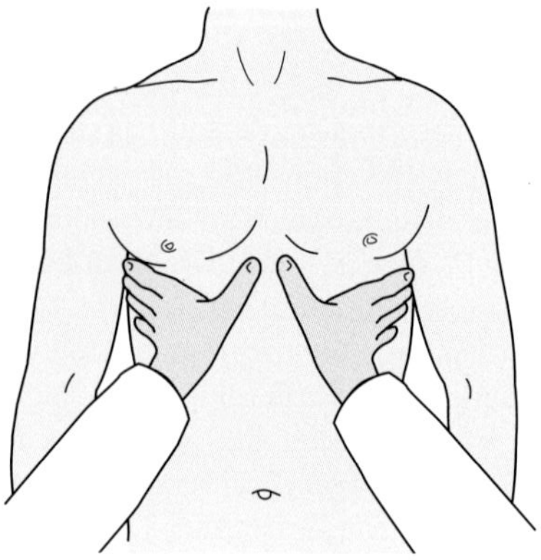

Figure 16.2 Checking for chest expansion

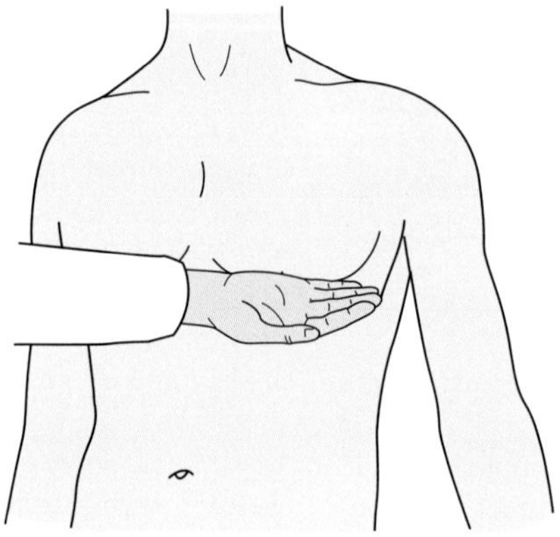

Figure 16.3 Tactile fremitus

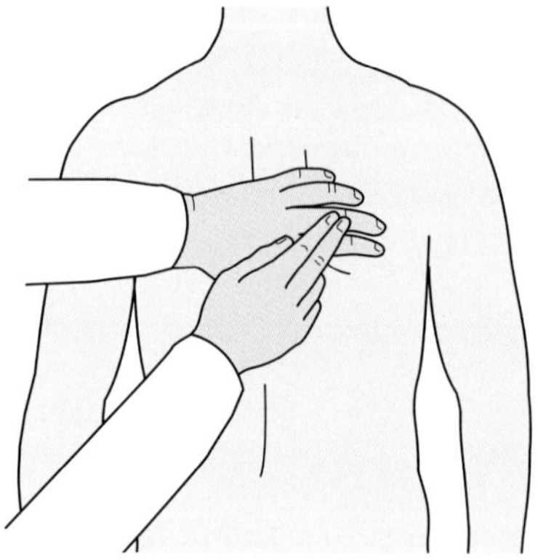

Figure 16.4 Example of percussion

Figure 16.5 Example of the order of percussion and auscultation

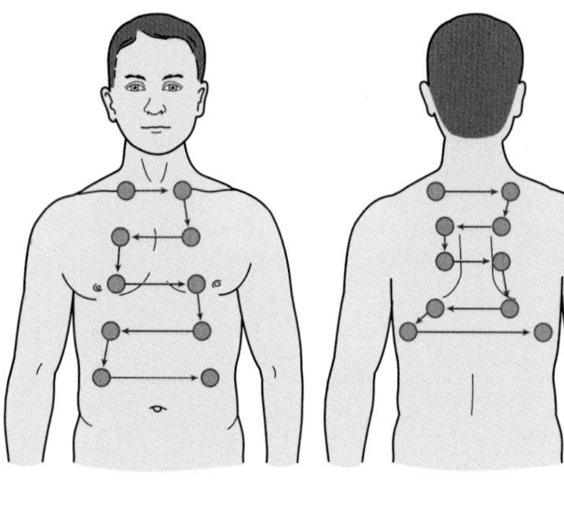
Anterior view
Posterior view

Table 16.2 Respiratory patterns

Normal (eupnoea)	Regular and comfortable at 12–20 breaths/minute
Tachypnoea	20 breaths/minute
Bradypnoea	<12 breaths/minute
Hyperventilation	Rapid, deep respiration >20 breaths/minute
Apneustic	Neurological – sustained inspiratory effort
Cheyenne – Stokes	Neurological – alternating patterns of depth separated by brief periods of apnoea
Kussmaul's	Rapid, deep and labored – common in DKA*
Air trapping	Difficulty during expiration – emphysema

*DKA, diabetic ketoacidosis

A clinical examination should be undertaken by practitioners who are competent to do so within the scope of their own practice.

When undertaking a respiratory clinical examination of a patient it is recommended to use a recognised examination tool to enable a systematic review. For this chapter the tool selected is that of inspection, palpation, percussion and auscultation (IPPA; Table 16.1).

It is essential to introduce yourself, wash your hands and gain consent before commencing the examination. Explain what each stage of the examination will involve and ensure a chaperone is available if needed. Consider privacy, modesty and dignity together with cultural and gender sensitivity.

First, undertake a general assessment of the patient – looking at the patient's breathing pattern (check the rate rhythm, symmetry and depth Table 16.2). Are there any signs of respiratory distress? Observe for accessory muscle use and intercostal recession. Observe for signs of audible wheeze, stridor, hypoxaemia or hypercapnoea (drowsy, shaking, flapping tremor, confusion and agitation) as any of these signs can alert the examiner to the acuity of the patient's condition. Assess the patient's ability to speak in full sentences. Assess for pain; this may be contributing to changes in the above and can require more prompt review to reduce discomfort. Is the patient producing any sputum (colour, consistency, volume and smell)? Also assess for weight loss or evidence of muscle wastage as this can indicate other more serious pathologies.

Inspection

At this point it is necessary to expose the patient's chest. Look at the shape (assess both the anterior and posterior view), check for symmetry, barrel chest, deformity (e.g. kyphosis) or tracheal tugging. Assess if the patient's chest rises and falls equally; this can be observed when assessing the respiratory rate and depth. Observe for any noticeable scars from previous surgery or evidence of radiological tattoos. Check the skin and peripheries for any evidence of cyanosis or flushing (both can be acute signs). Also check the hands for clubbing and undertake the Schamroth's window test (Figure 16.1) which can indicate advanced respiratory disease. At this stage check for tar staining as this indicates nicotine use.

Palpation

If the patient expresses pain or discomfort then ask them to locate the area then inspect this in more detail. Check the position of the trachea; locate the heads of the two clavicles as any deviation can suggest a pneumothorax or tumour. Is the chest expanding equally? To assess this place your hands on the chest wall with your thumbs meeting at the midline (Figure 16.2), ask the patient to take a deep breath in and note the distance between the thumbs and any asymmetry of movement. It is important to assess for any enlarged lymph nodes specifically supraclavicular, fossae and axilla (refer to a clinical examination text for the location of these). Feel for tactile fremitus by placing the medial edge of your hands bilaterally and ask the patient to say '99'. Start at the apex above the clavicle, move downwards from upper to lower lobes, checking for symmetry between left and right. You are feeling for transmission of sound vibration (Figure 16.3). Jugular venous pressure (JVP) needs to be assessed with the patient reclined at a 45° angle, with the head turned to the opposing side, observe above the clavicle for a superficial pulsation and the height of this is noted if seen.

Percussion

Percussion is a practised skill and involves placing the middle finger of the non-dominant hand flat on the chest wall then striking the finger placed on the patient's skin with the end of the finger of your dominant hand. Figures 16.4 and 16.5 give an example of a systematic way of examining the chest wall which can be also used for auscultation. When tapping the finger on the intercostal space listen for dullness or resonance, the former can indicate density associated with a solid such as fluid or a tumour and the latter can be heard in hyperinflated lungs or a pneumothorax (can be drum-like).

Auscultation

Auscultation is undertaken by listening with a stethoscope for the intensity and character of breath sounds. The recognition of sounds comes with experience. Each side is compared symmetrically (Figure 16.5) (top to bottom then axilla) and any added sounds are noted such as rubs, wheezes, crackles. The location of the sound is also documented (Table 16.1). It is good practice to ask the patient to cough before listening with a stethoscope and to breathe in and out with their mouth open, to help with transmission of sounds.

While these points are frequently assessed, dependent on the patient's presenting symptoms and the outcome of your examination, additional exploratory examination or assessment may be needed. There are a range of clinical examination texts and websites available for guidance on this subject.

Further reading

Douglas G, Nicol F, Robertson C. (eds.) (2013) *Macleod's Clinical Examination*, 13th edn. Churchill Livingstone.

17 Measuring dyspnoea

Figure 17.1 Downward spiral of inactivity and dyspnoea

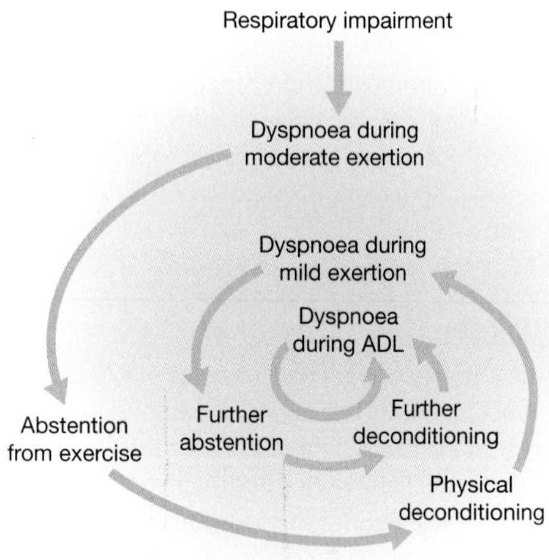
Respiratory impairment
Dyspnoea during moderate exertion
Dyspnoea during mild exertion
Dyspnoea during ADL
Further deconditioning
Physical deconditioning
Further abstention
Abstention from exercise

ADL = activities of daily living

Figure 17.2 Anxiety–dyspnoea–anxiety

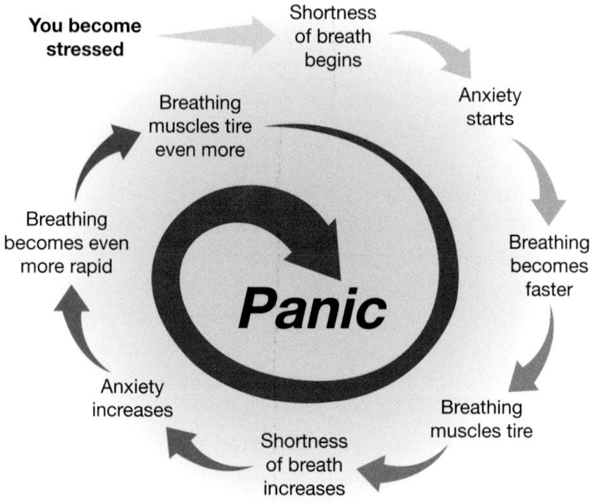
You become stressed
Shortness of breath begins
Anxiety starts
Breathing becomes faster
Breathing muscles tire
Shortness of breath increases
Anxiety increases
Breathing becomes even more rapid
Breathing muscles tire even more
Panic

Box 17.1 Descriptors for dyspnoea
Source: Adapted from Parshall et al. (2012).

- Urge to breath
- Hunger for air
- Unsatisfied inspiration
- Breath does not go in all the way
- Like breath hold
- Breaths felt too small
- Feeling of suffocation
- Cannot get enough air
- Need for more air
- Starved for air

Box 17.2 Borg scale

Borg rating of perceived exertion

6	No exertion at all
7	Extremely light
8	
9	Very light
10	
11	Light
12	
13	Somewhat hard
14	
15	Hard (heavy)
16	
17	Very hard
18	
19	Extremely hard
20	Maximal exertion

Table 17.1 Domains of dyspnoea measurement. VAS, visual analogue scale
Source: Adapted from Parshall et al. (2012).

Domain	Definition	Examples
Sensory-perceptual experience	Measures of what breathing feels like to the patient or research subject	• Single item ratings of intensity (e.g. Borg scale, VAS) • Description of specific sensations/clusters of related sensations
Affected distress	Measures of how distressing breathing feels. Focus can be either immediate (e.g. unpleasantness) or evaluative (e.g. judgements of meaning or consequences)	• Single-item ratings of severity of distress or unpleasantness • Multi-item scales of emotional responses such as anxiety
Symptom impact or burden	Measures of how dyspnoea/breathlessness affects functional ability, employment (disability), quality of life, or health status	• Unidimensional rating of disability or activity limitation (e.g. MRC scale) • Unidimensional or multidimensional ratings of functional ability • Multidimensional scales of quality of life/health status

Dyspnoea

Dyspnoea, or breathlessness, is one of the most distressing, disabling and prevalent symptoms that patients with respiratory disease experience. It is defined as a subjective experience of breathing discomfort. It has also been described as a complex and distressing experience of both body and mind and identified as a potent predictor of mortality and use of health care resources. It is associated with a real or impending threat to life and can be terrifying for the individual and those caring for them. Dyspnoea is therefore considered to be most appropriately assessed by the patient.

It should not be overlooked that breathlessness is a normal familiar sensation that occurs with physical exertion. However, in the presence of disease or sub-optimal physical fitness, the threshold for experiencing dyspnoea is lowered. Refractory dyspnoea is that which persists at rest or with minimal activity despite optimal therapy of the underlying condition. Dyspnoea can therefore be described as a heightened level of awareness of the uncomfortable sensation of feeling breathless.

Causes

Dyspnoea is a common symptom affecting up to 50% of all patients in acute care and 25% of patients in ambulatory settings (Parshall et al., 2012). The symptom may be experienced as a consequence of a wide range of diseases, commonly, but not exclusively, cardiopulmonary and neuromuscular. In addition, it may be seen as a manifestation of poor cardiovascular fitness and obesity, both which can pre-exist with clinical conditions serving to exacerbate the symptom. This is particularly common in patients with chronic lung conditions, where a fear of breathlessness itself contributes to a sedentary lifestyle, which in turn results in a loss of muscle mass and functioning; the ultimate consequence is general physical deconditioning which requires increased work of breathing and in turn enhances the sensation of dyspnoea (Figure 17.1). Overlaid with fear and anxiety of mortal danger, a vicious cycle of worsening dyspnoea often ensues which is extremely difficult to break or control. This emotional response to dyspnoea often manifests in panic and can be responsible for increased health care utilisation in addition to the negative impact on quality of life (Figure 17.2).

Assessing dyspnoea

In order to treat dyspnoea it is important to undertake a thorough assessment of the patient including a measure of dyspnoea. This can be difficult: attempting to make an objective measurement of a subjective phenomenon.

Dyspnoea has been described as several qualitatively distinctive sensations (Box 17.1). Assessment is by an individual's verbal description but there are also numerous validated tools (too many to outline here). It is important when considering the choice of instrument to understand that the various tools measure different domains of dyspnoea (Table 17.1).

These tools require different levels of input from the nurse or health care professional assessing the patient and are appropriate for different circumstances. For example, the Borg scale (Box 17.2) can be used to assess symptom severity while a patient is undertaking activities as a means of assessing exertional dyspnoea. Symptom intensity can be assessed using the Medical Research Council (MRC) breathlessness scale (see Table 15.3). This is a quick and easy-to-use tool that can be self-administered or administered by another person. It comprises five easily understood statements, which describe a range of levels of respiratory disability, from none (Grade 1) to almost complete incapacity (Grade 5). The score is the number that best fits the patient's level of activity. The score correlates well with the results of other breathlessness scales; however, it lacks sensitivity to changes in dyspnoea, for example during an activity. This is when more complex scales can be useful. The MRC dyspnoea scale, however, is a quick and easy-to-use tool and, as such, is recommended for use assessing dyspnoea in the initial diagnosis of chronic obstructive pulmonary disease (COPD), follow-up and as part of the referral criteria for pulmonary rehabilitation (NICE, 2011).

It is also worth noting that for many patients with chronic respiratory disease, dyspnoea and anxiety are inextricably linked. For these patients, in order to intervene to break this vicious dyspnoea–anxiety–dyspnoea cycle, it will be necessary to assess anxiety and depression in addition to dyspnoea (Chapter 23). With the morbidity of psychological characteristics, in particular moderate to high levels of anxiety, interventions to break this cycle can impact on dyspnoea and are worth targeting.

Treatment of dyspnoea

The treatment of dyspnoea is considered in more detail in Chapter 57 in the context of supportive and palliative care. These treatments involve a number of approaches, with both pharmacological and non-pharmacological therapies.

Needless to say, diagnosis and treatment of the underlying pathologic causes of dyspnoea is the recommended initial approach but, for many patients the cause may not be known, or dyspnoea becomes refractory and trying to improve the symptom can be challenging.

Summary

Dyspnoea is clearly a complex phenomenon that impacts on morbidity, mortality and health care utilisation. While physiological mechanisms are important, it is also clear that psychological, social and environmental factors are also pivotal in the way that dyspnoea is experienced and controlled. Only the person experiencing dyspnoea can perceive it as such.

Whatever the cause, there is little doubt that dyspnoea is extremely uncomfortable and has a profound negative impact on quality of life. The measurement and assessment of dyspnoea is therefore a vital aspect of caring for the patient with respiratory disease. This assessment allows treatments and therapies to be tailored to the patient on an individual basis and ensure that ineffective interventions are stopped if and when appropriate.

18 Sputum assessment

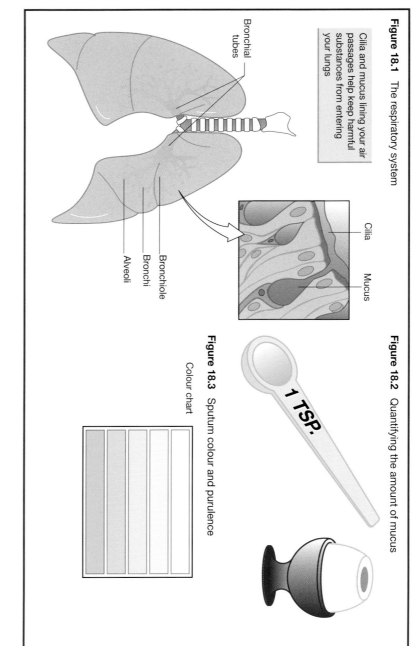

Figure 18.1 The respiratory system

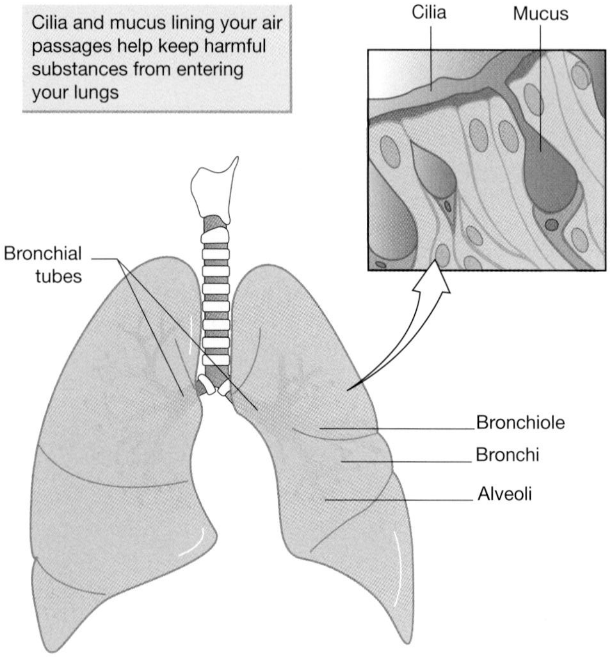
Cilia and mucus lining your air passages help keep harmful substances from entering your lungs
Cilia
Mucus
Bronchial tubes
Bronchiole
Bronchi
Alveoli

Figure 18.2 Quantifying the amount of mucus

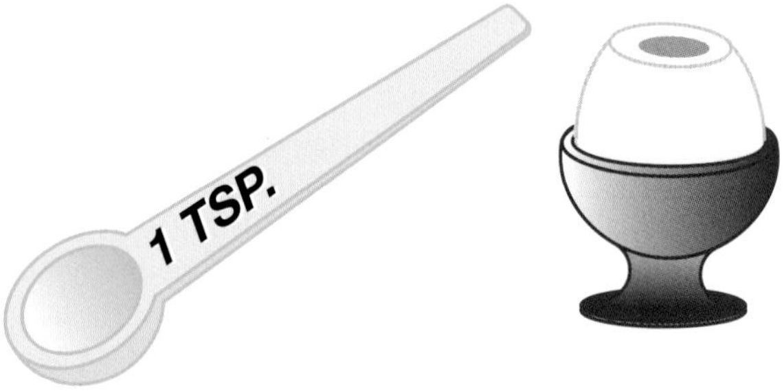
1 TSP.

Figure 18.3 Sputum colour and purulence

Colour chart

Sputum

Sputum or mucus is naturally produced in the lungs in order to catch tiny inhaled particles. Mucus is produced by cells in the trachea and bronchial tubes to keep air passages moist and aid in stopping dust, bacteria and viruses and other substances from entering the lungs. Impurities that do reach the deeper parts of the lungs can often be moved up by mucus utilising tiny hairs called cilia and coughed out or swallowed (Figure 18.1).

In many chronic respiratory conditions mucus can be over-produced and the goblet cells that produce the mucus can become stretched. In these conditions the mucus hypersecretion can limit the airflow and increase breathlessness and cough. If the mucus or sputum becomes particularly thick and sticky it can cause 'plugs' or blockages in the small airways, which can cause acute breathlessness and impact on ventilation. Excess sputum in the lungs encourages bacterial growth and patients with mucus hypersecretion are prone to infection.

Importance of clinical history in sputum assessment

Understanding the normal daily sputum production for the patient is a key component of respiratory clinical history to ascertain if the symptoms and or sputum production have changed recently. Questions to the patient should include the normal colour and consistency of the sputum, indicting purulence and signs of infection. Furthermore, sputum examination can also support clinical diagnosis: the amount, colour and consistency over how long, and for how many days in a month or year? Patients with copious sputum production may lean towards a more bronchitic phenotype; however, this requires a medical opinion and CT examination to verify.

Further respiratory consultation should include questioning on cough and sputum production. How often does the patient cough, is it productive, how much sputum is produced a day?

Answers can be diagnostically relevant and so it is helpful for patients to have guidance so they can quantify the amount of sputum more accurately (Figure 18.2).

Obtaining a sample

Clear the nose and the back of the throat. Gargle, spit and rinse to clear the mouth of any debris. Sputum should be taken from the lungs after a deep cough.

If sputum cannot be obtained in this way, chest clearance or sputum induction with inhaled saline can be performed. Caution is required to avoid cross-infection.

Samples need to be clean to ensure that any microbiology or laboratory test is accurate, and the correct antibiotic recommended. Sputum can be a useful tool to understand airways inflammation using cell counts of eosinophils and neutrophils.

Sample observations

Examining sputum is clinically important for:

- Diagnosis
- Signs of infection.

Sputum colour can aid in determining the purulence of the sputum. Purulence is indicative of bacterial load. Stockley et al. (2001) and his team have developed a sputum colour chart, which can be correlated directly to sputum purulence (Figure 18.3). This tool can be used with patients to assist them to recognise respiratory infections.

Excess sputum can encourage bacterial growth and can restrict normal ventilation; therefore an assessment of the ease of expectoration is required. This can be achieved by assessing the consistency or the thickness/viscosity of the sputum, by inverting the specimen in a container or holding to a light source to assess opaqueness. The more opaque, or the slower the sputum travels, the more viscos it is.

Medications such as carbocysteine can be prescribed to reduce the viscosity of the sputum and make it easier to expectorate. Dehydration can also make mucus thicker and stickier, encouraging fluids (note any co-morbidities indicating fluid restriction) can loosen sputum.

Troubleshooting haemoptysis

Medical opinion and further specimens are required to screen for mycobacteria. Note that haemoptysis can also be a sign of respiratory infection.

Further reading

Tangedal S, Aanerud M, Persson LJP, et al. (2014) Comparison of inflammatory markers in induced and spontaneous sputum in a cohort of COPD patients. *Respir Res* 15: 138.

19 Pulse oximetry

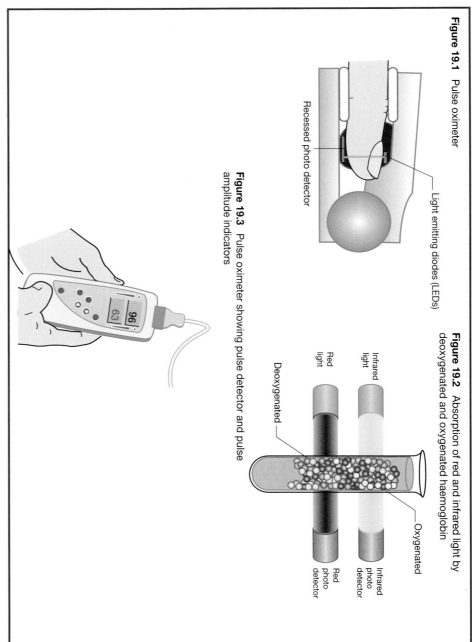

Figure 19.1 Pulse oximeter

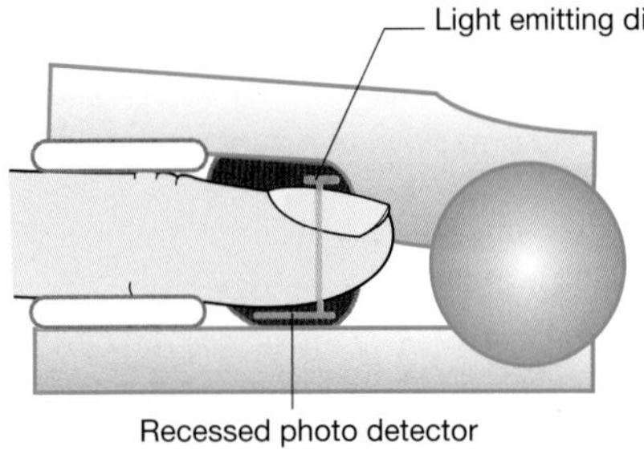
Light emitting diodes (LEDs)
Recessed photo detector

Figure 19.2 Absorption of red and infrared light by deoxygenated and oxygenated haemoglobin

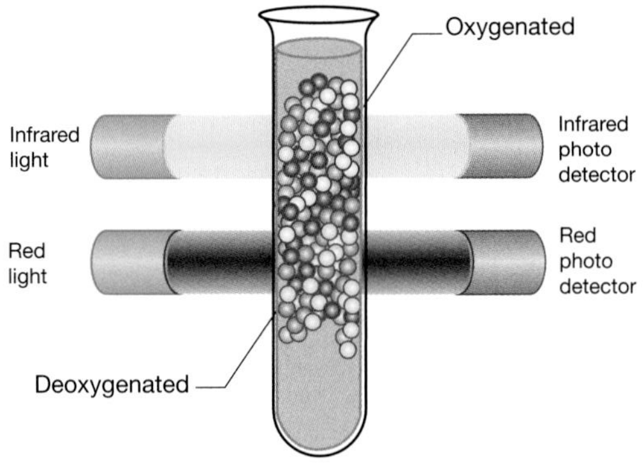
Oxygenated
Infrared light
Infrared photo detector
Red light
Red photo detector
Deoxygenated

Figure 19.3 Pulse oximeter showing pulse detector and pulse amplitude indicators

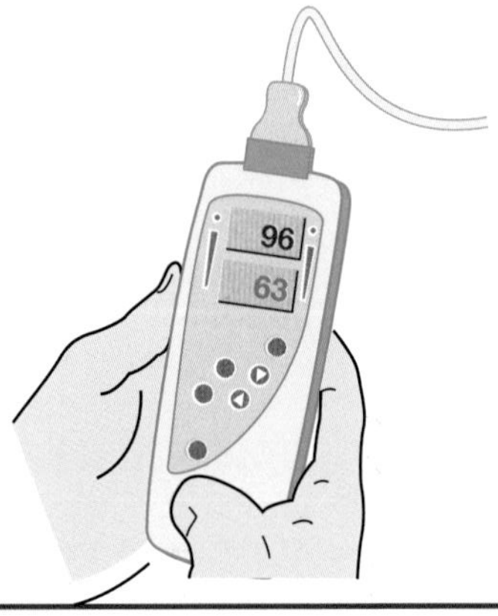
96
63

Pulse oximetry is a simple non-invasive method of measuring oxygen levels which can be useful in a variety of clinical settings to enable oxygenation to be monitored continuously or intermittently. An oximeter is a device that emits red and infrared light, shone through a capillary bed (usually fingertip or ear lobe) on to a sensor (Figure 19.1). Deoxygenated haemoglobin absorbs more red light and oxygenated haemoglobin absorbs more infrared light. Multiple measurements are made every second and the ratio of red to infrared light calculated to determine the peripheral oxygen saturation (SpO_2) (Figure 19.2).

Indications for use

Traditionally, observation of cyanosis was the primary clinical sign of hypoxaemia but early studies found that even skilled observers are not consistently able to detect central cyanosis (a blue tinge to the lips, tongue and mucus membranes) until oxyhaemoglobin saturation is below 80% (Hanning et al., 1995). Factors such as ambient light, skin pigmentation and peripheral perfusion all impact on ability to identify cyanosis. Pulse oximetry enables the earlier identification of clinically important low tissue oxygenation and current guidelines recommend that it should be available in all clinical settings where emergency oxygen is used (O'Driscoll et al., 2008). It also provides a useful monitoring and screening tool in the assessment of breathless patients in primary care.

However, pulse oximetry supports rather than replaces comprehensive assessment and examination. It is essential that inspired oxygen (FiO_2) and delivery device are recorded alongside oxygen saturations and that the effect of any changes to FiO_2 is monitored and documented. Results should be interpreted with clinical judgement in the context of the patient's existing diagnosis, presenting symptoms and other findings (PCRS-UK, 2009; Kelly, 2008).

Pulse oximetry should be available for use in all clinical settings where hypoxaemia can occur:

- Assessment of breathless/acutely ill patients including acute confusion
- To provide objective indication of severity of an acute respiratory episode and need for hospital admission such as exacerbation of chronic obstructive pulmonary disease (COPD) or asthma (NICE, 2010; BTS/SIGN 141, 2014), pneumonia (NICE, 2014)
- To determine need for emergency oxygen therapy in acute illness (O'Driscoll et al., 2008)
- Continuous recording such as during anaesthesia or sedation or in the assessment of oxygenation during sleep studies

- Routine monitoring in chronic respiratory disease to screen for suitability for assessment for domiciliary oxygen therapy (NICE, 2010; BTS, 2015)
- To guide titration of oxygen therapy during acute illness (O'Driscoll et al., 2008) or for domiciliary use (BTS, 2015). Additional monitoring with arterial blood gas sampling may be required where patients are at risk of type 2 (hypercapnic) respiratory failure.

It should be noted that pulse oximetry does not give a measure of arterial blood oxygen content or ventilation; oxygen delivery to the tissues is dependent on adequate ventilation and circulation but oximetry can add to the clinical picture to aid diagnostic and treatment decisions.

Limitations of oximetry

Pulse oximetry requires a good pulsatile blood flow and no interference with measurement of light absorption and detection. Pulse strength can be checked by ensuring the recorded heart rate correlates with a manual pulse rate; some devices have a pulse amplitude indicator in addition to a pulse detector (Figure 19.3).

Common causes of inaccuracies include:

- Poor peripheral circulation:
  - Cold peripheries
  - Constriction (e.g. from BP cuff, tight clothing or tight oximeter probe)
  - Poor perfusion due to hypovolaemia, marked hypotension or cardiac arrhythmias, peripheral vascular disease
  - Raynaud's syndrome
- Motion artefact
- Gross movement can cause loss of signal
- Fine vibration can interfere with accuracy
- Carbon monoxide/smoke inhalation/intravenous dyes used in diagnostic tests (e.g. methylene blue)
- Carboxyhaemoglobin (from carbon monoxide) is detected as oxyhaemoglobin and will overestimate true oxygen saturation
- Ambient light interference – light emitters and detectors must be directly opposite each other and light should only reach the detector via tissues. Inappropriate sized probes or excessive ambient light can result in inaccuracies
- Interference with transmission/detection of light signals
- Dirty probe sensors
- Nail varnish/synthetic nails
- Anaemia/skin discoloration (very dark skin/jaundice) can affect readings but is rarely clinically significant.

Optimising accuracy of pulse oximetry readings

Oxygen saturations measured by pulse oximetry contribute to clinical decision making and some simple steps can reduce the risk of erroneous readings.

- Consider choice of device – fingertip devices with integrated sensor and display may be appropriate for spot checks of SpO_2, handheld devices with detachable sensor allow for selection of most appropriate probe, wrist-worn devices have sensor attached by a short cable and are useful for overnight oximetry and exercise testing, desktop/bedside devices may be more appropriate in the acute setting for continuous monitoring.
- Ensure the oximeter is in good condition and probe sensor cleaned according to local infection control policy/manufacturer's guidance.
- Explain the procedure to the patient and gain consent where possible.
- Ensure the chosen site is warm and well-perfused; select the most appropriate probe for the site chosen; in adult patients the most common sites are the fingertip and ear lobe. Using the incorrect probe will lead to inaccuracies in the readings obtained.
- Position probe correctly so that the LEDs are opposite the sensor; probes that are too small or two large for a digit can affect the ability of the device to calculate the light absorbed accurately.
- When using a finger probe, ask the patient to rest the hand down gently to reduce motion interference.
- Check the pulse strength signal and ensure pulse rate reading correlates with manual pulse.
- Allow pulse oximeter to remain in situ for at least 5 minutes to ensure the device equilibrates.

Interpreting results

Oxygen saturation readings should be recorded alongside documentation of whether the patient is breathing room air or oxygen and the oxygen delivery device (e.g. Venturi mask, nasal cannulae, simple face mask), flow rate or percentage oxygen being used. Any other factors that can influence accuracy such as movement, cold hands and so on should also be recorded.

In the acute setting, patients should have a target oxygen saturation range prescribed and resting oximetry readings should be compared with this, with appropriate actions taken if the readings fall outside the target (Chapter 46).

It may also be useful to record saturations during exercise testing to determine exertion desaturation; in this case, results should be interpreted with reference to resting saturations and those recorded during/after activity in addition to any supplementary oxygen therapy.

Nursing considerations

It is important to note that patient comfort and safety must be considered when using pulse oximetry. Pressure damage can occur with medical devices such as pulse oximetry, together with burns, especially if continuous monitoring is employed. In addition, attention to infection control is necessary if using the same probe for many patients.

Further reading

Primary Care Respiratory Society UK (PCRS-UK) (2009) Pulse Oximetry in Primary Care: Opinion Sheet No 28 (revised 2013). https://www.pcrs-uk.org/system/files/Resources/Opinion-sheets/os28_pulse_oximetry.pdf (accessed 23 February 2016).

20 Blood gas sampling and analysis

Figure 20.1 Alveolar ventilation

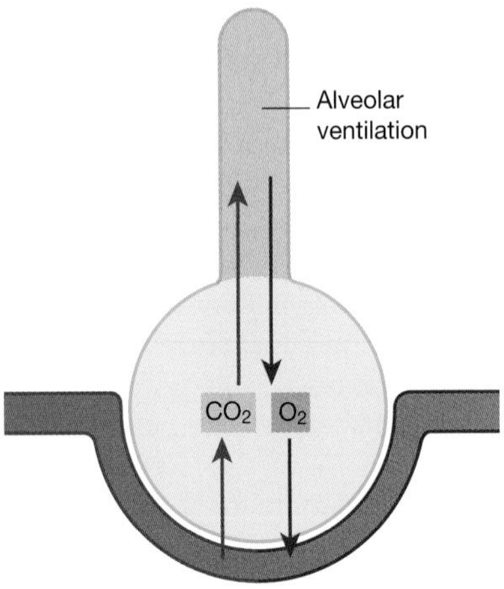
Alveolar ventilation
CO2
O2

Figure 20.3 Allen's test

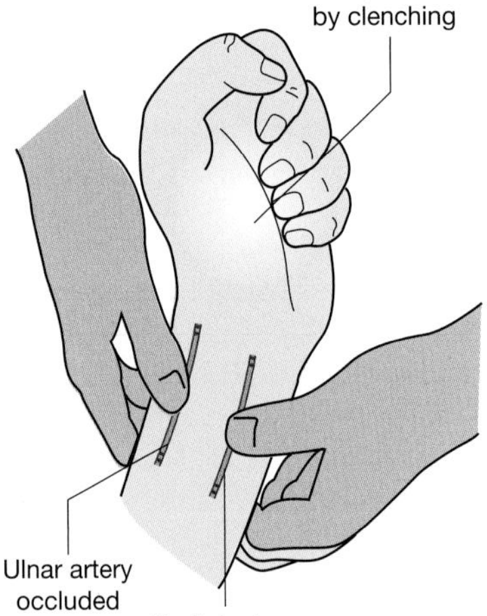
Pallor produced by clenching
Ulnar artery occluded
Radial artery occluded

Figure 20.4 Correct positioning for obtaining sample from radial artery

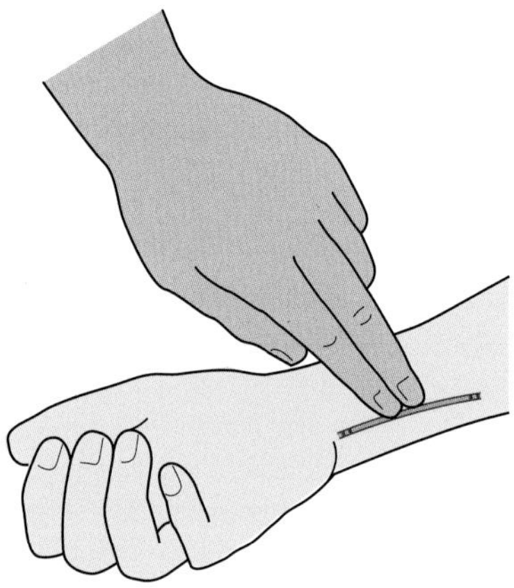

Figure 20.5 Correct position for needle insertion

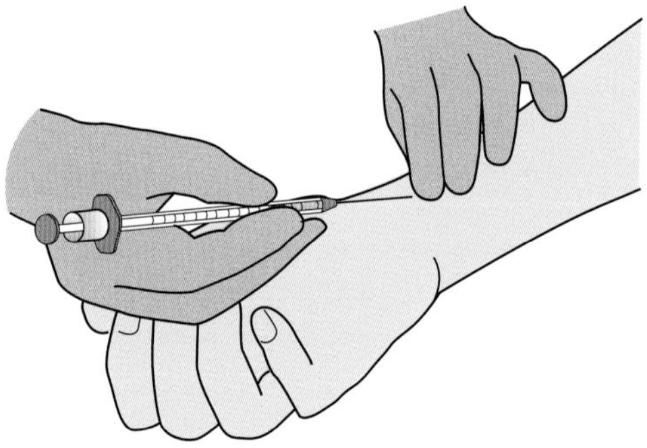

Table 20.1 Normal blood gas values

pH	7.35–7.45
PaO_2	>10.6
$PaCO_2$	4.7–6.6
(HCO_3)	22–28
Base excess (BE)	−2–+2
SaO_2	>96%

Figure 20.2 pH scale

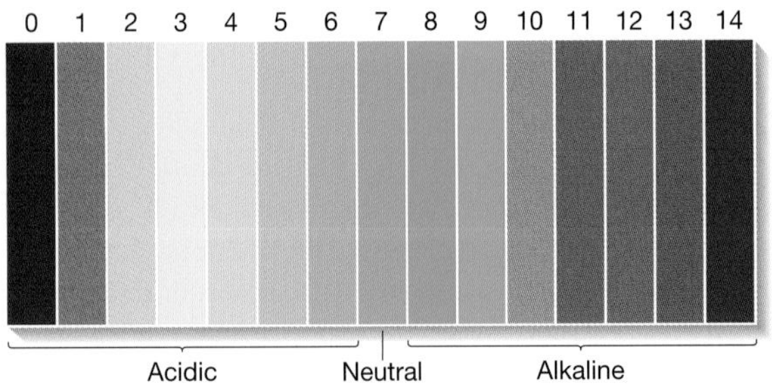
0
1
2
3
4
5
6
7
8
9
10
11
12
13
14
Acidic
Neutral
Alkaline

Figure 20.6 Normogram depicting areas of compensated acid-base balance
Source: Leach R. *Critical Care Medicine at a Glance*, 3rd edn. Reproduced with permision of John Wiley & Sons Ltd.

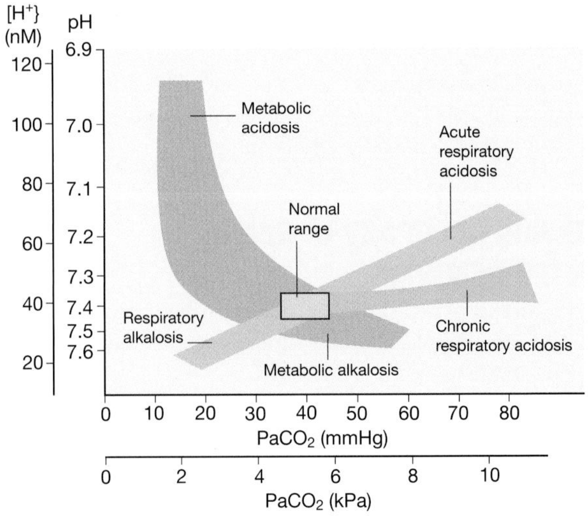
[H+} (nM)
pH
120
100
80
60
40
20
6.9
7.0
7.1
7.2
7.3
7.4
7.5
7.6
Metabolic acidosis
Acute respiratory acidosis
Normal range
Respiratory alkalosis
Chronic respiratory acidosis
Metabolic alkalosis
0 10 20 30 40 50 60 70 80
PaCO2 (mmHg)
0 2 4 6 8 10
PaCO2 (kPa)

Arterial blood gases refer to the measurement of pH and the partial pressure of oxygen (O_2) carbon dioxide (CO_2) and bicarbonate (HCO_{3-}) in arterial blood.

Once we have these values we are able to assess the internal environment and the acid–base balance in blood to monitor how well the lungs are able to ventilate the alveolus to maintain internal homeostasis (Figure 20.1).

Any deviation from the normal values (Table 20.1) results in the failure of internal respiration system. The correct assessment of the blood gas results improves patient outcomes and allows clinicians to provide optimum levels of care.

It is important to look at the patient and assess his/her condition and use this along with the blood gas results to make an objective decision around treatment options. When initiating, discontinuing or adjusting oxygen prescription there should be a minimum of 20 minutes before obtaining a sample to allow for adjustment and improve accuracy.

Acid–base balance

This is important to maintain normal cellular reactions to support life. Arterial blood pH is essential for life and is closely regulated by various mechanisms including bicarbonate, other plasma buffers and the renal system. Depending on the number of hydrogen ions (H^+), a solution can become acidic or alkaline. Blood pH is normally between 7.35 and 7.45 (Figure 20.2), therefore indicating a slightly alkaline reading.

If the blood pH falls below 7.35 it is termed acidic. If it is above 7.45 it is termed alkaline. It is important to remember that when CO_2 dissolves in the blood it becomes more acidic. The more CO_2 in the blood the more H_2CO_{3-} (carbonic acid) is produced which releases free H^+. These free H^+ are then excreted in urine by the kidneys to maintain the internal pH levels.

Disorders of acid–base balance

There are many causes for disturbance of acid–base balance.

- Pulmonary causes – emphysema, pneumonectomy, pneumonia and hypoventilation (amongst many others)
- Cardiovascular – decreased cardiac output and pulmonary oedema
- Haematological – anaemia and polycythaemia
- Gastrointestinal – vomiting, nasogastric drainage and diarrhoea.

In order to correct any changes in acid–base balance the body attempts to rectify the change by utilising the lungs to adjust the respiratory rate to exhale or retain more CO_2. The renal system excretes hydrogen ions, therefore reducing the concentration in the blood and lowering CO_2 levels.

Obtaining a blood gas sample

Prior to obtaining a blood gas sample it is recommended that both the ulnar and radial artery are checked using Allen's test (Figure 20.3). The hand is held up and the patient is asked to squeeze the hand into a fist. Both arteries are occluded by both thumbs and then the thumb released from one side then the other.

If the hand flushes red after the release of each artery, there is sufficient blood supply to the hand and it is safe to obtain the sample. If the hand flushes with only the release of one artery then it is not recommended to take the sample from that site because of poor blood supply, and increased risk of hand ischaemia.

After performing Allen's test and gaining consent from the patient, prepare to take the sample by palpating the artery (Figure 20.4). When you are happy insert the needle (bevel up) into the radial artery (Figure 20.5). The syringe should fill under pressure. If you have to draw back on the syringe you may have a venous sample and interpretation of the results should be treated with caution. If there are any discrepancies the sample should be repeated.

Capillary blood gas

Blood can also be taken from the ear lobe or a digit for occasional blood gas monitoring. It is considered less painful and invasive than arterial sampling. A small tube is used to collect the sample. If the ear lobe is used a vasodilator cream is applied. This increases the blood flow through the capillary.

Interpretation

This four-step method of interpretation is easy to utilise and provides the basics for interpreting blood gas samples.

- *Step 1:* Oxygen. Examine oxygenation – pO_2 and SpO_2. Determine the oxygen status of the patient (normal for patient, over-oxygenated, hypoxic?).
- *Step 2*: Acidity. Note the pH value:
  - Determine the presence of acidosis or alkalosis
  - Refer back to the normal values and the pH scale
  - Remember that <7.35 denotes acidosis and >7.45 alkalosis.
- *Step 3*: Carbon and bicarbonate:
  - Study the $PaCO_2$ and HCO_{3-} values. If the CO_2 level is abnormal and the bicarbonate (HCO_{3-}) and base excess are normal, it indicates a respiratory problem.
  - If the HCO_{3-} and base excess are abnormal and the CO_2 is normal, it points to a metabolic problem.
- *Step 4*: Check if there is any compensation taking place. Are the respiratory and renal systems working to maintain the pH levels? Are the pH, HCO_{3-} and CO_2 levels all abnormal? Examine which has produced the change in pH? If the pH is more acidic, this suggests a primary acidotic process. If the pH is more alkaline, this suggests a primary alkalotic process.

Figure 20.6 provides an overview of acid–base balance. The coloured areas demonstrate respiratory acidosis, metabolic acidosis, respiratory alkalosis and metabolic alkalosis. The box denotes normal range values.

Further reading

BMJ (2013) Interpreting arterial blood gas results. *BMJ* 346: f16.

21 Spirometry

Table 21.1 Contrindications to spirometry AFB, acid-fast bacilli

Contraindication to spirometry	
Absolute	Relative
• Active infection e.g. AFB positive TB until treated for 2 weeks • Dissecting unstable aortic aneurism • Current pneumothorax • Recent ophthalmic surgery • Recent cardiac or thoracic surgery • Recent abdominal surgery • Recent neurosurgery	• Suspected respiratory infection in last 6 weeks • Haemoptysis • Any history that may be aggravated by forced blow e.g. history of MI, stroke, uncontrolled hypertension • Patient too unwell to perform forced blow • Communication issues such as confusion or learning disability

Box 21.1 Common technical errors in spirometry

- Failure to breathe out fully
- Taking an extra breath in during the blow
- Not putting enough effort into the blow
- Coughing
- Not blowing out quickly enough at the start of the blow (slow start)
- Stopping blowing out too soon

Table 21.2 Interpretation of spirometry results

	Normal	Obstructive	Restrictive	Combined
FEV_1	>80%	Any value	<80%	<80%
FVC	>80%	>80%	<80%	<80%
Ratio	>70%	<70%	>70%	<70%

Figure 21.1 Patterns of flow-volume curves in obstruction and restriction

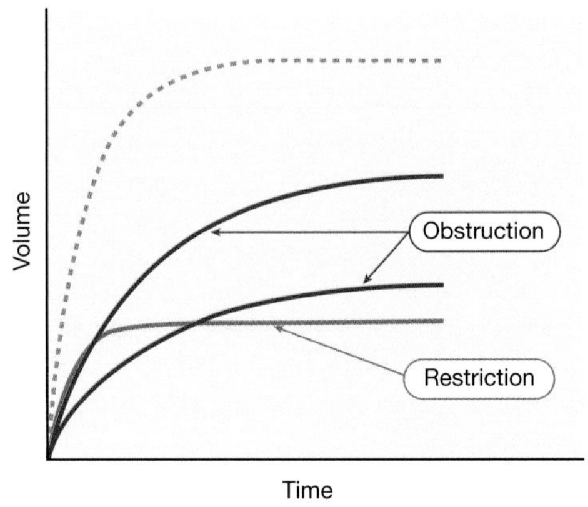

Volume
Obstruction
Restriction
Time

Figure 21.2 Patterns of volume-time curves in obstruction and restriction

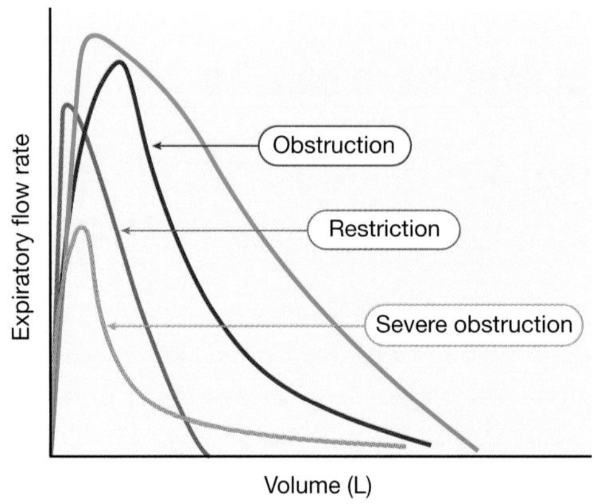

Expiratory flow rate
Obstruction
Restriction
Severe obstruction
Volume (L)

Spirometry measures how fast and how much air can be breathed out of the lungs. It is a painless but essential test to aid diagnosis and monitor severity of obstructive and restrictive lung conditions. Health care professionals should be trained to undertake the test and should have been assessed to Association for Respiratory Technology and Physiology (ARTP) or equivalent standards to undertake diagnostic spirometry.

The spirometer should meet ISO standard 26782, should be serviced annually, cleaned according to manufacturer's guidelines, calibrated regularly and calibration should be verified before each clinic session or after every tenth patient. A cleaning and calibration log should be maintained together with a record of servicing and any problems.

Undertaking the test

Ensure there are no contraindications to undertaking the test (Table 21.1). The patient's age, height, gender and ethnicity are required in order to interpret the results. The patient should be sitting upright, comfortably. The test should be explained and demonstrated before starting. The patient should be encouraged verbally throughout the test.

The patient should be asked to apply a nose clip and then to fill his/her lungs with air and expel the whole volume steadily into the spirometer mouthpiece until the lungs are completely empty (relaxed vital capacity, VC). This should be repeated until at least three results are obtained of which the maximum two should be within 100 mL or 5% and the third highest at least within 20%.

After resting, the patient should be asked to repeat the test (without the nose clip), filling his/her lungs fully but this time forcing all of the air out of their lungs with maximum effort (forced vital capacity blow, FVC). Again, the results should be within 100 mL of each other (150 mL if unable to achieve 100 mL in a highly variable patient).

Observe carefully for errors in technique (Box 21.1).

Interpreting results

After confirming that the correct patient details are entered and results are technically acceptable (within 100 mL or 5%), review the best result.

The VC and FVC are measures of lung size – the largest value of the two results should be used as the measure of VC.

The FEV_1 is a measure of the portion of the vital capacity that can be expelled in 1 second and allows us to estimate how well the airways are carrying air.

An FEV_1/FVC or VC (ratio) of less than 70% indicates airflow obstruction. The severity of the obstruction would be demonstrated by the FEV_1 as a percentage of predicted value for the person being tested. A ratio of more than 70% would reflect normal lung volumes if the FEV_1 and the FVC and VC are all above 80% of predicted. A ratio of more than 70% with FEV_1 and FVC or VC less than 80% would be seen in restrictive defects (Table 21.2). Interpretation of results should also include reviewing and interpreting both the flow volume and volume time courses (Figure 21.1 and Figure 21.2).

National standards for undertaking and interpreting diagnostic spirometry should be followed.

Other pulmonary function tests

Peak expiratory flow rate measurement

This test is undertaken using a peak flow meter and measures the maximum flow of air that a patient can expel from his/her lungs following a full inspiration. The patient should blow into the peak flow meter as forcibly as possible and the peak flow is measured after a tenth of a second in litres per minute. (Advise the patient to blow as if they are blowing out a candle from a metre away to gain good technique.) The test should be repeated until the patient has achieved at least three results, the best of which should be within 100 mL or 5% of each other.

A single peak flow test cannot be used as a diagnostic tool; however, repeated tests that vary by more than 20% can help towards making a diagnosis of asthma; for example testing before and after administering a bronchodilator with an improvement of 20% or more, or testing daily morning and evening over 2–3 weeks and showing more than 20% diurnal variation on at least 3 days per week.

Lung volume measurement

The residual volume (RV) of the lungs cannot be measured using spirometry because a volume of air remains in the lungs after full expiration – in health this represents approximately 30% of the total lung capacity. An increased RV is seen in obstructive lung disease where air trapping causes hyperinflation.

Lung function laboratories carry out one of three tests available (nitrogen washout, helium dilution or plethysmography) to measure residual volumes and therefore measure total lung capacity.

Gas transfer

The main role of the lungs is to exchange gasses between the alveoli and the blood. The diffusing capacity of the lungs can be estimated by using carbon monoxide (DLCO) as a surrogate measure as this has similar properties to oxygen in terms of its solubility and ability to diffuse across membranes.

This test is usually carried out in the lung function laboratory and measures the amount of gas exchanging surface area that is available. The patient breathes in a gas mixture containing CO, holds his/her breath for 10 seconds and then exhales. The amount of CO that has disappeared across the alveolar capillary membrane is calculated and corrected using the patient's haemoglobin levels.

A reduced DLCO can occur in a variety of parenchymal diseases (e.g. emphysema, pulmonary fibrosis) and also in vascular diseases (e.g. pulmonary oedema, pulmonary hypertension).

Further reading

Shiner RJ. (2012) *Lung Function Tests Made Easy.* Churchill Livingstone. www.peakflow.com (accessed 23 February 2016).

22 Measuring quality in healthcare

Figure 22.1 The five domains of NHS England
Source: Reproduced with permission of NHS.

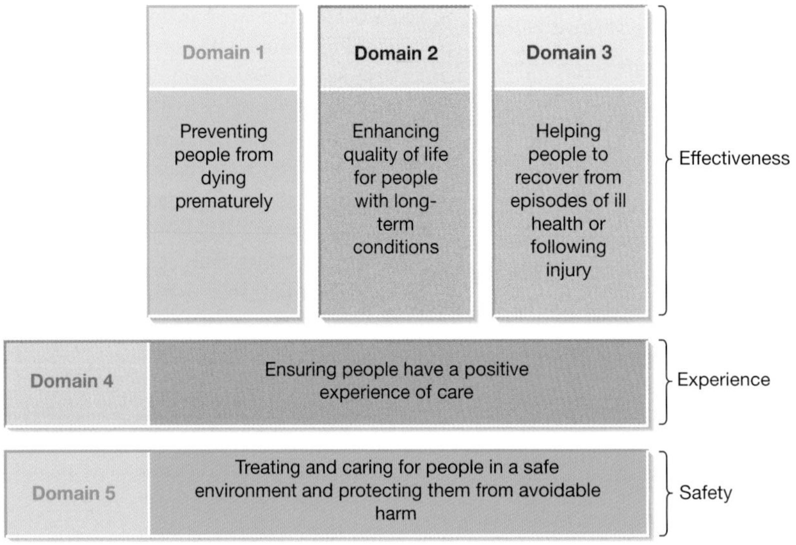
Domain 1
Preventing people from dying prematurely
Domain 2
Enhancing quality of life for people with long-term conditions
Domain 3
Helping people to recover from episodes of ill health or following injury
Effectiveness
Domain 4
Ensuring people have a positive experience of care
Experience
Domain 5
Treating and caring for people in a safe environment and protecting them from avoidable harm
Safety

Table 22.1 Methods of patient feedback
Source: The Health Foundation. No.18 Measuring Patient Experience (2013). Reproduced with permission of The Health Foundation.

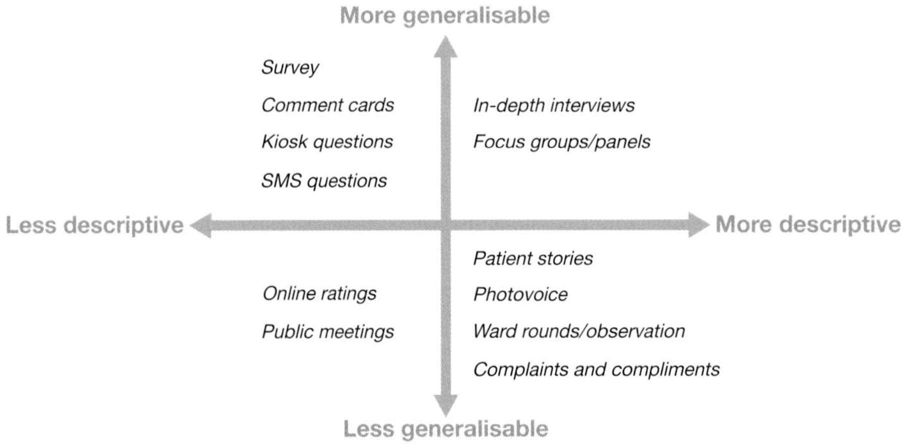
More generalisable
Survey
Comment cards
Kiosk questions
SMS questions
In-depth interviews
Focus groups/panels
Less descriptive
More descriptive
Online ratings
Public meetings
Patient stories
Photovoice
Ward rounds/observation
Complaints and compliments
Less generalisable

The national drive to improve the quality of care for patients by putting people at the heart of their own care is not just about being involved in the decisions around care, but also being involved in the experience of health care. Being able to record and report the experience alongside the experience of living with the illness or disease is a key factor. But how does the NHS capture this and what does the bigger picture look like and how can we start to measure quality in respiratory care?

Within the many new changes in the NHS structure and formation of health policy, a domain lead for patient experience along with a further four domains within the newly created NHS England were created (Figure 22.1). The vision of the new NHS (2013) is that everyone has greater control of their health and their well-being, supported to live longer, healthier lives by high quality health and care services that are compassionate, inclusive and constantly improving. The main focus for health care providers in delivering this vision is that of a 'high quality' service, and built into this is the need for a 'positive patient experience'.

A common marker of measurement in health care has been the recording of patient satisfaction surveys as now routinely used in hospitals in many European countries as a benchmark of how well services are performing from the 'patient's perspective' (Säilä et al., 2008). In a range of NHS hospitals and general practices in the UK, it is possible to complete satisfaction surveys at electronic booths in hospital foyers or as you leave the building at GP practices, moving towards real-time patient satisfaction feedback. These data are then used to describe the 'patient experience' in quality accounts or Trust reports for example, and also are commonly used within respiratory teams to gauge an understanding of the service provided by the team or individual.

The Health Foundation (2013) undertook a comprehensive evidence scan which explored further the concept of patient experience in the health service. The Health Foundation Report (2013) like others (Cornwell, 2012; Black et al., 2014) advocates that the measurement of experience could potentially enhance patients' expectations, experience and satisfaction of health care. The evidence scan explored 328 empirical studies and gives a comprehensive overview of the current literature, but, most importantly, understands and highlights that there are a number of different ways in which health care can be measured (Table 22.1) such as postal surveys, questionnaires, email and face-to-face interviews.

It has become clear that the different measurements and the collection of health care experience cannot be undertaken simply by one specific measure or measurement, because health care remains complex and varied, and there are a number of different elements that potentially impact on the measurement of experience in multi-faceted health systems such as the NHS (Beattie et al., 2014). Terminology can therefore be confusing.

The following gives a brief overview of some examples of how this may relate to respiratory care.

Patient reported experience measures

Patient reported experience measures (PREMs) are a measurement of patients' perceptions of their personal experience of the health care they have received. PREM instruments should focus on the aspects of the care that matter to patients (Coulter et al., 2002). PREMs results can be used to improve services and provide the patients' views on these improvements and moves away from the technological or economic model that is often employed in service design. The PREM COPD-9, for example, is a validated instrument to benchmark practice and quality used in routine chronic obstructive pulmonary disease (COPD) care and as an outcome measure in services such as pulmonary rehabilitation.

Patient reported outcome measures

Patient reported outcome measures (PROMs) are self-report questionnaires or scales, and seek to measure patients' perceptions of their health status or health-related quality of life, normally completed by patients (Hodson et al., 2013). PROMs are familiar research tools and are widely accepted, but are now increasingly used to direct individual patients as a measure of an intervention and to provide patient-related comparative data across health care providers. They are potentially a useful measure of quality from the health care provider or clinician (Black et al., 2014). Examples of respiratory PROMS include the St George's Respiratory questionnaire and COPD Assessment Test. Both instruments have all been designed to seek a patient-centred perception of disease or impact.

Quality of life

The measurement of quality of life has been reported on for many years. Quality of life is also being measured by the vast number of PROMs which were identified as ways in which to interpret the views of patients in everyday activity or through the impact of intervention. This leads to a broader understanding of terminology used to describe quality of life measurement. An example of this is the use of the Dyspnoea-12 (Yorke et al., 2010) which was developed to give a global score of breathlessness and encompasses both 'physical' and 'affective' aspects but critically over a number of different lung diseases such as COPD, interstitial lung disease and heart failure.

The national UK mandate and focus on quality of measurement is complex but there has been a real clear shift within the NHS and NHS England to ensure that services, staff and patients have an integral role in the future of the NHS, and that patient experience is central to the measurement of quality, alongside patient safety and clinical effectiveness.

Further reading

Hodson M, Andrew S, Roberts CM. (2013) Towards an understanding of PREMS and PROMS in COPD. *Breathe* 9: 358–364. doi:10.1183/20734735.006813

23 Assessing anxiety and depression

Figure 23.1 DSM descriptors: depression

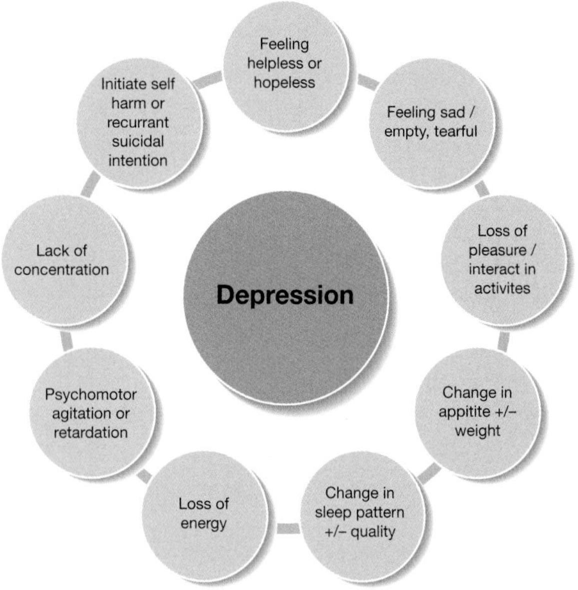
Depression
Feeling helpless or hopeless
Feeling sad / empty, tearful
Loss of pleasure / interact in activites
Change in appitite +/– weight
Change in sleep pattern +/– quality
Loss of energy
Psychomotor agitation or retardation
Lack of concentration
Initiate self harm or recurrant suicidal intention

Box 23.1 DSM descriptors: anxiety

Autonomic arousal symptoms
- Palpitations or pounding heart/accelerated heart rate
- Trembling or shaking/sweating
- Dry mouth (not due to medication or dehydration)

Symptoms involving chest and abdomen
- Difficulty breathing/feeling of choking
- Chest pain or discomfort
- Nausea or abdominal distress (such as churning in stomach)

Symptoms involving mental state
- Feeling dizzy, unsteady, faint or light-headed
- Feeling that objects are unreal (derealisation) or that the self, in not really here, (depersonalisation)
- Feeling of losing control, fear of dying

General symptoms
- Hot flushes or cold chills/numbness or tingling sensations
- Muscle tension or aches and pains/restlessness and inability to relax
- Feeling keyed up, on edge or mentally tense
- A sensation of a lump in the throat or difficulty in swallowing
- Exaggerated response to minor surprises or to being startled

Figure 23.2 Interrelationship of self and environment

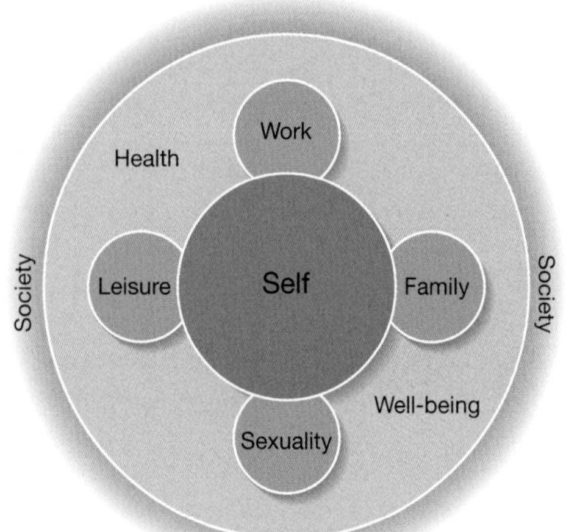
Self
Work
Leisure
Family
Sexuality
Health
Well-being
Society
Society

Figure 23.3 PHQ-9 and GAD-7
Source: Spitzer, RL, Williams, JBW Kroenke K, et al. (2006) *Arch Intern Med* 166: 1092-1097.

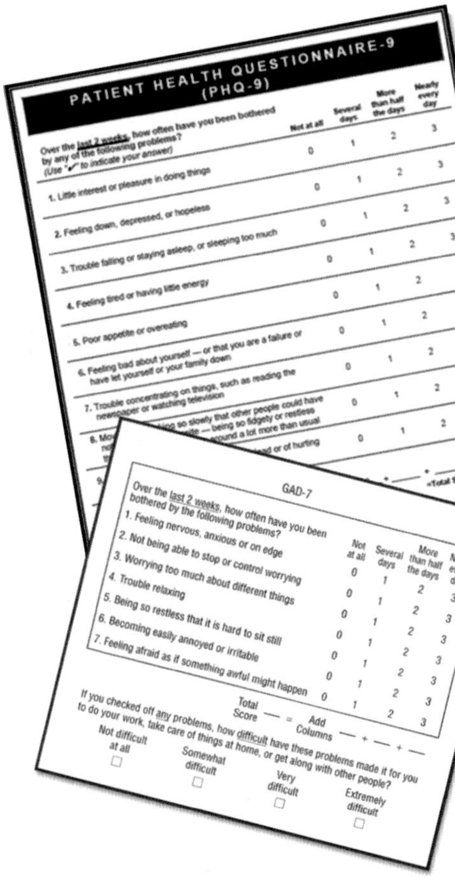
PATIENT HEALTH QUESTIONNAIRE-9 (PHQ-9)
GAD-7
Over the last 2 weeks, how often have you been bothered by the following problems?
Not at all
Several days
More than half the days
Nearly every day
1. Feeling nervous, anxious or on edge
2. Not being able to stop or control worrying
3. Worrying too much about different things
4. Trouble relaxing
5. Being so restless that it is hard to sit still
6. Becoming easily annoyed or irritable
7. Feeling afraid as if something awful might happen
If you checked off any problems, how difficult have these problems made it for you to do your work, take care of things at home, or get along with other people?
Not difficult at all
Somewhat difficult
Very difficult
Extremely difficult

Figure 23.4 Emotional thermometer

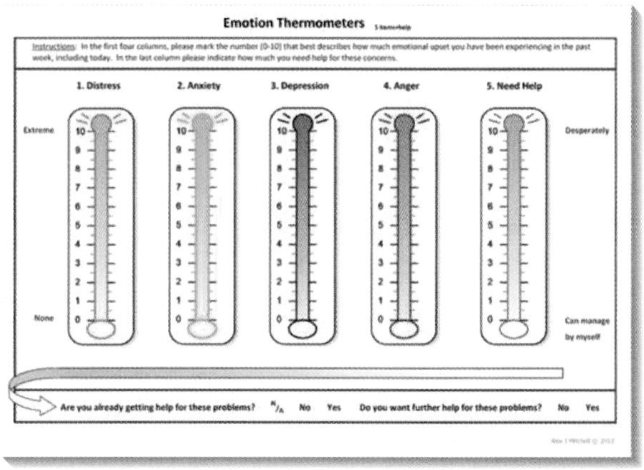
Emotion Thermometers
1. Distress
2. Anxiety
3. Depression
4. Anger
5. Need Help
Extreme
None
Desperately
Can manage by myself
Are you already getting help for these problems?
Do you want further help for these problems?

Screening

Recognising signs of mental ill health is not always easy in patients with acute or chronic respiratory disorders and may go undetected. Two simple screening questions: in the last few weeks, have you:

- Felt low, depressed or hopeless?
- Had little interest or pleasure in doing things?

Signs and symptoms

Signs and symptoms indicative of depression (Figure 23.1) and anxiety (Box 23.1) are classified by the Diagnostic and Statistical Manual of Mental Disorders (DSM-V) criteria. The greater number of symptoms experienced, the greater the degree of severity which will impact treatment decisions.

Discussing signs and symptoms requires a trusting relationship and a sensitive awareness of possible stigma and discrimination associated with depression. A detailed history includes not only how the patient is feeling, but also how long he/she has been feeling this way. Explore patterns of behaviour both established and new; the ability to cope with symptoms of respiratory disease, exacerbation and progression and the perceived impact of this. Review the health record with the patient to ascertain if he/she has an existing co-morbid or a history of mental health conditions; has received or is currently receiving treatment, including non-prescribed therapies/substances. Assess any functional, interpersonal or social difficulties; how the balance of the four basic elements depicted in Figure 23.2 impinge on the patient's well-being in the context of their society.

Organic causes

Consider organic causes of low or altered mood such as hypothyroidism, anaemia, vitamin D deficiency or drug side effects, particularly in patients taking high dose or prolonged courses of steroids. Prednisolone significantly enhances mood in some patients.

Many patients with chronic respiratory conditions are cared for in the community with nurse-led care. There should be clear agreement between practitioners especially the GP, regarding responsibilities for assessing, monitoring and treating these patients.

NICE have issued specific guidance regarding depression in adults with a chronic physical health problem. The pathways for chronic respiratory diseases recommend screening using validated measures in people who:

- are hypoxic
- are severely breathless
- have recently been seen or treated at a hospital for an exacerbation.

Self-report measures

Self-report symptom measures are useful to establish emotional distress but while helpful in staging they must not be relied upon exclusively to make a diagnosis. 'Emotional distress' can be a response to a new diagnosis or significant transition on the disease trajectory; part of a 'normal' adaptive process. While chronic physical illness is known to increase the risk of depression and depression is significantly associated with breathlessness severity (Katon et al., 2007), not every patient with respiratory disease will develop clinically significant anxiety or depression.

Frequency of assessment

All individuals with chronic respiratory illness should complete a relevant self-report assessment of their health *at least* every 6 months. This enables earlier detection of mental ill health, and prompt management and referral. A baseline assessment at the outset of treatment is helpful but it must also be repeated at follow-up, within 6–12 weeks if new treatment has been initiated. Weekly assessments should be considered for patients undergoing frequent treatment (e.g. chemotherapy and radiotherapy for lung cancer). This level of monitoring helps evaluate whether interventions are effective and can facilitate modification of treatment plans.

Which patient reported outcome measure?

It is preferable to select a validated patient reported outcome measure (PROM) specific for the particular respiratory disease where possible or a validated generic measure. Here we give examples of the Patient Health Questionnaire (PHQ) (Figure 23.3), a diagnostic tool that measures depression and is quick and easy for patients to complete. The PHQ-9 scores each of the nine DSM-IV criteria now superseded by DSM-V (Figure 23.1) (2013). The GAD-7 (Figure 23.3) is a valid and efficient tool for screening for Generalised Anxiety Disorder and assessing the severity of the anxiety in both clinical practice and research. The Emotion Thermometer Visual analogue scale (ET VAS) (Figure 23.4) is a simple screening tool for the detection and monitoring of emotional disorders in clinical practice. It has been validated for evaluation of distress in cancer and is undergoing evaluation in interstitial lung disease. The ET VAS is easy to understand, quick to administer and score. These tools have the advantage of being free for clinical use subject to permissions.

Inclusivity

Patients with extreme breathlessness who find it difficult to leave the house should have access to adapted means of completing questionnaires electronically or via other means. Patients with learning disabilities must also be accommodated and independent interpreters available to assist when necessary. Information and access to self-help resources must be suitable for the recipient.

Using PROMs in clinical practice creates an opportunity to open up a dialogue; discuss patients concerns and priorities for care; facilitate appropriate referral; improve health outcomes and patient satisfaction. A flexible approach that takes account of the differing needs and personalities is needed. We must be sensitive to diverse cultures, ethnicities and religious practices and how this influences the presentation of anxiety and depression. The more holistic our approach then the more likely we are to build rapport and be able to support desired changes in negative thoughts or behaviours.

Family

Where appropriate involve family members or carers, with the patient's consent, to obtain third-party history if appropriate, particularly if there are signs of self-neglect or severe agitation. Offer the carer an assessment of their caring and mental health needs too.

This section focuses on the assessment of anxiety and depression. Information on treatments and education can be found in the National Institute for Health and Care Excellence (NICE) guidelines.

Further reading

NICE Guidance (2009) Depression in adults with a chronic physical health problem: Treatment and management. NICE guidelines CG91. NICE.

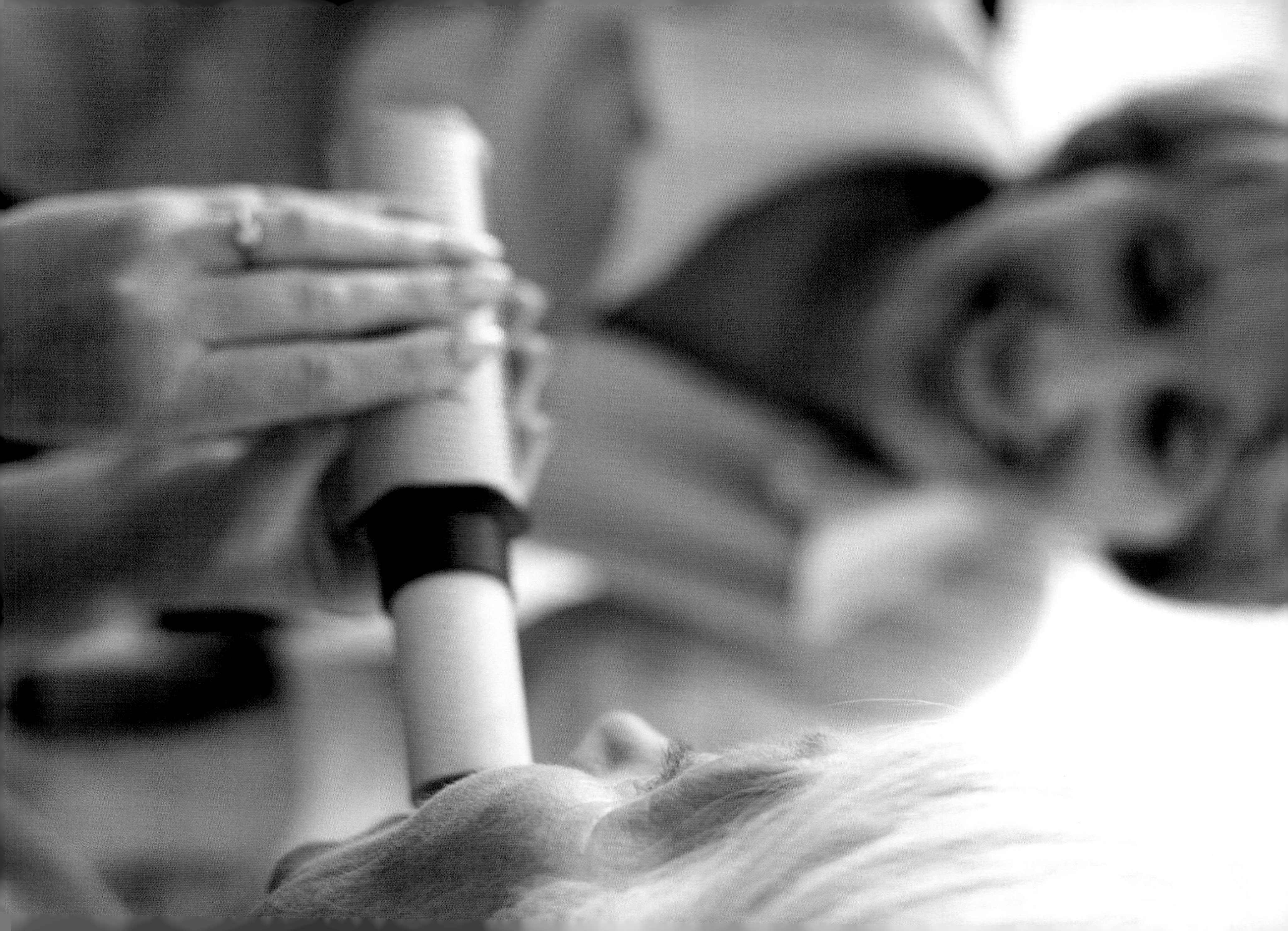

Respiratory diseases

Part 4

Chapters

Overview

In order to provide the necessary care and management for patients with respiratory conditions, nurses need to be familiar with a variety of conditions and diseases. While it is not possible to include all presentations here, some of the more common respiratory diseases are discussed and the main management strategies outlined.

24 Asthma

Figure 24.1 The airways and asthma

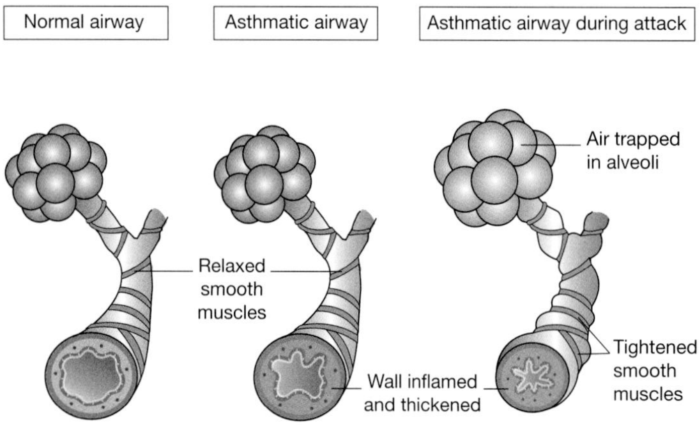
Normal airway
Asthmatic airway
Asthmatic airway during attack
Air trapped in alveoli
Relaxed smooth muscles
Wall inflamed and thickened
Tightened smooth muscles

Figure 24.2 Common triggers
Source: BTS SIGN. *Thorax* 2014; 69:i1-i192. Reproduced with permission of BMJ Publishing Ltd.

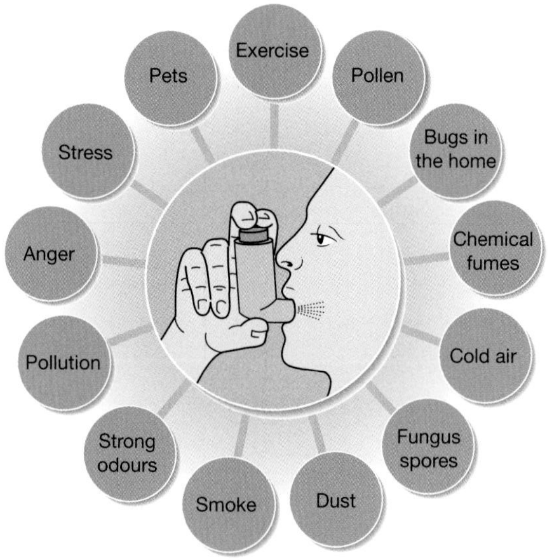
Exercise
Pets
Pollen
Stress
Bugs in the home
Anger
Chemical fumes
Pollution
Cold air
Strong odours
Fungus spores
Smoke
Dust

Figure 24.3 Stepwise approach to asthma. SR, slow release
Source: BTS SIGN. *Thorax* 2014;69:i1-i192. Reproduced with permission of BMJ Publishing Ltd.

Patients should start treatment at the step most appropriate to the initial severity of their asthma. Check concordance and reconsider diagnosis if response to treatment is unexpectedly poor

Move up to improve control as needed

Move down to find and maintain lowest controlling step

Step 1
Mild intermittent asthma
Inhaled short-acting O$_2$ agonist as required:

Step 2
Regular preventer therapy
Add inhaled steroid 200–800 mcg/day*:
400 μg is an appropriate starting dose for many patients

Start at dose of inhaled steroid appropriate to severity of disease

Step 3
Initial add-on therapy
1. Add inhaled long-acting ⊠$_3$ agonist: (LABA)
2. Assess control of asthma:
- **good response to LABA**
  - continue LABA
- **benefit from LABA but control still inadequate**
  - continue LABA and increase inhaled steroid dose to 800 μg/day* if not already on the dose
- **no response to LABA**
  - stop LABA and increase inhaled steroid to 800 μg/day.* If control still inadequate institute trial of other therapies leukotriene receptor antagonist or SR theophyline

Step 4
Persistent poor control
Consider trials of:
- increasing inhaled steroid up to 2000 μg/day*
- leukotriene receptor antagonist. SR theophyline, ⊠$_2$ agonist tablet

Step 5
Continuous or frequent use of oral steroids
Use daily steroid tablet in lowest dose providing adequate control

Maintain high dose inhaled steroid at 2000 μg/day*

Consider other treatments to minimise the use of steroid tablets

Refer patient for specialist care

*BDP or equivalent

Symptoms VS Treatment

Asthma is a respiratory condition affecting the airways. It is a disease that may be diagnosed at any age and currently over 5 million people in the UK are receiving treatment.

The British Thoracic Society (BTS) defined asthma as: 'A common and chronic inflammatory condition of the airways, whose cause is not completely understood. As a result of inflammation, the airways are hyper responsive and they narrow easily in a response to a wide range of stimuli … narrowing of the airways is usually reversible' (BTS, 2014).

The National Institute for Health and Clinical Excellence (NICE) published quality standards in 2013 for the management of asthma, stating: 'The goal of management is for people to be free from symptoms and able to lead a normal active life. This is achieved partly through treatment, tailored to the person, and partly by people getting to know what provokes their symptoms and avoiding these triggers as much as possible.'

Symptoms

A pathological response to an irritant in the airways (Figure 24.1) causes muscle tightening and narrowing of the lumen, additionallythe lining becomes subject to an inflammatory response and increasing mucus production. This leads to the clinically recognised symptoms of:

- Shortness of breath
- Wheeze
- Tightness of chest
- Cough.

A wheeze may not always be present, some asthmatics experience a simple cough or feel breathless and thereforewhen exacerbating the presence of a wheeze should be documented in the health records.

Diagnosis

Accurate history taking is arguably the most important aspect of patient assessment and can provide a great deal of the information required for a diagnosis. Clinical diagnosis is based on the recognition of a characteristic pattern of symptoms and signs and the absence of an alternative explanation for them in order to establish the level of probability of asthma.

A history of atopy and allergic conditions in the patient and family members, such as eczema and rhinitis, increase the probability of asthma.

Spirometry is the preferred initial test to assess the presence of airflow obstruction (NICE, 2013), in order to establish the probability of asthma: high, intermediate or low and treatment and management of symptoms. Serial peak expiratory flow (PEF) can also be used to identify variable airflow obstruction; however, it only looks at the large airways and therefore underestimates the level of obstruction when using this method in diagnosing asthma.

From the identification of probability of asthma a treatment pathway can be established as per NICE quality standards 2013.

Treatment

The severity of asthma is dynamic, and therefore it is important to treat according to the current level of severity using the Stepwise Approach (Figure 24.2) as guided by NICE quality standards 2013. This approach aims to achieve early control and step up or down treatment on individual need basis.

Pharmacological management is in the form of inhaled medication, as per the Stepwise Approach. Reliever and preventer inhalers are used to control symptoms, with regular monitoring in order to assess the effectiveness of the treatment which involves always checking adherence to inhalers and inhaler technique to ascertain if a referral to a specialist centre is indicated.

Non-pharmacological management should always include smoking cessation advice and lifestyle advice taking into consideration the individual's identified asthma triggers (Figure 24.2). This enables the patient to reduce exposure to triggers, reducing the impact of asthma on their daily lives.

Management

The goal of management is for people to be free from symptoms and able to lead normal active lives.

Patients with asthma whose lung function (PEF) declines over a few days or weeks sometimes significantly underestimate the severity of their condition prior to seeking medical help. Asthma is responsible for a large number of accident and emergency attendances and hospital admissions, mostly emergencies, where as many as 70% of these could have been preventable with appropriate early intervention. There are around 1000 deaths a year from asthma, about 90% of which are associated with preventable factors (Levy, 2014).

Therefore, as asthma is a long-term condition it requires ongoing proactive management and regular professional review in order to ensure the symptoms are well controlled. With self-management emphasising the importance of recognising and acting on the signs and symptoms of deterioration, education should include a written Personalised Asthma Action Plan (PAAP) as such direction improves health outcomes in a proactive environment. The PAAP can be based on symptoms and/or PEF with clear indications given as to what to do when symptoms worsen and peak flow declines so seeking medical advice in a timely manner (Chapter 39).

Further reading

Levy M. (2014) Why asthma still kills asthma still kills. The National Review of Asthma Deaths. https://www.rcplondon.ac.uk/sites/default/files/why-asthma-still-kills-full-report.pdf (accessed 24 February 2016).

NICE (2013) Asthma: diagnosis and monitoring. https://www.nice.org.uk/guidance/indevelopment/gid-cgwave0640 (accessed 24 February 2016).

25 Chronic obstructive pulmonary disease

Figure 25.1 Chronic obstructive pulmonary disease (COPD)

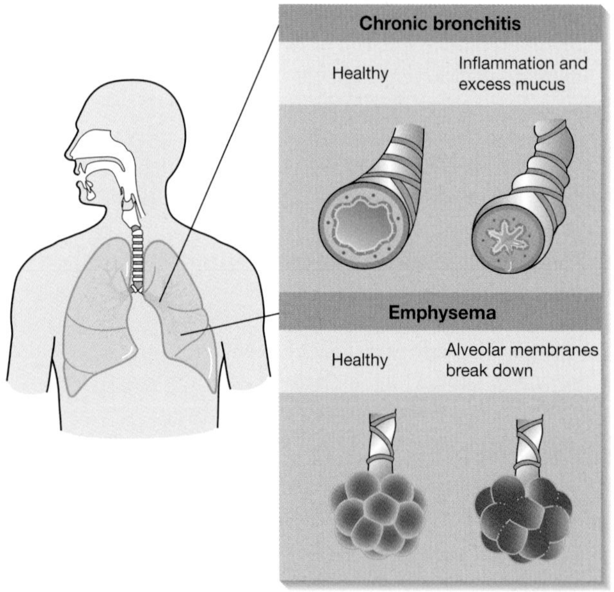
Chronic bronchitis
Healthy
Inflammation and excess mucus
Emphysema
Healthy
Alveolar membranes break down

Figure 25.2 Time-volume curve for patients with COPD compared with healthy subjects

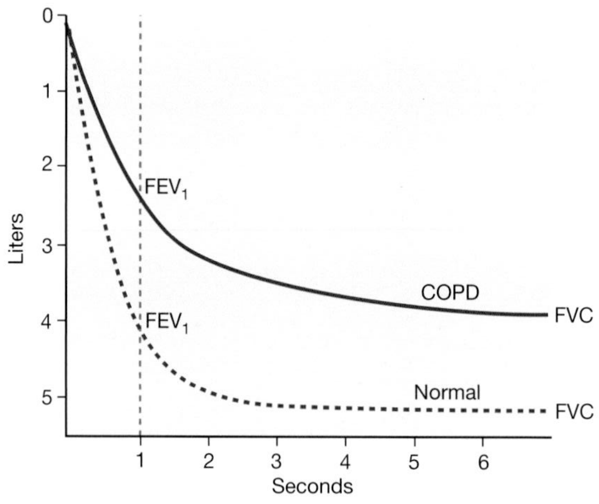
Liters
0
1
2
3
4
5
FEV1
FEV1
COPD
FVC
Normal
FVC
1
2
3
4
5
6
Seconds

Box 25.1 The four classification of severity of COPD based on FEV_1%

Stage I: Mild
Spirometry shows mild airflow limitation (FEV_1 ≥80% predicted: FEV_1/FVC <0.70). Primary symptoms are chronic cough and sputum production

Stage II: Moderate
Spirometry shows worsening airflow limitation (FEV_1 ≥50% and <80% predicted: FEV_1/FVC <0.70). Patients often experience dyspnoea, which can interfere with their daily activities

Stage III: Severe
Spirometry shows severe airflow limitation (FEV_1 ≥30% and <50% predicted: FEV_1/FVC <0.70). Symptoms of cough and sputum production typically continue, dyspnoea worsens, and repeated exacerbations occur

Stage IV: Very severe
Spirometry shows very severe airflow limitation (FEV_1 <30% predicted or FEV_1 <50% predicted. FEV_1/FVC <0.70 plus chronic respiratory failure). Complications such as respiratory failure or heart failure can develop

Chronic obstructive pulmonary disease (COPD) is a long-term condition of the airways, characterised by progressive breathlessness, cough and sputum production. It is a major cause of mortality and mortality and COPD is the second highest reason for emergency admission to acute care. Progressive breathlessness for people living with COPD limits exercise and activities of daily living resulting in a reduced quality of life. COPD is incurable but there are a number of interventions and medications to slow the progression of the disease. It is thought that COPD affects those people over the age of 35 though it is a latent disease and often symptoms are not reported until much later in life; however, there are exceptions. It affects both males and females, and more recently there has been an increase in female diagnosis, probably because of an increase in smoking in women post 1950.

It is thought that there are over 3 million people in the UK living with COPD; however, only approximately 1 million people are diagnosed. It has been suggested that this is because many people live with symptoms of COPD but do not seek help because it is associated with normal ageing processes or smoking.

Definition of chronic obstructive pulmonary disease

COPD is an umbrella term given to describe a number of lung conditions including emphysema and chronic bronchitis (Figure 25.1). COPD is characterised by airflow obstruction which is caused by increased airway narrowing which is not fully reversible post bronchodilatation.

Cigarette smoking is a major cause of COPD. This is because smoking causes irritation and inflammation in the airways resulting in tissue damage and scaring of the lung. The walls of the airways become thicker and excess mucus is produced. There is also destruction of the alveoli in the small airways causing emphysema with a loss of elasticity so the lungs are unable to work normally. This progressive damage to the airways can result in permanent narrowing and scaring which ultimately results in the symptoms associated with COPD. These symptoms most commonly present as shortness of breath (dyspnoea), cough and sputum production.

Causes of COPD

There are a number of reasons why people develop COPD. The major cause of COPD is smoking. Approximately 80% of people diagnosed with COPD have a significant smoking history; the duration and number of cigarettes smoked can affect onset and severity. There are also a number of other causes such as occupational (dust), environmental (air pollution) and genetic factors, the later being rarer and in a younger population.

Diagnosis

There is no single test to confirm a diagnosis of COPD so it should always be made in combination with a good clinical history including the recording of smoking history, onset and current symptoms along with occupational and other risk factors. A spirometry test should be performed to determine if airflow limitation is present and confirm obstruction.

The following definition of COPD should be used:

- 35 years or over (this is a guide).
- Airflow obstruction is defined as a reduced FEV_1/FVC ratio (FEV_1 is forced expired volume in 1 second and FVC is forced vital capacity), when the FEV_1/FVC ratio is less 0.7 (70%).
- The $FEV_1\%$ should be ≤80% predicted unless there is presence of respiratory symptoms such as breathlessness or cough. Severity is classified according to $FEV_1\%$ (Figure 25.2).

Assessment

Once a confirmed diagnosis of COPD is made, the assessment is initially to classify the severity against which medications and recommended management are planned.

Assessment of severity

Currently, there are four classifications of severity in COPD (NICE, 2010). Assessment is made by measuring and reporting on the FEV_1 (Box 25.1).

Assessment of breathlessness

Breathlessness is subjective and in some cases the severity of COPD and a patient's reported breathlessness do not correlate. The MRC dyspnoea scale (see Table 15.3) is a simple to administer assessment that can be used to grade the effect of dyspnoea on daily activities (Chapter 17).

Management of stable COPD

Flu vaccination

Because of the risks associated with exacerbations and COPD, the influenza vaccination should be offered to every patient with COPD (unless contraindicated) as part of routine management.

Smoking cessation

Smoking cessation advice and support is the responsibility of every health care professional and should be asked at every contact. It is the only evidenced-based intervention that has been demonstrated to slow progression of lung function and thus help to reduce the burden of symptoms associated with the disease (Chapter 10).

Pulmonary rehabilitation

Pulmonary rehabilitation is an evidence-based non-pharmacological intervention for patients with COPD (Chapter 11). It is an individualised physical activity programme together with supported education covering a number of areas, such as the management of breathlessness and oxygen therapy. It is recommended for patients with COPD with a MRC score 3 or above, but there is also evidence that anyone with breathlessness and a lack of physical activity would benefit.

Education and self-management

A key component of management of COPD is the understanding of the lung disease itself. It is key to ensure that patients understand that COPD is a long-term condition and that this includes the need for assessment of oxygen, anxiety and depression and regular review within primary care.

Self-management, including teaching and checking inhaler technique and warning signs of an acute exacerbation, are paramount at every contact. All patients should have a self-management plan informing them of tips and prompts including what to do in an acute exacerbation (Chapter 39).

Medicines optimisation

Once a patient has been diagnosed with COPD there are a number of pharmacological therapies and interventions available. Current guidance is to follow the NICE COPD 2010 guidelines; however, many areas will also have local medicines management guidelines. Medicines management tends to be used for breathlessness and exacerbation management. Inhaler technique is critical and should be assessed at every contact.

Oxygen therapy can be indicated in more advanced COPD and a referral for oxygen assessment should be considered in patients with a stable SpO_2 ≤92% on air.

Further reading

National Institute Clinical Excellence (NICE) (2010). *Chronic obstructive pulmonary disease: management of chronic obstructive pulmonary disease in adults in primary and secondary care.* London: National Clinical Guideline Centre.

26 Pleural disease

Figure 26.1 Pneumothorax

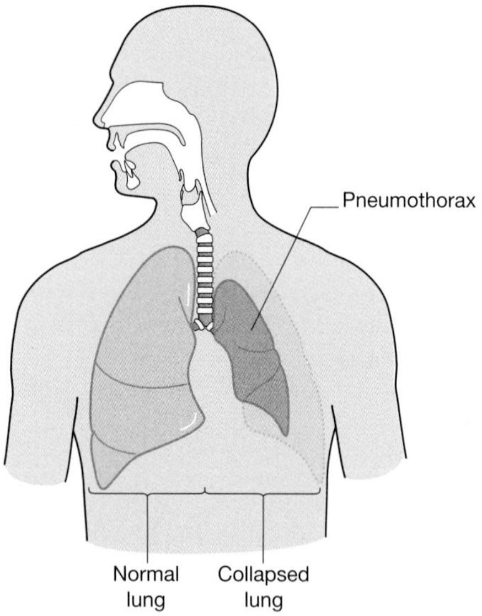
Pneumothorax
Normal lung
Collapsed lung

Figure 26.2 X-ray showing left pneumothorax

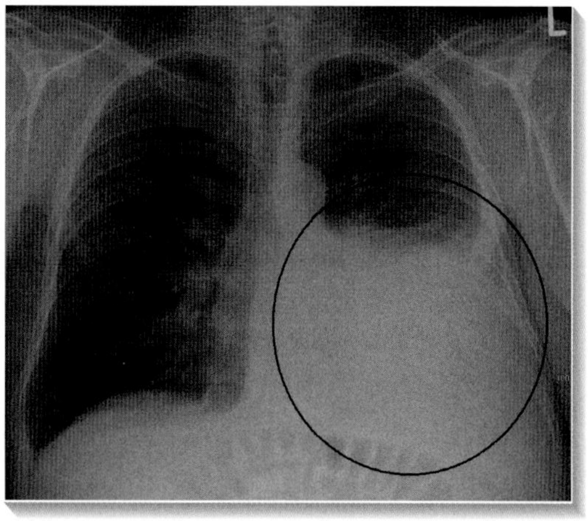
L

Table 26.1 Criteria to assess pleural effusion LDH, lactate dehydrogenase

Pleural fluid analysis		
	Exudate	**Transudate**
Pleural fluid protein/serum protein ratio	>0.5	<0.5
Pleural fluid LDH	>200 U/L or >2/3 upper limit of normal	<200 U/L or <2/3 upper upper limit of normal
Pleural fluid LDH/serum LDH ratio	>0.6	<0.6
*If any on of the above criteria is positive the effusion is exudative		

Pleural disease is a collective term used for a group of conditions affecting the pleura. The aim of this chapter is to briefly define and discuss the common types of pleural disease.

Pneumothorax

A pneumothorax is defined as the collection of air between the visceral and parietal pleura (Figure 26.1). It is colloquially referred to as a 'collapsed lung'. Pneumothoraces can be induced by trauma, surgery or occur spontaneously. Common symptoms include chest pain and shortness of breath. Diagnosis can sometimes be made of physical examination alone; however, a chest X-ray is required to confirm presence (Figure 26.2).

Types of pneumothorax

Primary

A primary pneumothorax occurs in the absence of any lung disease or trauma. The cause of such pneumothoraces is unknown but risk factors include male gender, smokers (especially cannabis) and family history.

Secondary

A secondary pneumothorax occurs as a result of a variety of lung diseases. The diseases that significantly increase the risk of pneumothorax include cancer, connective tissue disease, chronic obstructive pulmonary disease (COPD) and interstitial lung diseases.

Traumatic

A traumatic pneumothorax occurs as a result of trauma, such as a penetrating injury or blunt trauma to the chest wall. Sudden changes in atmospheric pressure, such as in deep sea diving, can also cause this type of pneumothorax.

Complications

A tension pneumothorax is a particular type of pneumothorax where air enters the pleural cavity on inspiration but cannot escape on expiration, causing further compression of the lung. This should be treated as a medical emergency.

A haemothorax is where blood accumulates in the pleural cavity. This usually results from traumatic or penetrating injury to the chest wall. Each side of the thorax can hold up to 40% of the body's blood volume so blood loss can be very significant.

Empyema

Empyema is a collection of pus in the pleural cavity that often develops when bacteria invade the pleural space. Risk factors for empyema include underlying lung disease, malignancy, HIV infection and drug use.

Small pleural effusions often occur during pneumonia, with many collections being small and resolving with simple antibiotic therapy. However, if empyema develops, additional interventions can be required.

Pleural effusion

A pleural effusion is the accumulation of fluid between the visceral and parietal pleura. The most common symptom is shortness of breath. Diagnosis is often made by chest X-ray (Figure 26.2).

The fluid can either be a transudate or an exudate. The criteria to assess this is shown in Table 26.1.

- *Transudate effusions:* most commonly caused by congestive cardiac failure, liver cirrhosis or end stage renal disease, although there are multiple other conditions.
- *Exudate effusions:* commonly caused by malignancy, infection or inflammation. Lung cancer, breast cancer and lymphoma are responsible for 75% of malignant effusions.

Pleural fluid should ideally be sent off for further analysis, such as Gram staining, culture and cytology.

Treatment

Treatment of pneumothorax and pleural effusion depends on size and severity of the respective air–fluid in the cavity and the symptom profile of the patient. If a pneumothorax or pleural effusion is relatively small, no invasive treatment is necessarily required and disease can resolve with treatment of the underlying case and close monitoring.

If a pneumothorax or pleural effusion is small to moderate, air–fluid can be aspirated using a needle or aspiration kit. This is known as thoracentesis. Fluid samples can be obtained this way to aid diagnosis. However, in cases where pleural disease is significant, chest drainage and pleurodesis may be required (Chapter 53).

Pleuritis

Pleuritis, also known as pleurisy, is a condition affecting the pleura. Pleuritis is characterised as the inflammation of pleura which can cause sharp pain when breathing. Other symptoms include shortness of breath and tachycardia.

Pleuritis is often caused by viral infections spreading from the lungs to the pleural cavity. The inflamed pleural layers rub against each other every time the lungs expand to breathe in air. Other causes include lung cancer, pulmonary embolism, bacterial infections and cardiac problems.

Treatment consists of treating the underlying condition such as infection. Anti-inflammatory drugs such as indomethacin have shown some benefit in relief of symptoms.

Further reading

British Thoracic Society (BTS) (2010) Pleural Disease Guidelines.

27 Lung cancer

Figure 27.1 Incidence of types of cancer

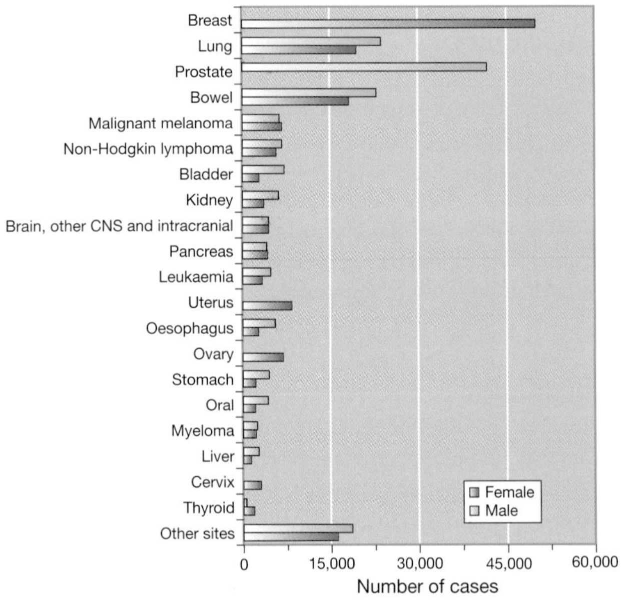
Breast
Lung
Prostate
Bowel
Malignant melanoma
Non-Hodgkin lymphoma
Bladder
Kidney
Brain, other CNS and intracranial
Pancreas
Leukaemia
Uterus
Oesophagus
Ovary
Stomach
Oral
Myeloma
Liver
Cervix
Thyroid
Other sites
0
15,000
30,000
45,000
60,000
Number of cases
Female
Male

Box 27.1 31/62 day pathway

62 days

- Relates to new suspected cancer referrals (NSC) from GP
- Have 62 days from receiving referral to investigate, diagnose and give first treatment

31 days

- Applies to all cancers diagnosed regardless of referral route
- Patient to receive first treatment with 31 days of agreeing treatment plan

Box 27.2 Signs and symptoms of lung cancer

Common signs and symptoms of lung cancer

- Cough for >3 weeks/altered cough
- Unresolving chest infection/repeated chest infections
- Increasing breathlessness
- Coughing up blood
- Hoarse voice
- Unresolving chest/shoulder pain

Other possible symptoms

- Losing weight for no obvious reason
- Increasing tiredness/fatigue
- End of fingers becoming larger/rounded (clubbing)

Box 27.3 Investigations

Radiology

- CXR
- CT thorax*
- PET scan*

Diagnostic

- Bronchoscopy
- EBUS – Endobronchial ultrasound scan*
- CT guided lung biopsy
- Pleural tap/aspiration
- Mediastinoscopy*
- Thoracoscopy – VATS/medical
- Image guided liver biopsy – (if abnormal tissue in liver)*

(*can assist with staging the cancer)

Box 27.4 Types of lung cancer

2 main types of lung cancer

(a) Non small cell lung cancer (NSCLC)
- Squamous
- Adenocarcinoma
- Large cell

(b) Small cell lung cancer (SCLC)

Other cancers affecting the lung
- Mesothelioma
- Carcinoids
- Soft tissue sarcomas

Box 27.5 TNM staging

- **T** Tumour size/position: 1a, 1b, 2a, 2b, 3, 4
- **N** Lymph nodes: depends on position/lymph node station (1, 2, 3)
- **M** Metastasis: If present within the chest (1a) or outside chest (1b)
- The greater the TNM stage the more advanced the cancer
- Stage 4–T4 N3 M1b

Lung cancer is the second most common cancer in the UK (Figure 27.1). In 2012, 44,488 new cases of lung cancer were diagnosed (CRUK). Many patients present in an advanced stage of their disease. Patients referred from their GP with suspected lung cancer should be seen, investigated and treated on a 31/62 day pathway (Box 27.1).

Symptoms

Patients can experience varying symptoms (Box 27.2).

Though smoking can increase the risk of developing lung cancer it is important to remember that those people who have never smoked can also be diagnosed with the disease.

Diagnosis

Investigations are undertaken to confirm a diagnosis, but will depend upon the patient's general condition. Radiology (X-ray and scans) help to identify where there may be abnormal tissue. Samples of the tissue or cells are taken to confirm and distinguish which type of lung cancer (Box 27.3). This is important as treatment and management are determined by where the cancer is and its type. Often, a sample is taken from the lungs; however, radiology can identify abnormal tissue outside the lungs which may be easier and safer to sample. Patients sometimes require more than one or different procedures. Some diagnostic procedures also help to stage the cancer (see Staging).

When samples of tissue/cells are processed in the laboratory special 'stains' (immunohistochemistry/immunocytochemistry) can be used to help identify where the cancer cells have originated from.

Types of lung cancer

There are two main types of primary lung cancer: non small cell lung cancer (NSCLC) and small cell lung cancer (SCLC) (Box 27.4). They behave in different ways and respond differently to treatment.

Other cancers that affect the lungs are mesothelioma, which affects the lining (pleura) and rarer types of lung cancer known as carcinoid tumours or soft tissue sarcomas.

Staging

Staging is based on knowledge of the way cancers progress. It describes the size, position and whether the cancer has spread (TNM staging) (Box 27.5). Radiology is used to help stage cancers but some diagnostic procedures can also help with this (Box 27.3). Staging can help to determine appropriate treatment options and estimate prognosis (prediction on how the disease will affect an individual's chance of recovery).

The higher the stage the more advanced the cancer:

- *Stage 1:* early or localised cancer
- *Stage 2–3:* locally advanced cancer
- *Stage 4:* metastatic and secondary cancer.

Treatment

Treatment includes surgery, radiotherapy, chemotherapy, targeted therapies or a combination of treatments. The type of treatment depends on staging and the patient's fitness for treatment. Other illnesses (co-morbidities) also need to be considered when planning treatment options.

Surgery

Surgery is considered in NSCLC when there is no evidence of spread. The intention is cure. Surgery can involve removing a whole lung (pneumonectomy), lobe (lobectomy) or part of a lobe (wedge resection).

Radiotherapy

Radical radiotherapy

This is considered when surgery is not an option because of co-morbidities. Intention is cure but there is a lower success rate than for surgery. It can be given with chemotherapy.

Radical radiotherapy can also be given following surgery to reduce risk of recurrence.

Palliative radiotherapy

This can be used following chemotherapy and can help to manage symptoms when the cancer is more advanced or has spread to other parts of the body. It can be used for both types of lung cancer.

Radiotherapy can affect healthy lung tissue and can therefore affect lung function.

Chemotherapy

Chemotherapy (anticancer drugs) can be used in both types of lung cancer. It can shrink cancers, improve symptoms and may increase survival. However, it is unlikely to cure lung cancer. It is often the first choice of treatment in SCLC. It works by disrupting the way cancer cells grow and divide. However, chemotherapy can also affect normal cells and renal function. Therefore, during treatment, the patient's blood profile and renal function are carefully monitored.

Targeted therapies

These are usually used to treat NSCLC. Chemical processes within cells send a signal to start the division process that allows the cancer cells to grow and spread. If a mutation is present on the cancer cells, drugs (targeted therapies) can be used to block this signal. Although all lung cancers are tested for this mutation, only a small percentage are positive.

Other treatments:

- *Stereotactic radiotherapy:* specialised radiotherapy used for small cancers where surgery is not possible.
- *Radiofrequency ablation:* for very early cancers. Uses heat to destroy cancer cells.

Symptom management

Patients with lung cancer experience various symptoms but the three most common are breathlessness, cough and pain.

Breathlessness

It is important to treat and exclude other causes of breathlessness. Breathlessness caused by lung cancer can improve with treatment. It can also improve with medication, breathing exercises, breathlessness management interventions and complementary therapies.

Cancer in the lung can cause fluid to collect in the lining (pleura) of the lung (pleural effusion). Aspirating the fluid or inserting a chest drain can improve breathing.

Cough

This is often distressing and can be difficult to address. Sometimes, radiotherapy can help as can analgesics containing codeine.

Pain

Assessment of cause and type of pain is important. Analgesics can relieve many types of pain and are often used in combination with other medications. Radiotherapy often helps with bone pain.

Further reading

NICE guidelines. (2011) Lung cancer: diagnosis and management. https://www.nice.org.uk/guidance/cg121 (accessed 24 February 2016).

28 Obstructive sleep apnoea syndrome

Figure 28.1 Anatomy of obstructive sleep apnoea

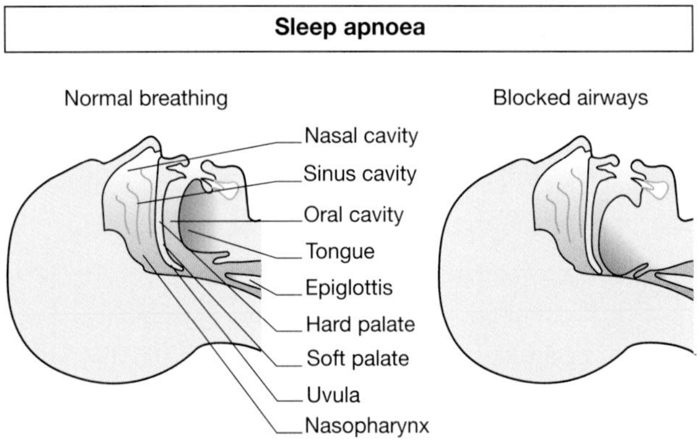
Sleep apnoea
Normal breathing
Blocked airways
Nasal cavity
Sinus cavity
Oral cavity
Tongue
Epiglottis
Hard palate
Soft palate
Uvula
Nasopharynx

Box 28.2 Symptoms of obstructive sleep apnoea

- Unrefreshed sleep
- Daytime sleepiness
- Loud snoring
- Witnessed apnoeas
- Morning headaches
- Nocturia
- Poor libido

Box 28.3 Treatment options for obstructive sleep apnoea

- Continuous positive airway pressure (CPAP)
- Mandibular advanced device (MAD)
- Positional training
- Surgery-ENT/bariatric
- Weight loss
- Electrical stimulation (research)

Figure 28.4 Factors affecting compliance with CPAP

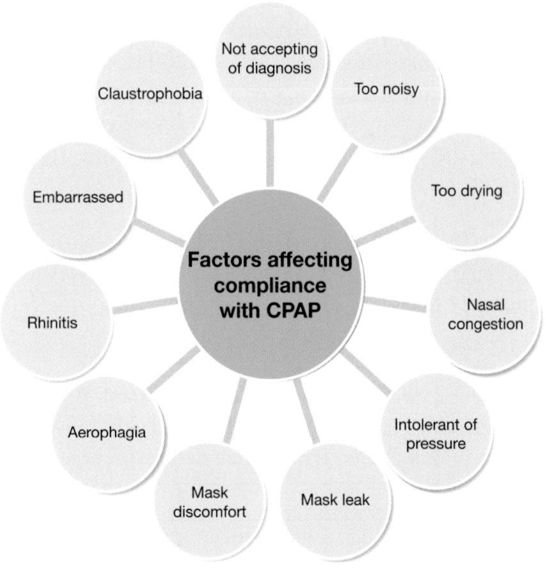
Factors affecting compliance with CPAP
Not accepting of diagnosis
Too noisy
Too drying
Nasal congestion
Intolerant of pressure
Mask leak
Mask discomfort
Aerophagia
Rhinitis
Embarrassed
Claustrophobia

Box 28.1 Risk factors for obstructive sleep apnoea

- Obesity
- Male
- Over 40 years old
- Smoking
- Use of alcohol
- Use of sedatives
- Large neck <43 cm
- Retronathic
- Nasal congestion
- Narrowed airway
- Hypothyroidism

Figure 28.2 Examples of respiratory limited polysomnography (PSG)

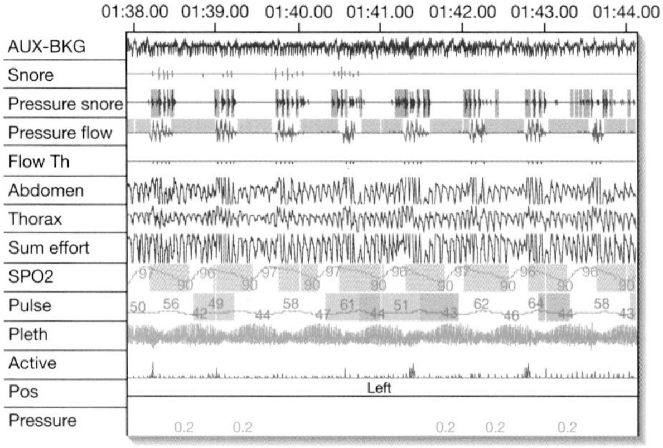
01:38.00 01:39.00 01:40.00 01:41.00 01:42.00 01:43.00 01:44.00
AUX-BKG
Snore
Pressure snore
Pressure flow
Flow Th
Abdomen
Thorax
Sum effort
SPO2
Pulse
Pleth
Active
Pos
Pressure
Left

Figure 28.3 A selection of continuous positive airway pressure (CPAP) equipment

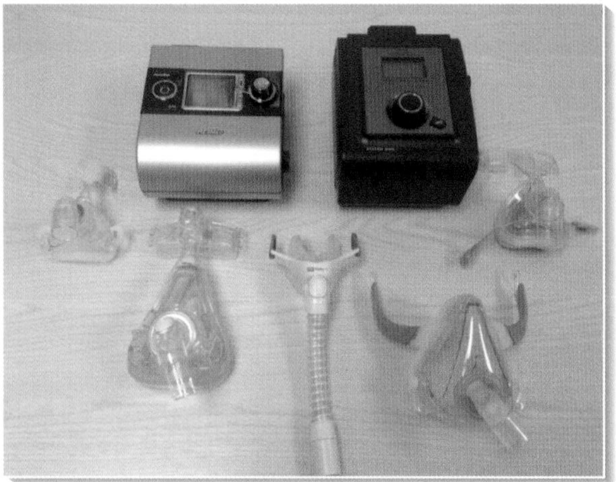

What is obstructive sleep apnoea syndrome?

Obstructive sleep apnoea (OSA) is a condition in which breathing during sleep is interrupted by closure of the upper airway (pharynx) for a minimum of 10 seconds (Figure 28.1). Most people with OSA have a combination of apnoeas (a complete cessation of breathing) and hypopnoeas (a partial obstruction of the upper airway). The apnoeas or hypopnoeas are accompanied by oxygen desaturation and are terminated by transient and brief awakening.

Many healthy people will have occasional periods of apnoea and/or hypopnoea during sleep without any symptoms and this is known as OSA. However, the constant fragmentation of sleep often results in the characteristic symptom of daytime somnolence. The combination of sleep disordered breathing with sleepiness is known as obstructive sleep apnoea syndrome (OSAS). OSAS is sometimes called obstructive sleep apnoea hypopnoea syndrome (OSAHS).

Predisposing factors

The literature suggests that around 4% of men and 2% of women have OSA; however, these data come from 15 years ago and it is now thought to be more likely that around 10% are affected and possibly up to 30% in the elderly. The majority of those affected are not diagnosed.

The risk factors for OSA are listed in Box 28.1. The main risk factor is obesity in around 70% of people, and neck size. This means that 30% have other predisposing factors and it is important that this differential diagnosis should not be ignored in someone of normal weight.

Symptoms of OSAS and associated problems

The most common symptom that patients present with is somnolence. However, snoring and the impact that this has on a domestic harmony is also a major complaint. Other symptoms are listed in Box 28.2.

There is increasing evidence that untreated OSA(S) can lead to increased risk of cardiovascular disease (independent of the effects of coexistent obesity) particularly hypertension, cardiac arrhythmia and stroke.

Diagnosis

Investigations used to diagnose OSA vary from simple overnight oximetry to full polysomnography. Oximetry alone, however, will miss other sleep disordered breathing patterns and can underestimate OSA severity, and therefore respiratory studies are the preferred investigation. Figure 28.2 is an example of a respiratory study showing OSA. The desaturations and changes in air flow can be clearly seen. Other sleep disordered breathing conditions can also occur separately or with OSA and these include hypoventilation, Cheyne–Stokes respiration and complex OSAS.

To be able to make an informed decision on appropriate treatment, a sleep study should be used in conjunction with a full medical history. It is essential to have information on symptoms, sleep hygiene, parasomnias, medical history, including medication and lifestyle issues such as alcohol, smoking and the use of recreational drugs.

Classification of OSA

The severity of OSA is based on the frequency of apnoeas and hypopnoeas per hour (the Apnoea Hypopnoea Index, AHI). The classification generally used is that recommended by the American Academy of Sleep Medicine. An AHI of 0–5 is normal, 5–15 mild, 15–30 moderate and greater than 30 severe.

The relationship between the severity of OSA and symptoms is generally weak.

Treatment

The most effective treatment for OSAS is continuous positive airway pressure (CPAP) but other treatments are listed in Box 28.3.

CPAP is administered using a flow of air generated by a compressor and delivered to the pharynx via a nasal or oro-nasal mask. CPAP can be delivered by fixed pressure and autopressure machines and also machines that can be accessed remotely, enabling increased input from sleep services thus potentially improving compliance. Figure 28.3 shows various machines and masks but many more are available.

CPAP is highly effective and few other medical treatments have such profound effects on quality of life, social functioning and relationships.

If CPAP is not tolerated, the use of a mandibular advancement device (MAD) can be effective for patients with mild or moderate OSAS. Positional training can also be effective for patients who have symptoms only when they lie supine; however, there is evidence to show that people do not continue long term with this treatment.

Lifestyle advice is also important in the treatment of OSAS.

Compliance with CPAP can be challenging for many reasons (Figure 28.4) but for treatment to be effective it requires considerable input from expert staff with education, support, choosing an appropriate interface, dealing with discomfort and monitoring compliance.

Driving and the DVLA

The diagnosis of OSAS increases the risk of having a road traffic accident. In the UK, people with a diagnosis of OSAS must inform the DVLA. This is why a distinction must be made between OSA and OSAS. Patients should refrain from driving until their symptoms are under control. Professional drivers (including HGV and PSV) are permitted to drive with this diagnosis once they have been adequately treated.

In summary, OSAS is a common chronic condition which it is important to diagnose for improved quality of life for the patient, and their family and long-term health. The treatment is effective but requires commitment from the patient.

Further reading

NICE (2015) http://cks.nice.org.uk/obstructive-sleep-apnoea-syndrome (accessed 24 February 2016).

29 Acute respiratory infections

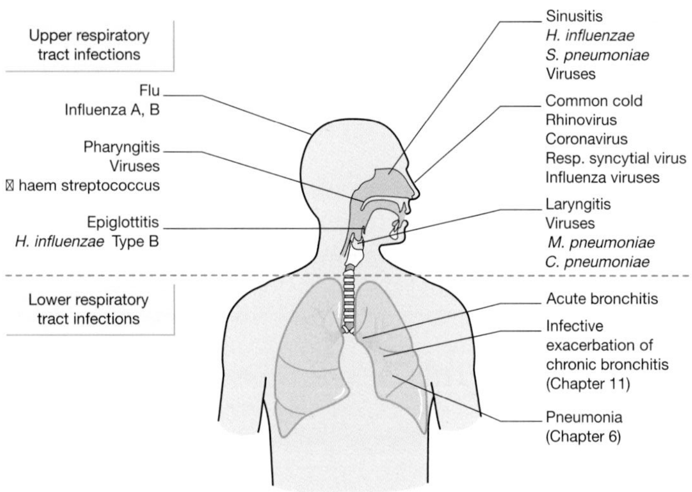

Upper respiratory tract infections
Flu
Influenza A, B
Pharyngitis
Viruses
β haem streptococcus
Epiglottitis
H. influenzae Type B
Lower respiratory tract infections
Sinusitis
H. influenzae
S. pneumoniae
Viruses
Common cold
Rhinovirus
Coronavirus
Resp. syncytial virus
Influenza viruses
Laryngitis
Viruses
M. pneumoniae
C. pneumoniae
Acute bronchitis
Infective exacerbation of chronic bronchitis (Chapter 11)
Pneumonia (Chapter 6)

Figure 29.1 Acute respiratory infections
Source: Reproduced with permission of WHO.

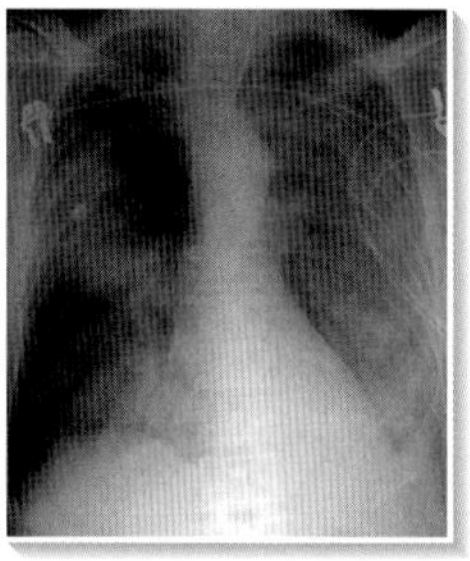

Figure 29.2 Chest X-ray showing pneumococcal pneumonia

Figure 29.3 Causes of pneumonia

Previously well infant 1 RSV 2 Adenovirus and other viruses 3 Bacterial	**Previously ill infant** 1 Staphylococcus 2 *E. coli* and Gram-negative bacteria 3 Viruses and opportunistic organisms
Children 1 Viruses 2 Pneumococcus 3 Mycoplasma 4 Others	**Previously fit adults** 1 Pneumococcus 2 Mycoplasma 3 *H. influenzae* 4 Viruses 5 Staphylococcus 6 *Legionella* 7 Others
Previous respiratory illness; elderly and debilitated 1 Pneumococcus 2 *H. influenzae* 3 Staphylococcus 4 *Klebsiella* and Gram-negative organisms	**If no response think of:** TB, Mycoplasma, *Legionella*, carcinoma
Severely immunocompromised and AIDS 1 Pneumocystis pneumonia 2 Cytomegalovirus 3 Adenovirus 4 Herpes simplex 5 Bacteria (*Legionella*, Staphylococcus, Pneumococcus) 6 Opportunistic mycobacteria; tuberculosis	**Hospital-acquired pneumonia** 1 Gram-negative bacteria (*Pseudomonas, Klebsiella, Proteus)* 2 Staphylococcus 3 Pneumococcus 4 Anaerobic bacteria, fungi 5 NB aspiration pneumonia 6 Others

Figure 29.4 CURB-65 severity score

- Confusion
- Urea >7 mmol/L
- Respiratory rate ≥30/min
- Blood pressure (systolic <90 mmHg or diastolic <60 mmHg)
- Age ≥65 years

Score 1 point for each feature present

CURB-65 Score

0 or 1 → **Likely suitable for home treatment**

2 → **Consider hospital supervised treatment**
Options include:
(i) short stay inpatient
(ii) hospital supervised outpatient

3 or more → **Manage in hospital as severe pneumonia**
Assess for ITU admission especially if CURB-65 score = 4 or 5

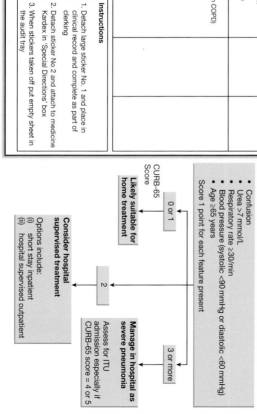

Figure 29.5 Care bundle

Date Time Ward	Name DOB Hospital number NHS number **(Affix patient label)**

Community acquired pneumonia (CAP)

1.

Action	Time completed, or reason for variation	Signed
Investigation and Diagnosis Arrange the following investigations for all suspected cases of AP: CXR (must have consolidation) FCB, U&Es, LFTs, CRP SaO_2– check ABG if <92% on air Blood cultures if febrile/severe CAP Sputum for MC&S if able to expectorate Serology for respiratory pathogens in severe CAP, or at particular risk for atypical pathogens (e.g. travel) Urine for legionella and pneurmococcal Ag in all cases of CAPS		
Assess severity (CURB65 score + 1 pt for each): Confusion Urea >7 mmols/l Respiratory rate >30/min BP: SBP <90 mmHg or DBP <60 mmHg Age >65 years **Low severity** – CURB65 0–1, <3% mortality. Consider treating at home (ambulatory pathway available). Admission maybe considered for reasons other than pneumonia severity e.g. Social reasons/unstable comorbid illness **Moderate severity** – CURB652, 9% mortality. Consider admission (non ITU/HUD wards): review on PTWR **High severity** – CURB65 3–5, 15–40% mortality. Consider critical care review–patients admitted to HDU/ITU		
Treatment Prescribe oxygen on medicine Kardex – Goal = SaO_2 >94% (88–92% in COPD) Administer antibiotics according to guidelines based on severity **0–1: Oral antibiotics** Follow guidelines available on intranet **2: Antibiotics to be administered within 4 hours** Oral antibiotics if possible – Follow guidelines on intranet **3–5: Antibiotics to be given ASAP** IV (review at 48 hrs) Follow guidelines on GEH intranet Clarithromycin oral unless NMB/gastric disturbance **Note:** Microbiology advice is available if needed via switchboard **Refer to smoking cessation if current smokers – x 1342**		

2.

CAP CARE BUNDLE
Antibiotic review – 48 hours

	Sign	Date	Time
Team reminded			
Antibiotics reviewed			
Lab reports reviewed			
Deviation from pathway? If yes document	Yes?	No?	
Discussed with mirobiology	Yes?	No?	

Instructions

1. Detach large sticker No. 1 and place in clinical record and complete as part of clerking
2. Detach sticker No 2 and attach to medicine Kardex in 'Special Directions' box
3. When stickers taken off put empty sheet in the audit tray

Acute respiratory infections remain a major cause of mortality worldwide. This chapter summarises some of the most common types.

Upper respiratory tract infection

Upper respiratory tract infection (URTI) is the most common respiratory complaint and in general practice accounts for approximately 9% of all consultations (Bourke and Burns, 2015). Most are viral in origin (Figure 29.1); however, they are often difficult to distinguish from more serious lower respiratory tract infections. Most URTIs are mild and self-limiting.

Bronchitis

Bronchitis is usually viral and affects the bronchial tree causing acute or chronic inflammation and typically causes coughing and bronchospasm. Extension of bronchial infection into the lung parenchyma is called bronchopneumonia.

Lower respiratory tract infection

Lower respiratory tract infection (LRTI) is where the infection is located below the larynx (which is normally sterile). Infections can reach the lungs by a number of routes:

- Inhalation
- Aspiration
- Direct inoculation (e.g. stab wound to chest)
- Blood-borne.

LRTIs include acute bronchitis, infective exacerbation of bronchitis and pneumonia. They are often bacterial and symptoms include productive cough, yellow or green sputum and fever. NICE guidelines 2014 recommend considering a C-reactive protein (CRP) test (there is a point of care – pin prick – test that can be used in the community) and not to give antibiotic therapy if less than 20 mg/L. A delayed antibiotic prescription can be provided if 20–100 mg/L, to be taken if symptoms worsen. Immediate antibiotics are given if over 100 mg/L. Local guidelines ensure consistent antibiotic prescription to reduce the increasing prevalence of multi-resistant bacteria.

Pneumonia

Pneumonia is a general term denoting inflammation of the gas exchange region of the lung and usually parenchymal lung inflammation caused by infection and causing consolidation on a chest X-ray (Figure 29.2). There are multiple causes which vary according to age, background and clinical location (Figure 29.3).

In the UK, one-quarter of all deaths in the elderly population is related to pneumonia and is often the terminal illness of serious concomitant disease.

Community-acquired pneumonia

This is acquired outside of hospital; this includes residential or nursing homes. Diagnosis can be made in primary care without an X-ray based on signs and symptoms, for example:

- Focal chest sounds
- Fever
- Productive cough – green sputum
- Pleuritic pain
- Breathlessness.

In hospital, a chest X-ray must show consolidation to confirm diagnosis. The severity can be determined using a CURB-65 score which can help decide if treatment can be given in the community, hospital ward or whether intensive care support is required. The score is based on key parameters that are associated with increased mortality (Figure 29.4):

- Confusion (new onset)
- Urea (>7 mmol/L)
- Respiratory rate (≥30/min)
- Blood pressure (systolic <90 mmHg or diastolic <60 mmHg)
- Age ≥65 years.

Hospital-acquired pneumonia

Hospital-acquired (nosocomial) pneumonia is defined as developing either 2 days or more after admission for another cause, or if a patient develops pneumonia who had a hospital stay within the previous 10 days of this admission. Local antibiotic guidance should be followed and is often different from those used for community acquired infection.

Pneumonia is caused by a variety of organisms, with 50% being caused by Gram-negative bacteria.

Aspiration pneumonia

Aspiration pneumonia is likely to occur in people with impaired swallow often resulting from reduced conscious levels, oesophageal or neuromuscular disease. The most common cause is dementia and strategies such as thickened fluids are used to reduce this risk. The clinical features are usually found in the base of the right lung and are not infectious.

Ventilator-associated pneumonia

This is defined as pneumonia occurring more than 48 hours after the patient has been intubated and received mechanical ventilation. This nosocomial infection increases morbidity and mortality as well as the cost of health care.

Treatment

Antibiotics should be prescribed when the cause is suspected or proven to be bacterial and local guidance used to reduce resistance. Guidance should be given on completing the course. When sputum samples are taken the results should be taken into account and antibiotic prescription reviewed.

Care bundles are a systematic and simple approach to care delivery that standardises care to provide evidence-based practice. Figure 29.5 shows an example of a community-acquired pneumonia care bundle (Chapter 38).

The recovery period will vary depending on the type of acute respiratory infection and its severity. The length of time taken and the effect on function and co-morbidities are often underestimated. It often takes weeks for symptoms to settle and months for a person to feel back to 'normal'. In a frail or elderly person this may never happen fully. For current smokers brief intervention advice and a smoking cessation referral should be offered (Chapter 10).

Vaccinations are available for influenza and pneumococcal pneumonia (Chapter 6). The pneumococcal vaccine is recommended for all people over 65 years of age and those with long-term conditions (especially chronic lung disease) and those who are asplenic or immunodeficient. *Haemophilus influenza* type B (Hib) is a virulent bacteria that can cause epiglottitis, bacteraemia, meningitis and pneumonia. A Hib vaccine is given to children.

Further reading

NICE (2014) Pneumonia in adults: diagnosis and management. NICE Guidelines CG191. https://www.nice.org.uk/guidance/cg191 (accessed 24 February 2016).

30 Cystic fibrosis

Figure 30.1 Main effects of cystic fibrosis GERD, gastro-oesophageal reflux disease

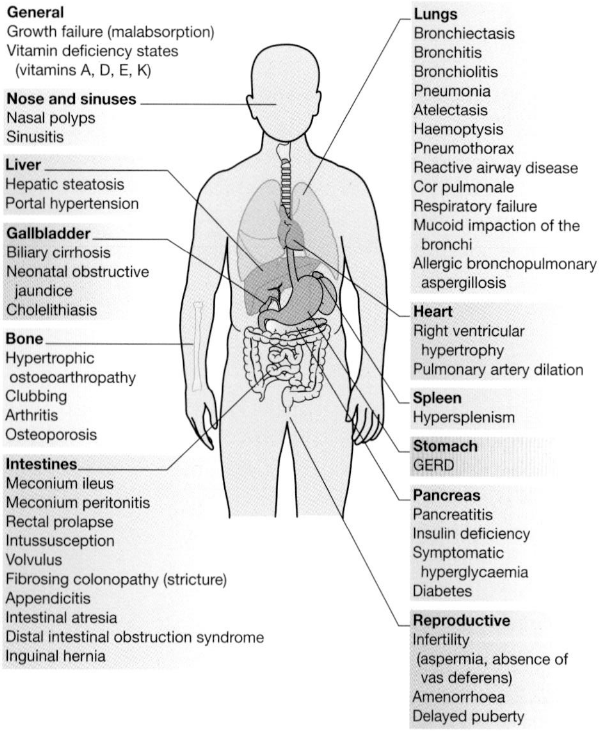
General
Growth failure (malabsorption)
Vitamin deficiency states (vitamins A, D, E, K)
Nose and sinuses
Nasal polyps
Sinusitis
Liver
Hepatic steatosis
Portal hypertension
Gallbladder
Biliary cirrhosis
Neonatal obstructive jaundice
Cholelithiasis
Bone
Hypertrophic ostoeoarthropathy
Clubbing
Arthritis
Osteoporosis
Intestines
Meconium ileus
Meconium peritonitis
Rectal prolapse
Intussusception
Volvulus
Fibrosing colonopathy (stricture)
Appendicitis
Intestinal atresia
Distal intestinal obstruction syndrome
Inguinal hernia
Lungs
Bronchiectasis
Bronchitis
Bronchiolitis
Pneumonia
Atelectasis
Haemoptysis
Pneumothorax
Reactive airway disease
Cor pulmonale
Respiratory failure
Mucoid impaction of the bronchi
Allergic bronchopulmonary aspergillosis
Heart
Right ventricular hypertrophy
Pulmonary artery dilation
Spleen
Hypersplenism
Stomach
GERD
Pancreas
Pancreatitis
Insulin deficiency
Symptomatic hyperglycaemia
Diabetes
Reproductive
Infertility (aspermia, absence of vas deferens)
Amenorrhoea
Delayed puberty

Figure 30.2 Pattern of cystic fibrosis genetic inheritance

- The faulty gene is carried by 1 in 25 people
- As shown in this diagram, if two carriers have a baby there is:

– a 25% chance the baby will have cystic fibrosis
– a 50% chance the baby will be a carrier of the faulty cystic fibrosis gene
– a 25% chance the baby will neither be a carrier nor have cystic fibrosis

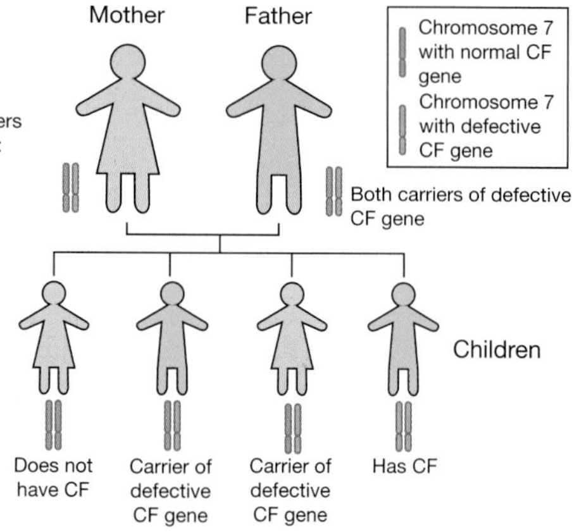
Mother
Father
Chromosome 7 with normal CF gene
Chromosome 7 with defective CF gene
Both carriers of defective CF gene
Children
Does not have CF
Carrier of defective CF gene
Carrier of defective CF gene
Has CF

Figure 30.3 (a) Cross-section of the lungs with healthy airways and widened airways. (b) Cross-section of a healthy airway. (c) Cross-section of an airway with bronchiectasis

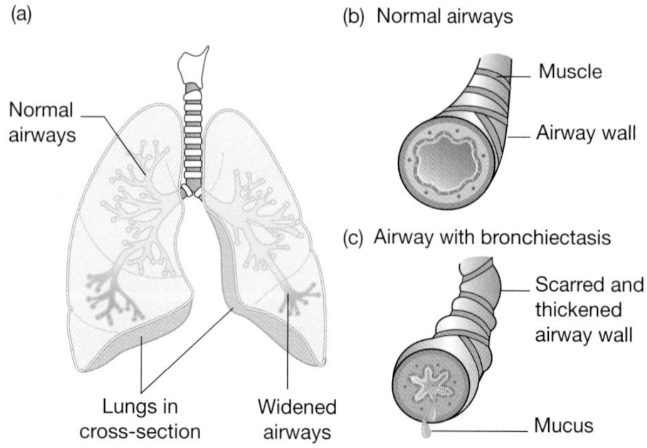
(a)
Normal airways
Lungs in cross-section
Widened airways
(b) Normal airways
Muscle
Airway wall
(c) Airway with bronchiectasis
Scarred and thickened airway wall
Mucus

Figure 30.4 Cystic fibrosis can lead to lung disease

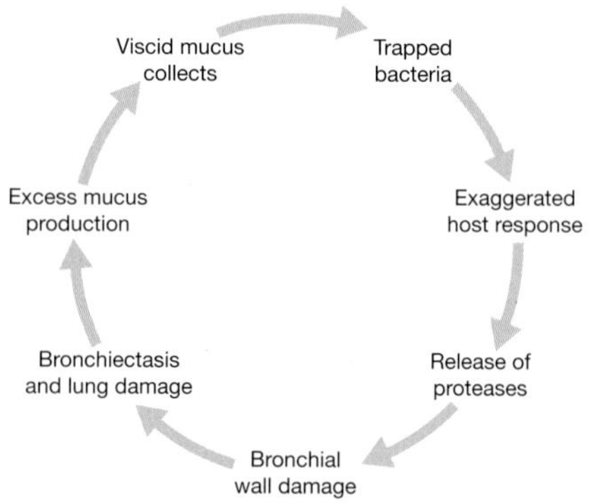
Viscid mucus collects
Trapped bacteria
Exaggerated host response
Release of proteases
Bronchial wall damage
Bronchiectasis and lung damage
Excess mucus production

Box 30.1 Common respiratory pathogens in cystic fibrosis MDR-PA, multi-drug-resistant *Pseudomonas aeruginosa*; MRSA, methicillin-resistant *Staphylococcus aureus*

Ages 1–10
Staphylococcus aureus
Haemophilus influenzae

Ages 10–adult
Pseudomonas aeruginosa

Other pathogens
Burkholderia cepacia complex

MRSA
Achromobacter
Stenotrophomonas maltophila
MDR-PA

History of cystic fibrosis

'Woe to the child who tastes salty from a kiss on the brow, for he is cursed and soon must die' (Busch, 1990)

In 1936 the first clinical description of cystic fibrosis (CF) as a distinct disease was put forward by Professor Fanconi (Swiss physician).

In 1938 Dorothy Hansine Anderson wrote about CF of the pancreas, and began to hypothesise that the lungs were involved.

In 1949 Professor di Sant' Agnese (USA) ascertained that mucous obstruction was the cause of CF lung disease. In 1952 he discovered abnormalities in sweat electrolytes; a sweat test to aid diagnosis was developed as a result.

In 1989 the CF gene *CFTR* (cystic fibrosis transmembrane conductance regulator) was isolated on the long arm of chromosome 7, by Lap-Chee Tsui et al. in Canada. Subsequent research has found over 1000 different mutations of the *CFTR* gene.

What is cystic fibrosis?

The name cystic fibrosis refers to the characteristic fibrosis and cysts that form within the pancreas, but it is also a multi-system disease resulting in many health issues (Figure 30.1).

CF is the most commonly inherited genetic disorder in the UK with over 10,000 people living with the disease. There is an incidence of 1 in 2500, with 1 in 25 being a carrier (Anderson, 1938). (There are approximately 2.5 million carriers.) It is a recessive condition which means that both parents need to be carriers to have a child with CF (Figure 30.2).

The normal function of the *CFTR* gene is to act as a chloride channel in the membranes of cells that line the passageways of the lungs, liver, pancreas, intestines, reproductive tract and skin. CF is usually diagnosed at birth to 12 months, and is now usually found during the UK newborn screening programme. Diagnostic indicators:

- Meconium ileus – inability of newborn to pass meconium, causing blockage of the small intestine (requires urgent surgery)
- Failure to thrive – malabsorption secondary to pancreatic insufficiencies
- Repeated chest infections/asthma – leading to bronchiectasis
- Infertility clinic – asymptomatic adults screened during fertility testing shows CF genes present
- Late diagnosis – as above, family history, diagnostic tests (blood tests, chest X-ray, CT).

Physiological effects

CF is a multi-system disease, but approximately 85% of patients die from respiratory disease. Lung disease develops from the clogging of the airways with a build-up of mucus and decreased mucociliary clearance, which results in inflammation. Inflammation and infection cause injury and structural changes to the lungs, leading to bronchiectasis (Figure 30.3).

CF eventually results in severe bronchiectasis in nearly all cases. Bronchiectasis is usually confirmed with a CT scan by determining the width of the bronchi (Figure 30.4).

The main symptoms include recurring chest infections, excessive sputum production, varying degrees of breathlessness, wheeze and occasional haemoptysis. There are many pathogens that leave the lungs of those with CF vulnerable to infection. Treatment options depend upon which pathogens are grown in the sputum. During the first decade of life of patients with CF, *Staphylococcus aureus* and *Haemophilus influenzae* are the most common bacterial pathogens isolated, but in the second and third decade of life, *Pseudomonas aeruginosa* is the prevalent bacteria (Box 30.1). Other pathogens appear, but appropriate segregation and isolation of patients based upon pathogens cultured from their sputum helps control and manage cross-infection.

Nutritionally, patients are often pancreatic insufficient – they do not produce the enzymes to digest fat and thus suffer the effects of malabsorption. Over the years, pancreatic damage leads to insulin deficiency and CF-related diabetes. This results from thick secretions that block ducts in the pancreas leading to scarring and fibrosis and then destruction and depletion of beta cells.

Treatment

The methods used for CF treatment have improved greatly in recent years. Common forms of treatment include antibiotics, exercise and chest physical therapy, with the aim of:

- Mucus clearance from the lungs
- Preventing and controlling pathogens in lungs
- Preventing blockages in the intestines
- Providing adequate nutrition.

Intravenous antibiotics are given via a Port-a-cath or mid-line for 2 weeks to eradicate or control symptoms produced in the lungs by the pathogens cultured from sputum samples. There is also emphasis on prevention of exacerbations by promoting patients to keep well in the community with the use of oral prophylactic antibiotics, nebulised antibiotics, self-physiotherapy and exercise.

Regular clinic attendance with access to a full CF team including consultant, nurse specialist, dietitian, physiotherapist, pharmacist, psychologist and social worker help to encourage the patient to lead as 'normal' a lifestyle as possible.

Further reading

Flume PA, Mogayzel PJ Jr, Robinson KA, et al. (2010) Cystic fibrosis pulmonary guidelines: pulmonary complications: hemoptysis and pneumothorax. *Am J Respir Crit Care Med* 182: 298–306. doi:10.1164/rccm.201002-0157OC. PMID 20299528.

31 Bronchiectasis

Figure 31.1 Dilated bronchi and mucus pooling
Source: Boyton RJ. (2008). Bronchiectasis. *Medicine*. 36: 315–320. (2008). Reproduction with permission of Royal Brompton & Harefield NHS Trust.

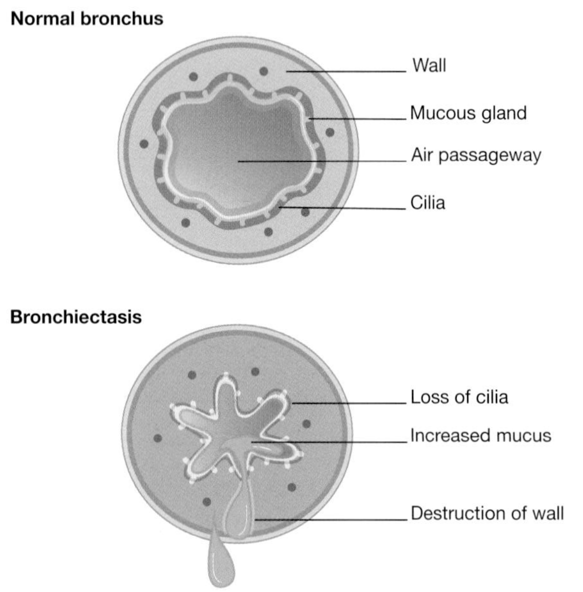
Normal bronchus
Wall
Mucous gland
Air passageway
Cilia
Bronchiectasis
Loss of cilia
Increased mucus
Destruction of wall

Table 31.1 Underlying causes of bronchiectasis
Source: Shoemark A, Ozerovitch L, Wilson R. (2007) *Respir Med* 101(6): 1163–70. Reproduced with permission of Elsevier.

Causes and association of bronchiectasis	
Deficient immune response	Primary immune deficiency e.g. CVID/XLA Specific polysaccharide antibody deficiency Secondary immune deficiency e.g. CLL
Infection	Pneumonia Tuberculosis Non-tuberculous mycobacteria
Deficient of mucociliary clearance	Cystic fibrosis Primary ciliary dyskinesia Young's syndrome (sinusitis and infertility)
Excessive immune response	Allergic broncho-pulmonary aspergillosis Rheumatoid arthritis
Airway insult	Smoke inhalation Foreign body Aspiration of gastric content
Congenital	Mounier–Kuhn syndrome and Williams–Campbell syndrome (defect of the bronchial wall structure)
Other	Yellow nail syndrome Pan bronchiolitis Inflammatory bowel disease Alpha–1–antitrypsin deficiency
Abbreviations	CLL, chronic lymphatic leukaemia CVID, common variable immune deficiency XLA, X–linked agammaglobulinemia

Figure 31.2 The cycle of infection and inflammation
Source: Ozerovitch L, Wilson R. Independent Nurse 2011; Aug 22:18–20. Reproduced with permission of MA Healthcare Ltd.

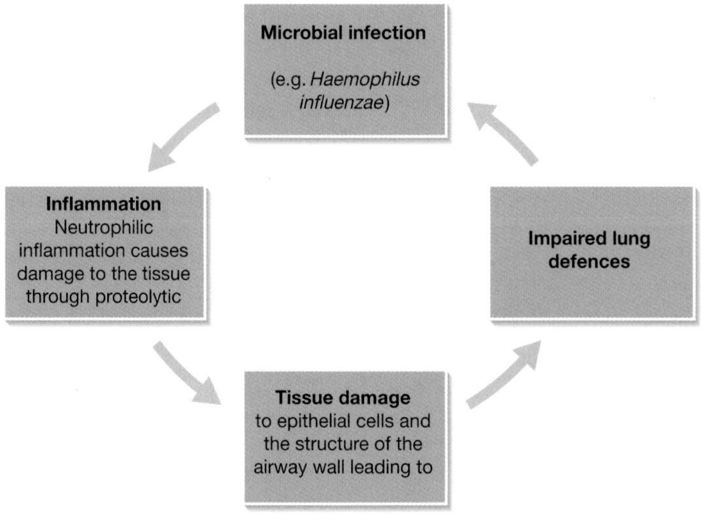
Microbial infection
(e.g. Haemophilus influenzae)
Inflammation
Neutrophilic inflammation causes damage to the tissue through proteolytic
Tissue damage
to epithelial cells and the structure of the airway wall leading to
Impaired lung defences

Patients with bronchiectasis experience chronic productive cough, recurrent respiratory infections and an impaired quality of life. Early diagnosis of bronchiectasis is important so that specific medical management can be instigated in order to establish control of symptoms, significantly improve health status and prevent progression.

What is bronchiectasis?

Bronchiectasis is defined as abnormal chronic dilatation of one or more bronchi (Bilton, 2003). The dilated bronchi are caused by weakness and destruction of structural components of the bronchial wall and this together with loss of ciliated epithelium causes mucus to accumulate. Damage to the surface epithelium leads to loss of ciliated cells which are replaced by mucus secreting cells and mucous gland hypertrophy causing increased mucous volume, which becomes more viscous when it is infected, impairing the clearance of secretions (Figure 31.1). The collection of stationary mucus acts as a conducive environment for bacteria to grow and this is the source of chronic infection.

Chronic inflammation is stimulated by bacterial infection which causes further damage to the walls of the bronchi, this sets up a vicious cycle with progressive lung damage (Figure 31.2). The consequence for the patient is chronic respiratory tract infection with acute exacerbations, sometimes provoked by viral infections that impair lung function, resulting in chronic morbidity and premature mortality.

What are the associated symptoms of an exacerbation of bronchiectasis?

Patients experience an increased cough and sputum production that appears thicker and darker in colour. Other common symptoms are wheeze, shortness of breath, chest tightness and/or pain, haemoptysis, fever, sinusitis, rhinitis, poor appetite and malaise. Patients often describe profound tiredness which is always a feature of poor disease control. Most patients with bronchiectasis experience an infection two to three times a year which is usually relieved by a course of oral antibiotics. For patients experiencing persistent respiratory infective symptoms despite oral antibiotics, admission to hospital to receive intravenous antibiotic therapy will be necessary.

Protocol of investigations

Diagnosis is confirmed by high resolution computed tomography scan to assess lung structure. Additionally, other investigations may be required: lung function tests; screening tests for primary ciliary dyskinesia (a relatively rare condition that affects lungs, sinuses and ears due to abnormal beating cilia); blood tests to screen for problems of immune function; skin prick tests for allergy; sweat test/blood tests (genetics) for cystic fibrosis; sputum examination for routine pathogens and fungi and prolonged cultures for slow growing mycobacteria; sputum cell count (neutrophils and eosinophils); physiotherapy assessment and, where appropriate, input from dietitians, psychologists, ENT and gastroenterology colleagues.

The role of the clinical nurse specialist within the work-up is to obtain a nursing assessment of the patient's lifestyle; measure exercise capacity and oxygenation (using the Shuttle/6 minute walk test and Borg breathlessness scale); report on quality of life (Chapter 22) and scheduling urgent and complex clinical reviews and hospital admissions.

Causes and association of bronchiectasis

In developing countries, bronchiectasis is usually the result of damage by serious infections especially tuberculosis. Prevalence is higher in areas with poor standards of living, nutrition and sanitation and limited access to health services, antibiotic treatment and immunisation programmes (Bilton, 2003). In the developed world, bronchiectasis is the end result of a number of pathologies. Some patients are born with a weakness of the lungs' innate defences (e.g. cystic fibrosis), or deficiency in their body's ability to fight infection (e.g. common variable immune deficiency), which renders them prone to catching repeated respiratory infections and leads to bronchiectasis (Table 31.1). Other patients are born with a normal host defence system but develop a severe infection (e.g. whooping cough or pneumonia) which damages the airways and causes bronchiectasis.

Prevalence

The true prevalence rate may be underestimated. Prevalence has been estimated to be 3.7–4.2 per 100,000 (Pasteur et al., 2010), and about 1000 people die from bronchiectasis each year in England and Wales, with the rate increasing year on year by 3% (Roberts and Hubbard, 2010). The prevalence of bronchiectasis in patients with chronic obstructive pulmonary disease (COPD) is high: 29% in primary care and 50% in hospital attendees (Pasteur et al., 2010).

Treatment

Chest physiotherapy is the bedrock of bronchiectasis management (BTS/ACPRC Guideline, 2009). Patients should have periodic reviews in their approach to using airway clearance techniques. Personalised techniques aim to remove secretions and reduce the risk of an exacerbation: active cycle of breathing; autogenic drainage and device adjuncts, such as the acapella and flutter.

Bronchodilators and inhaled steroids expand the airways in patients with an asthmatic component, making it easier to breathe and assist mucus clearance.

Nasal douching and use of steroid sprays or drops can help with post-nasal drip, runny nose and sinus pain as most patients with bronchiectasis develop chronic rhinosinusitis.

Antibiotics are commonly used to combat respiratory infections. The oral route is used to treat acute exacerbations; intravenous delivery is used when the oral route fails. Antibiotics can also be used continuously in patients with severe bronchiectasis to reduce bacterial load and therefore level of inflammation, and then the inhaled route is sometimes used. The route of administration will depend on frequency and severity of the exacerbation, bacterial sputum cultures and drug sensitivities. Long-term macrolide antibiotics can be of benefit because of their anti-inflammatory properties.

Surgery is considered an option for a few individuals who have localised bronchiectasis and experience frequent infective exacerbations.

Further reading

Ozerovitch L, Wilson R. (2011) Managing bronchiectasis. *Independent Nurse* August 22: 18–20.

Wilson CB, Jones PW, O'Leary CJ, Cole PJ, Wilson R. (1997) Validation of the St George's Respiratory Questionnaire in bronchiectasis. *Am J Respir Crit Care Med* 156: 536–541.

32 Occupational and environmental lung disease

Figure 32.1 Serial peak flows in occupational asthma

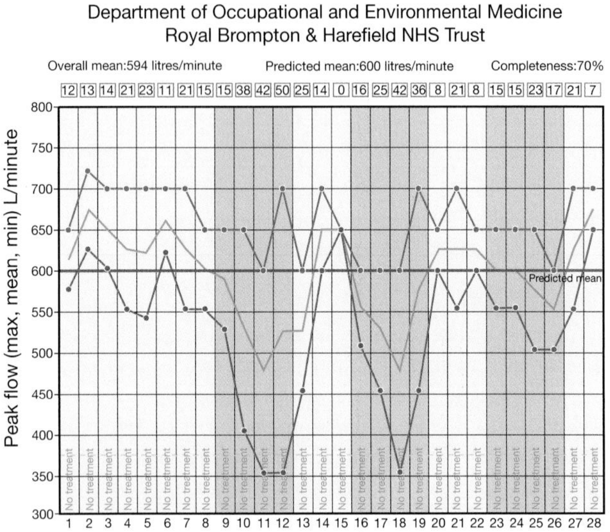
Department of Occupational and Environmental Medicine
Royal Brompton & Harefield NHS Trust
Overall mean:594 litres/minute
Predicted mean:600 litres/minute
Completeness:70%
12 13 14 21 23 11 21 15 15 38 42 50 25 14 0 16 25 42 36 8 21 8 15 15 23 17 21 7
Peak flow (max, mean, min) L/minute
800
750
700
650
600
550
500
450
400
350
300
Predicted mean
No treatment
1 2 3 4 5 6 7 8 9 10 11 12 13 14 15 16 17 18 19 20 21 22 23 24 25 26 27 28

Figure 32.2 A positive inhalation test to flour and enzymes in a baker

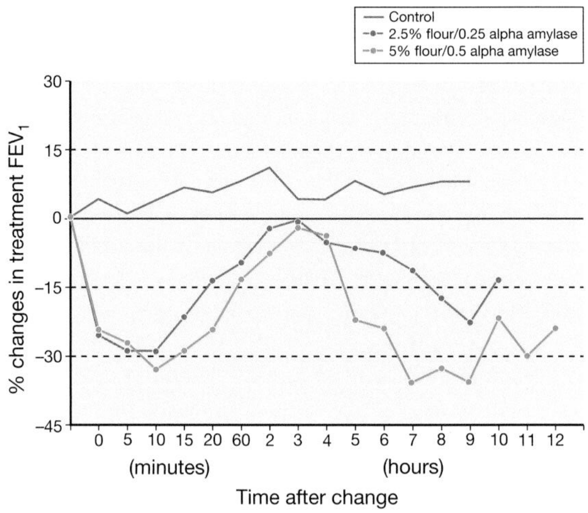
Control
2.5% flour/0.25 alpha amylase
5% flour/0.5 alpha amylase
% changes in treatment FEV1
30
15
0
−15
−30
−45
0 5 10 15 20 60 2 3 4 5 6 7 8 9 10 11 12
(minutes)
(hours)
Time after change

Figure 32.3 Working in an extremely dusty environment with high exposure to silica can cause silicosis in stonemasons

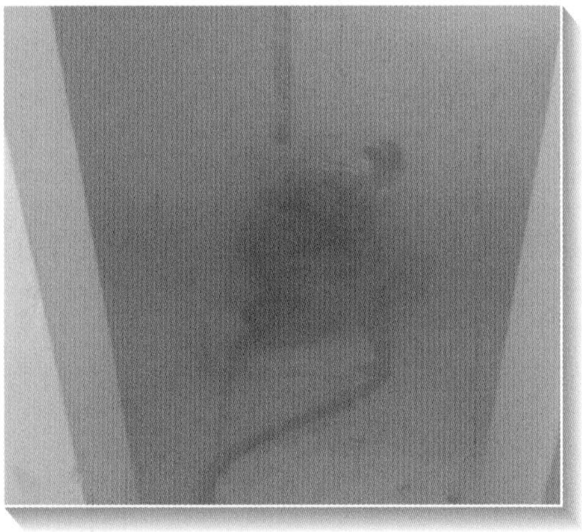

Figure 32.4 Long-term exposure to coal dust caused may miners to develop pneumoconiosis

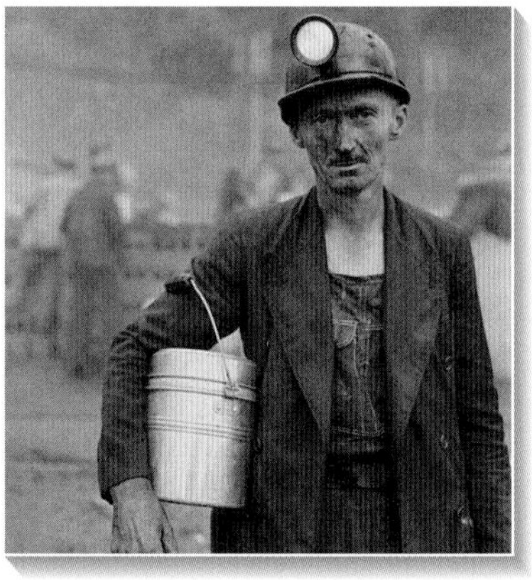

Figure 32.5 Chest X-ray showing benign pleural plaques from asbestos exposure

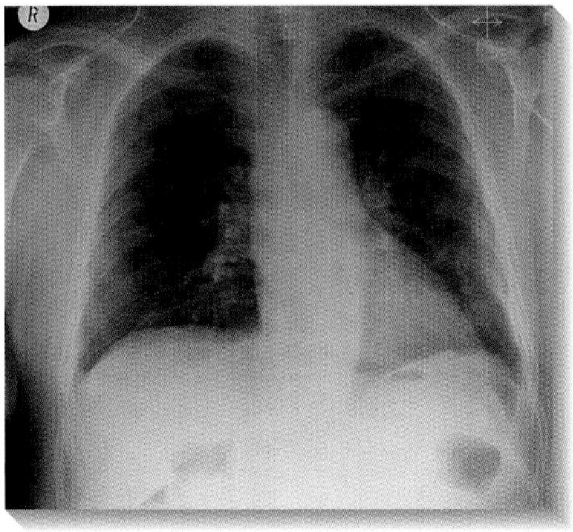

Figure 32.6 Regular exposure to avian proteins can lead to bird fancier's lung

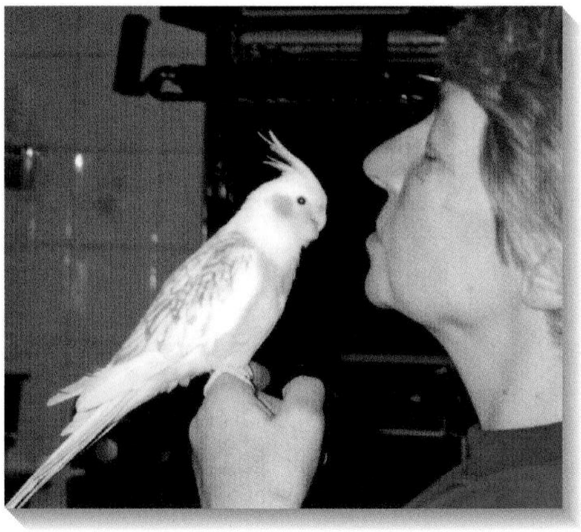

Lung diseases caused by the inhalation of allergenic or toxic dusts are often acquired in an occupational environment where the concentration and duration of exposure are far greater than in the general environment. A dusty or fume-filled working environment can also exacerbate an underlying respiratory disease. A total of 403,000 working days were lost in 2013–2014 due to work-related breathing or lung problems and there were 12,000 'occupational' respiratory deaths, predominantly from pneumoconiosis (HSE, 2014). There is a national reporting scheme for occupational lung disease in the UK (SWORD) but it is recognised that the conditions are markedly under-reported (Fishwick et al., 2008). Those diagnosed with an occupational lung disease are entitled to claim industrial injuries disablement benefit.

Occupational asthma

In adulthood, it has been estimated that asthma is related to work in about 10% of cases. *Occupational* asthma is caused by the inhalation of a specific substance in the work environment, leading to a respiratory hypersensitivity. This is to be distinguished from *work exacerbated* asthma, where non specific dust or fumes cause symptoms on a background of underlying asthma. Over 300 workplace agents are known to induce occupational asthma, although a smaller number occur commonly in high risk occupations (e.g. baking and detergent workers). Diagnosis should be undertaken in a specialist centre as the implications for health and employment are considerable and an erroneous diagnosis can be disastrous.

Investigations for occupational asthma

A detailed history of the onset and pattern of symptoms, as well as the work environment, is crucial. Symptoms can be additionally assessed by a series of 2-hourly peak flow recordings over a period of 4 weeks. This often shows a reduction in lung function when at work and an improvement on days off (Figure 32.1); increased variability in peak flow can be seen on days at work (blue columns).

Immunological testing is valuable in occupational asthma caused by high-molecular weight (protein) agents (e.g. flour or animal fur), by specialist skin prick tests and/or specific immunoglobulin E (IgE) measurement. In low-molecular weight (chemical) agents (e.g. isocyanates), immunological tests are less helpful.

Specific occupational inhalation testing is considered to be the gold standard in the diagnosis of occupational asthma; this should be carried out in a specialist centre. The workplace environment is recreated in a laboratory setting in carefully controlled conditions. The challenges are single blind, with an inert control day being compared with exposure to the suspected agent. Forced expiratory volume in 1 second (FEV_1) is then plotted over the remainder of the day (Figure 32.2). Daily measurement of bronchial hyperreactivity (histamine PC_{20}) is also measured. Management of those diagnosed with occupational asthma includes complete removal from further exposure to the sensitising material.

Pneumoconioses and asbestos-related diseases

The pneumoconioses are a group of lung diseases that are caused by the progressive accumulation of respirable toxic dust in the lungs, leading to inflammation and progressive fibrosis. The most common causes are asbestos fibres (asbestosis), crystalline silica (silicosis; Figure 32.3) and coal dust (coal worker's pneumoconiosis; Figure 32.4). These diseases have a long latency so symptoms appear many years after exposure. Symptoms are predominantly dyspnoea and cough. A detailed occupational history, going back over decades, is essential. Diagnosis is made by chest X-ray (Figure 32.5) or CT scan. Asbestos exposure often leads to pleural disease: benign pleural plaques, diffuse pleural thickening and, in some cases, malignant mesothelioma, as well as other lung cancers.

Hypersensitivity pneumonitis

Hypersensitivity pneumonitis (HP) is also known as extrinsic allergic alveolitis. It is caused by a hypersensitivity response in the small airways and alveoli to inhaled microbes or organic dust and moulds. Acute HP is similar in presentation to pneumonia with fever, chest tightness and cough, sometimes causing hypoxia and requiring hospital treatment. It can resolve fairly quickly once the patient is removed from exposure. Chronic HP has a similar presentation to idiopathic pulmonary fibrosis (IPF) with dyspnoea, cough, weight loss and fatigue.

There are many causes of HP, both occupational and environmental. Bird fancier's lung is caused by inhalation of avian proteins, and can be caused by keeping pet birds at home, particularly parrots, budgerigars and pigeons (Figure 32.6). There are many occupational causes of HP (e.g. metal worker's lung caused by inhalation of contaminated lubricating fluids during metal turning).

Diagnosis can be difficult – again, a careful history of exposures, in relation to onset of symptoms, is important. Measurement of serum precipitins in a specialist laboratory can be useful in some cases. Management requires avoidance of further exposure to the causative agent.

Environmental respiratory disease

Most of us spend much of our time indoors and when we are not at work we are at home or travelling between the two. Most of the evidence on non-occupational environmental exposures is epidemiological and difficult to apply to individual patients but there is strong evidence that exposure to pollution, especially that from traffic, causes reductions in lung growth in children, and in the elderly hastens hospitalisation and death from respiratory diseases such as chronic obstructive pulmonary disease (COPD). Exposure to tobacco smoke in the home increases the risk of wheezing and possibly the risk of asthma in children. Women who cook with gas have small reductions in their lung function. There is concern too over exposures to a huge variety of domestic chemicals, including volatile organic compounds, which are found in cleaning materials, paints or as emissions from furniture and fabrics but as yet there is little firm evidence that they cause respiratory disease.

Further reading

Fishwick D, Barber C, Bradshaw LM, et al. (2008) Standards of care for occupational asthma. *Thorax* 68: 240–250.

Health and Safety Executive (HSE) (2014) Work-related respiratory disease in Great Britain. http://www.hse.gov.uk/statistics/causdis/respiratory-diseases.pdf (accessed 25 February 2016).

33 Interstitial lung disease

Figure 33.1 Disorders of the lung interstitium

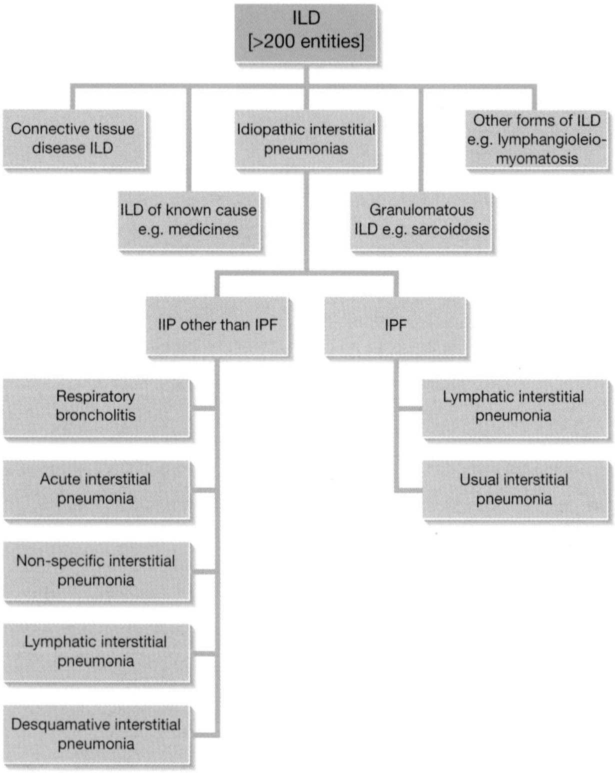
ILD
[>200 entities]
Connective tissue disease ILD
ILD of known cause e.g. medicines
Idiopathic interstitial pneumonias
Granulomatous ILD e.g. sarcoidosis
Other forms of ILD e.g. lymphangioleio-myomatosis
IIP other than IPF
IPF
Respiratory broncholitis
Acute interstitial pneumonia
Non-specific interstitial pneumonia
Lymphatic interstitial pneumonia
Desquamative interstitial pneumonia
Lymphatic interstitial pneumonia
Usual interstitial pneumonia

Figure 33.2 The interstitial space between the alveolar epithelium and capillary endothelium

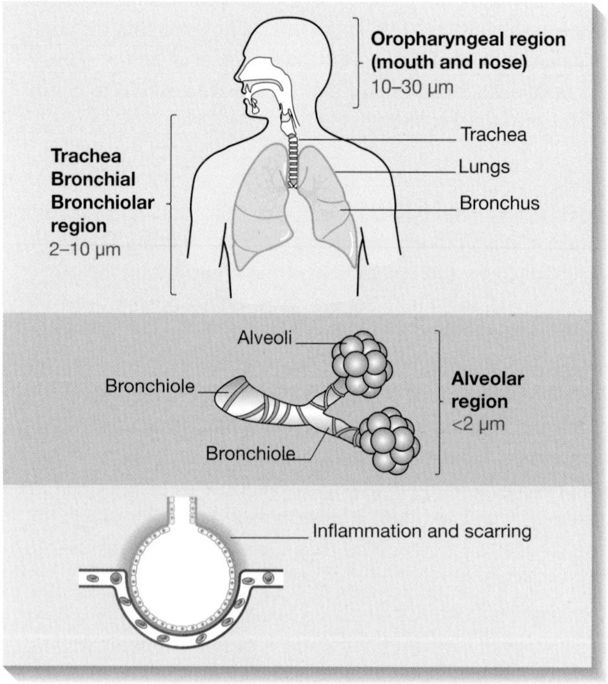
Oropharyngeal region (mouth and nose)
10–30 μm
Trachea
Lungs
Bronchus
Trachea Bronchial Bronchiolar region
2–10 μm
Alveoli
Bronchiole
Bronchiole
Alveolar region
<2 μm
Inflammation and scarring

Figure 33.3 High resolution CT: typical usual interstitial pneumonia – honeycomb lung

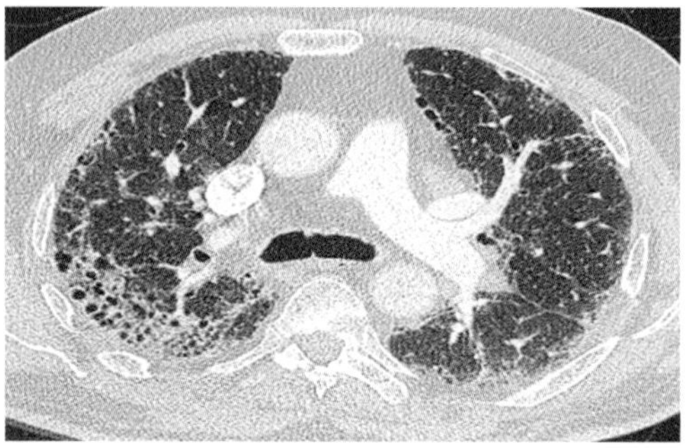

Figure 33.4 High resolution CT: non-specific interstitial pneumonitis. Note ground glass opacities

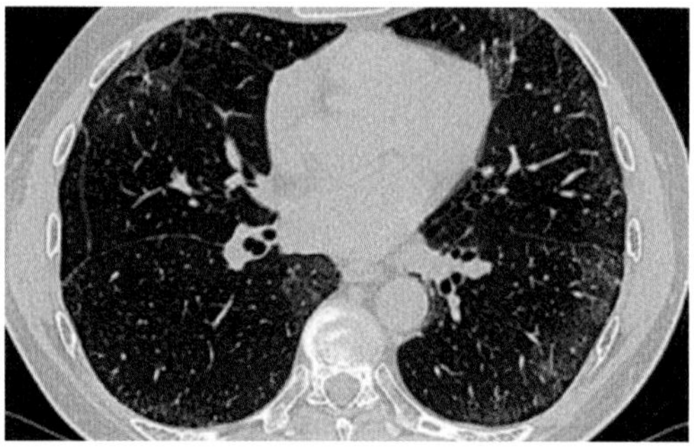

Figure 33.5 High resolution CT: non-acute hypersensitivity pneumonitis with mosaic pattern

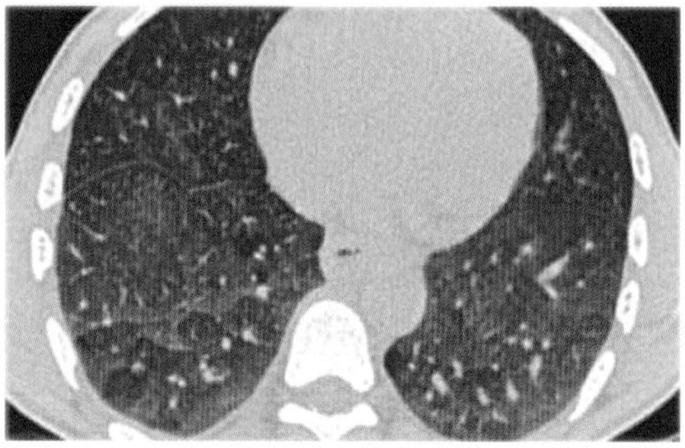

Figure 33.6 Potential clinical courses of idiopathic pulmonary fibrosis
Source: Image © 2011 The American Thoracic Society. in: Ley B, Collard HR, King TE Jr. *Am J Respir Crit Care Med* 2011,183, 431–440.

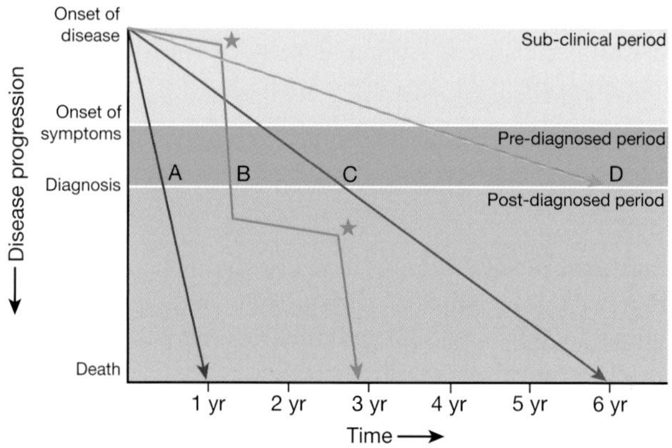
Onset of disease
Onset of symptoms
Diagnosis
Death
Disease progression
Sub-clinical period
Pre-diagnosed period
Post-diagnosed period
A
B
C
D
1 yr
2 yr
3 yr
4 yr
5 yr
6 yr
Time

Interstitial lung diseases (ILDs) are a diverse group of more than 200 entities (Figure 33.1). They are associated with fibrotic changes within the interstitium of the lung – the space between the alveolar epithelium and capillary endothelium (Figure 33.2). This inflammation or scarring distorts the basement membrane resulting in impaired gas exchange.

The most common ILDs are the idiopathic interstitial pneumonias (IIPs), predominantly idiopathic pulmonary fibrosis (IPF), connective tissue disease-related ILD (CTD-ILD); sarcoidosis (Chapter 34) and hypersensitivity pneumonitis (HP; Chapter 32).

The incidence of IPF in the UK is around 5 per 100,000 person years and is classified as rare disease. IPF is increasing, with 5000 new cases diagnosed each year. Non-specific interstitial pneumonitis (NSIP) is now recognised as a defined entity; other IIPs are rarer such as respiratory bronchiolitis (R-BILD), as are the other ILDs such as lymphangioleiomyomatosis (Figure 33.1).

Connective tissue disease-related ILD

CTD-ILD are more common in women: rheumatoid arthritis, systemic sclerosis, Sjögren's syndrome, polymyositis and dermatomyositis, systemic lupus erythematosus, undifferentiated and mixed connective tissue disease (MCTD) are associated with an ILD in approximately 30% of patients. While the majority of these patients remain stable, a significant minority will have progressive disease, most often characterised as NSIP. However, in patients with concomitant rheumatoid arthritis, usual interstitial pneumonia (UIP) is more common. A UIP pattern (Figure 33.3) is associated with a significantly better survival in CTD-related disease than idiopathic UIP.

Idiopathic interstitial pneumonias

Although familial IIPs have been reported in 2–20% of cases, the cause and course remain poorly understood. IIPs, in particular NSIP, are difficult to distinguish from HP, and vice versa (Figures 33.4 and 33.5). A detailed history is essential to identify possible exposures (Chapter 32).

NSIP is a disease entity in its own right although some patients will progress to end-stage fibrosis in keeping with UIP. The prognosis in IPF (UIP) is exceedingly poor: a median survival of 3 years from the point of diagnosis (Figure 33.6). Patients experience periods of relative disease stability punctuated by episodes of rapid decline, known as exacerbations, and are at higher risk of developing lung cancer. In the UK, 15,000 people currently have a diagnosis of IPF.

Symptoms

Patients present with one or more of the following: breathlessness (exertional), fatigue, gastric reflux and cough (usually dry and irritating). In CTD-ILD, patients also complain of joint pain and sicca symptoms. The focus of care is on symptom management in those ILDs where treatment is limited or associated with a significant side effect profile.

Diagnosis

NICE clinical guidelines (CG163:2013) and the Quality Standards (2015) provide a template to optimise the diagnosis and management of suspected IPF. NICE (2015) recommend that the differential diagnosis of IPF must be confirmed by the consensus of the expert ILD multi-disciplinary team. In suspected CTD-ILD a rheumatologist should be involved.

Pulmonary function tests

Monitoring patients relies on serial physiological measures. ILDs are restrictive rather than obstructive lung conditions characterised by a proportionally equal reduction in forced expiratory volume in 1 second (FEV_1) and forced vital capacity (FVC). FVC is the internationally accepted measure predicting survival and informing treatment. However, the diffusing capacity of carbon monoxide (DLCO), where it can be robustly measured in an accredited pulmonary function testing laboratory, is also used. A disproportionate reduction in DLCO could indicate coexistent emphysema or pulmonary hypertension. A DLCO level of less than 40% is indicative of advanced disease in IPF. A reduction of ≥10% in FVC or ≥15% in DLCO in the first 6–12 months is also associated with higher mortality.

Six-minute walk test

Desaturation during the six-minute walk test at diagnosis has stronger prognostic value in IPF than resting lung function. The modified MRC breathlessness score is also reliable in predicting survival and disease progression.

High resolution CT

High resolution CT scans help to diagnose IPF, particularly in complex cases where there is diagnostic uncertainly, and provide a measure of baseline severity.

Bronchoscopy and broncho-alveolar lavage

Broncho-alveolar lavage (BAL) can assist in diagnosis and can exclude infection. In IPF, neutrophils and eosinophils are present with usually ≤25% lymphocytes. Lymphocytes ≥40% is highly suggestive of HP. In RB-ILD, macrophages are increased and have a darker staining in smokers.

Treatment

Lung transplant is the only curative treatment. It is worth commenting on the issues related to transplantation: time of waiting; availability of donors; psychological support, and so on.

Pharmacology

Given the complexity of ILDs, some patients require an individualised treatment plan of either monotherapy or a combination of the following, depending upon the specific diagnosis, under the management of a specialist centre: immunosuppression; corticosteroids; antioxidant; chemotherapy; monoclonal antibodies; thalidomide for cough. Pirfenidone, an immunosuppressant with both anti-inflammatory and anti-fibrotic effects, is indicated for patients diagnosed with IPF (FVC between 50% and 80% predicted; NICE, 2013). Nintedanib, a tyrosine kinase inhibitor, approved by NICE for use in the UK in April 2016. Both pirfenidone and nintedanib reduce the decline in FVC, consistent with a slowing of disease progression in IPF. Clinical trials are ongoing.

Patients with ILD who are current smokers should receive smoking cessation advice. Patients should be assessed for oxygen therapy and all should have access to a pulmonary rehabilitation programme. Patients should have access to a clinical nurse specialist with disease-specific knowledge who is well placed to coordinate care and ensure prompt referral to palliative care, which is of great importance given the prognosis associated with ILDs.

While the approach is not standardised, thought must be given to managing and monitoring the patient's quality of life and optimising symptom management.

Further reading

British Thoracic Society (2008) www.brit-thoracic.org.uk/guidelines-and-quality-standards/interstitial-lung-disease-guidelines/ (accessed 25 February 2016).

34 Sarcoidosis

Figure 34.1 Sarcoid granuloma

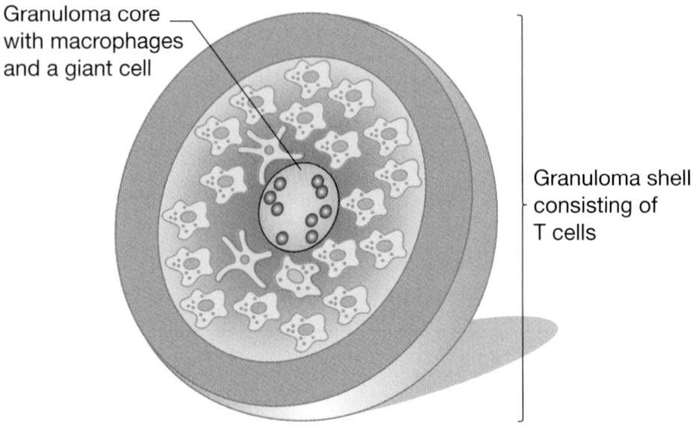
Granuloma core
with macrophages
and a giant cell
Granuloma shell
consisting of
T cells

Figure 34.2 Inflammatory phases in lung sarcoidosis

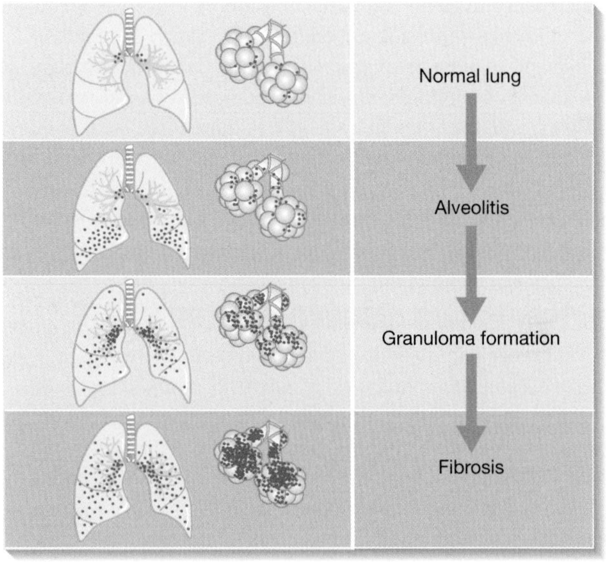
Normal lung
Alveolitis
Granuloma formation
Fibrosis

Figure 34.3 System involvement in sarcoidosis

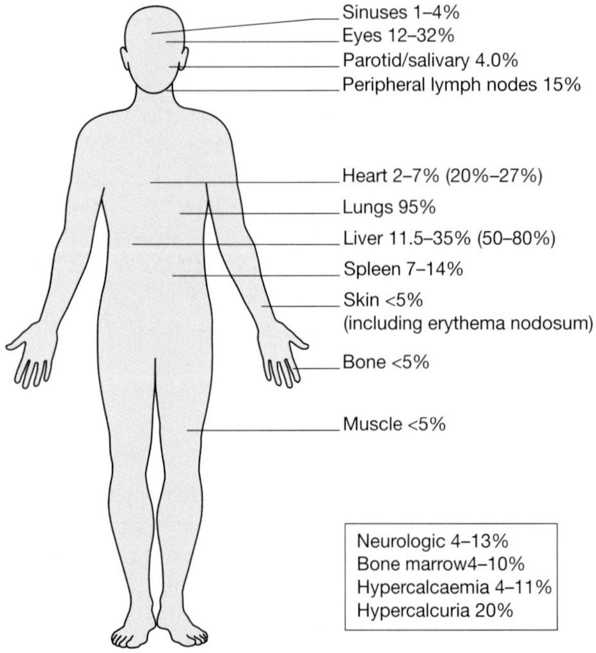
Sinuses 1–4%
Eyes 12–32%
Parotid/salivary 4.0%
Peripheral lymph nodes 15%
Heart 2–7% (20%–27%)
Lungs 95%
Liver 11.5–35% (50–80%)
Spleen 7–14%
Skin <5%
(including erythema nodosum)
Bone <5%
Muscle <5%

Neurologic 4–13%
Bone marrow4–10%
Hypercalcaemia 4–11%
Hypercalcuria 20%

Figure 34.4 Suspect causes of sarcoidosis

Infectious	**Non-infectious**
Mycobacteria	Dust
Tuberculous	Clay
Non-tuberculous	Pine
Bacteria	Pollen
Corynebacterium spp.	Talc
Propionibacterium acnes	Mixed
Tropheryma whipplei	Metals
Fungi	Aluminium
Cryptococcus spp.	Beryllium
Viruses	Zirconium
Cytomegalovirus	Silica
Epstein–Barr virus	
Herpes simplex virus	

Figure 34.5 Incidence of sarcoidosis per 100,000

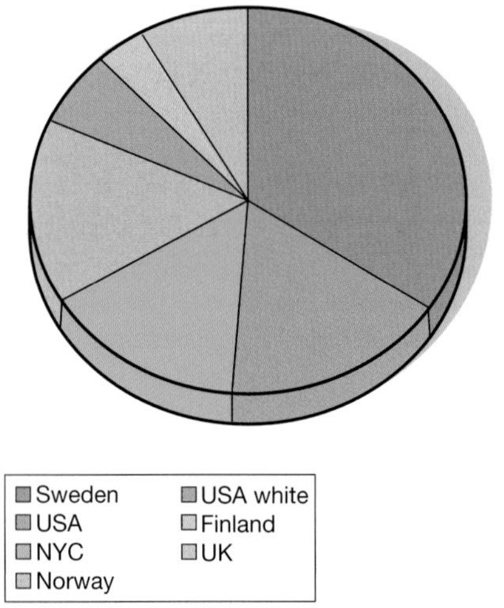
Sweden
USA
NYC
Norway
USA white
Finland
UK

Figure 34.6 Radiograph staging: prognostic value in sarcoidosis
Source: Scadding JG. (1961) *BMJ* 2: 1165–1172. Reproduced with permission of BMJ Publishing Ltd.

Pulmonary sarcoidosis can be classified on a chest radiograph into 5 stages (I–IV):

Stage 0: normal chest radiograph
5–10% of patients at presentation

Stage I: hilar or mediastinal nodal enlargement only
45–65% go on to complete resolution

Stage II: nodal enlargement and parenchymal disease
25–30% of patients at presentation

Stage III: parenchymal disease only
15% of patients at presentation

Stage IV: end-stage lung (pulmonary fibrosis)

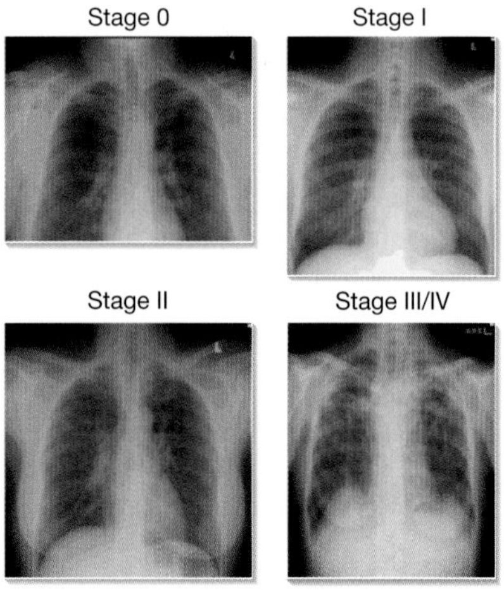
Stage 0
Stage I
Stage II
Stage III/IV

Sarcoidosis is a systemic granulomatous inflammatory disorder of unknown aetiology characterized by non-caseating granulomas (Figure 34.1) in multiple organs (Figure 34.2). These may resolve spontaneously; ≥60% of patients have a remission within 10 years or progress to fibrosis. Approximately 30% have continuing disease that progresses to clinically significant organ damage. Less than 5% of patients die from sarcoidosis, usually as a result of pulmonary fibrosis.

The lungs are the most frequently affected organ (90% of patients) leading to fibrosis of lung tissue (Figure 34.3). The next most common extrapulmonary sites affected are the skin, eye and lymphatics (Figure 34.2). Chronic sarcoidosis can cause significant morbidity but there is a paucity of data on patient-reported outcomes to determine the impact of impairment on health status.

It is thought that some antigens, especially particulate substances such as silica, beryllium or zirconium can form non-infectious granulomas (Figure 34.4).

Incidence

Sarcidosis is more common in women, with a peak age incidence of 20–40 years. It is more common in the USA and Sweden, occurring more often in Caucasians of European descent and in African-Americans. Ten to 40 out of every 100,000 people develop sarcoidosis (Figure 34.5).

Symptoms

Patients can present with only vague symptoms such as fatigue, weight loss and fever. Depression is not uncommon. Up to 50% of people with sarcoidosis have no symptoms when diagnosed. Symptoms can be associated with a specific organ (Figure 34.2):

- *Lungs:* shortness of breath, wheezing or cough (usually dry). Symptoms either resolve or persist and progress to fibrosis.
- *Lymph nodes:* enlargement of various lymph nodes – especially thoracic.
- *Eye:* inflammation, watering, redness, dry eyes and sensitivity to light; visual impairment can occur.
- *Skin:* raised, pink or purplish areas or painful nodules under the skin may appear. Deeper nodules are often found on the legs presenting as erythema nodosum (EN).
- *Bone:* nodules can be painful and cause pain in hands and feet.
- *Spleen and liver:* enlargement of the spleen or liver is possible as are abnormal liver function tests (LFTs).
- *Heart:* rare and difficult to diagnose, usually presenting as arrhythmia.
- *Brain and nervous system:* includes loss of sensation, loss of muscle strength, headaches and dizziness occurring in 1 : 100.
- *Salivary gland:* localised granulomas give rise to symptoms of dry mouth.

Löfgren's syndrome is an acute presentation of sarcoidosis occurring in up to 30% of the population; defined by arthritis, EN and bilateral hilar adenopathy. EN is seen predominantly in women and arthritis in men.

Diagnosis

Angiotensin converting enzyme (ACE) can be elevated but this is not disease-specific. ACE is found on vascular endothelium and other tissues and is produced by epithelioid cells of the sarcoid granulomata. Serum ACE is elevated in ≥70% patients with active sarcoidosis, particularly those with pulmonary involvement (80%).

Sarcoidosis is often a diagnosis attained by the exclusion of others. The Scadding scale can be helpful in interpreting chest X-rays and informing the need for high resolution CT ± positron emission tomography (PET) scan (Figure 34.6). When high reolution CT data generate uncertainty broncho-alveolar lavage (BAL) is useful.

Bronchoscopy and BAL

The diagnosis of sarcoidosis is less reliant on BAL analysis. Lymphocytosis is suggestive of sarcoidosis when the percentage of neutrophils and eosinophils is near normal whereas in classic HP lymphocytosis is likely to be associated with a marked increase in all cellular counts in active disease. The Kveim test (injecting an extract of sarcoid-affected tissue under the skin) is no longer used clinically in sarcoidosis evaluation.

Calcium and vitamin D

Vitamin D is partially activated in in the liver. The active form is produced by the kidneys resulting in 1,25 dihydroxy-vitamin D. This regulates serum calcium absorption from the gut and bone reabsorption.

Sarcoid granulomas contain macrophages (Figure 34.1), which may have the enzyme 1-alpha-hydroxylase, which converts vitamin D to its final active product. This increases serum calcium levels and/or urine. Approximately 5% of patients with sarcoidosis have elevated serum calcium, and approximately 15% have elevated urinary calcium levels. Chronically elevated calcium increases the risk of developing renal stones, renal dysfunction, predisposing to hypertension and cardiac anomalies.

Treatment

Some 50% of those diagnosed with sarcoidosis improve without treatment. Others require drug therapy to reduce inflammation and the majority will recover, but some will get worse despite treatment.

Medication

Corticosteroids reduce inflammation, decrease symptoms, improve lung function, and reduce granuloma formation. Methotrexate is an anti-inflammatory used as a second-line drug. It may be used with corticosteroids or after stopping corticosteroids. Other pharmacological options under specialist supervision include azathioprine, mycophenolate, hydroxychloroquine and clophosphamide.

The overriding goals of treatment:

- Maintain good lung function
- Relieve symptoms
- Prevent organ damage
- Prevent visual impairment through regular ophthalmology review
- Assess the need for oxygen therapy
- Provide pulmonary rehabilitation.

Further reading

British Lung Foundation (2016) Sarcoidosis. http://www.blf.org.uk/Page/Sarcoidosis (accessed 25 February 2016).

Judson MA. (ed.) (2014) *Pulmonary Sarcoidosis: A Guide for the Practicing Clinician Respiratory Medicine*, Vol. 17. Springer.

Mitchell DN, Wells AU, Spiroe SG, Moller DR, eds. (2012) *Sarcoidosis*. CRC Press, Taylor and Francis, FL.

35 Pulmonary tuberculosis

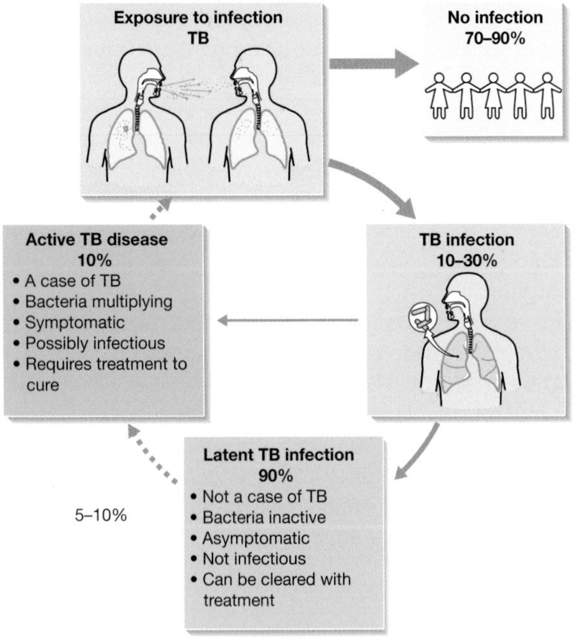
Exposure to infection TB
No infection 70–90%
TB infection 10–30%
Active TB disease 10%
• A case of TB
• Bacteria multiplying
• Symptomatic
• Possibly infectious
• Requires treatment to cure
Latent TB infection 90%
• Not a case of TB
• Bacteria inactive
• Asymptomatic
• Not infectious
• Can be cleared with treatment
5–10%

Figure 35.1 If untreated, an infectious person infects 10–15 others per year, early diagnosis and treatment stops onward transmission. Contact tracing identifies both active and latent TB infection and gives an opportunity for early treatment – not only improving individuals outcomes, but prevents onwards transmission. Treating latent TB reduces the reservoir of infection in the population

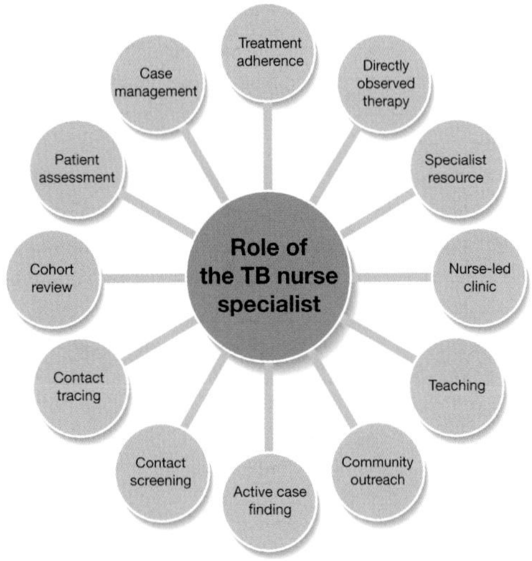
Role of the TB nurse specialist
Treatment adherence
Directly observed therapy
Specialist resource
Nurse-led clinic
Teaching
Community outreach
Active case finding
Contact screening
Contact tracing
Cohort review
Patient assessment
Case management

Figure 35.3 Role of the nurse specialist

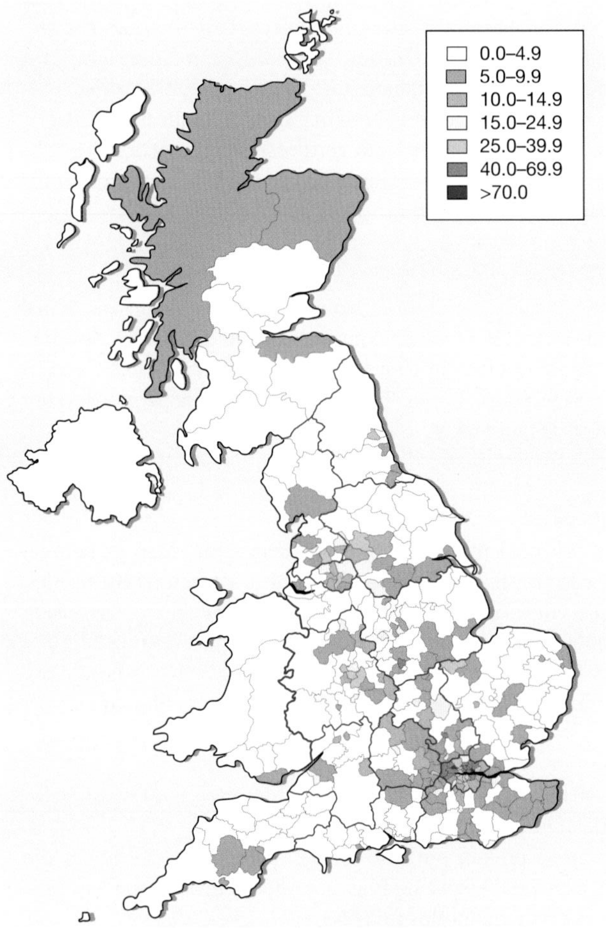
0.0–4.9
5.0–9.9
10.0–14.9
15.0–24.9
25.0–39.9
40.0–69.9
>70.0

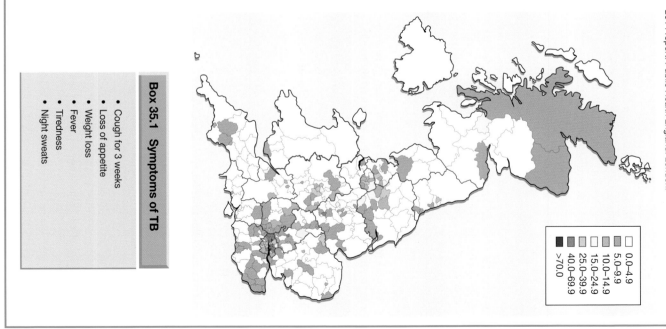

Figure 35.2 Three-year average tuberculosis case rates by local area per 100,000, UK, 2100–2013
Source: Public Health England. (2014) Tuberculosis in the UK: 2014 report. Public Health England: London.

Box 35.1 Symptoms of TB

- Cough for 3 weeks
- Loss of appetite
- Weight loss
- Fever
- Tiredness
- Night sweats

Tuberculosis (TB) is a serious but treatable and preventable infection caused by *Mycobacterium tuberculosis*. It is primarily a disease of the lungs (pulmonary TB), but it can infect any part of the body (extrapulmonary TB); commonly, lymph nodes, bones and central nervous system. The infection is spread through airborne transmission and only cases of the lungs, larynges or tonsils are considered infectious. TB is not usually highly contagious and people need to be in close and lengthy contact to have significant contact, such as living in the same household. If left untreated, a person with active infectious TB will infect 10–15 people each year. Figure 35.1 shows the transmission cycle of TB and identifies the two forms of TB: active TB disease and latent TB infection. Figure 35.2 shows the 3-year average rates of TB in the UK.

Signs and symptoms

Symptoms of active TB disease can develop weeks, or even years, after infection. They can develop slowly and vary depending on the site of the disease; Box 35.1 shows the most common symptoms.

Diagnosis

TB is diagnosed by a combination of clinical examination and diagnostic tests. The gold standard for TB diagnosis is microbiological culture. Investigations to diagnose pulmonary disease include sputum samples and chest X-ray. Sputum samples can be produced spontaneously, or by induced sputum. Gastric washings can be considered for children. At least three consecutive samples are required to increase the opportunity to detect the bacterium, which are often best collected in the morning, and sent for sputum smear microscopy and culture. Sputum microscopy provides a presumptive diagnosis and can indicate infectiousness. If acid–fast bacilli (AFBs) can be seen under the microscope, the sputum is called 'smear positive'. The absence of AFBs does not exclude a TB diagnosis, but indicates that the patient is less infectious. The sputum can then be cultured, taking up to 6 weeks, which confirms the diagnosis, drug sensitivities and informs public health assessment; this is called 'culture positive'.

Treatment and case management

Early diagnosis and prompt treatment is important as it not only improves the patient's outcomes, but reduces the possibility of onward transmission to others. Under the Health Protection Regulations (NICE, 2010), all forms of TB disease are statutorily notifiable on clinical suspicion and should be notified via the national surveillance systems.

Treatment for TB involves combination antibiotics and should be started following a presumptive diagnosis. Multi-therapy is required because resistance to anti-tuberculosis agents occur at a low, but constant rate. The World Health Organization's standard first-line treatment is 6 months of isoniazid and rifampicin, with the addition of ethambutol and pyrazinamide for the first 2 months, often written as: 2HRE/4HR. To ensure successful treatment completion, patients require a case management approach which includes a risk assessment to identify treatment adherence issues. Case management requires a collaborative multi-disciplinary team approach which is usually coordinated by a TB nurse specialist; Figure 35.3 highlights the roles of the TB nurse specialist. Patients with complex social or clinical needs might require enhanced case management (ECM) and directly observed therapy (DOT) to increase treatment adherence and completion. At the start of treatment, patients may struggle with the high pill burden or side effects. Once their symptoms resolve (within the first few months), patients may struggle to continue to take their medication and complete the regimen.

Drug resistance

The global spread of drug-resistant TB is undermining control efforts. Resistance has emerged as a result of interrupted, erratic or inadequate TB treatment. Patients can develop drug-resistance from poor adherence, or can be infected with drug-resistant strains. Drug resistance is categorised as mono-resistant, multi-drug resistant (MDR-TB) or extensively drug resistant (XDR-TB). Management of MDR-TB and XDR-TB is difficult and should be managed by specialist centres as treatment is required for longer.

All patients should be assessed for possible drug resistance. Risk factors for drug resistance include previous TB drug treatment; close contact with an MDR-TB case; birth or residence in a country with high TB rates; HIV infection; age 25–44; and male gender.

Infection control

Hospital

Most patients, regardless of site of TB, do not need to be hospitalised. However, if there are clear clinical or socio-economic needs, patients with suspected respiratory TB should be cared for in a single room ventilated to the outside and separated from immunocompromised patients. Usually after 2 weeks of appropriate treatment, a patient is considered non-infectious and does not require a single room.

Community

Patients in the community who are infectious should not attend work or school and should remain at home until they have completed 2 weeks of treatment. Visitors should be restricted to those who have already had recent contact and they will be offered contact screening.

Multi-drug resistant TB

All patients should have a risk assessment for drug resistance and HIV. If they have risk factors for MDR-TB, the patient should be cared for in a negative pressure room and requires closer monitoring of sputum. They are considered non-infectious after three negative culture results, which can take months of treatment.

Further reading

Royal College of Nursing (2012) Tuberculosis case management and cohort review. Guidance for health professionals.

36 Venous thromboembolism and pulmonary embolism

Figure 36.1 Virchow's triad

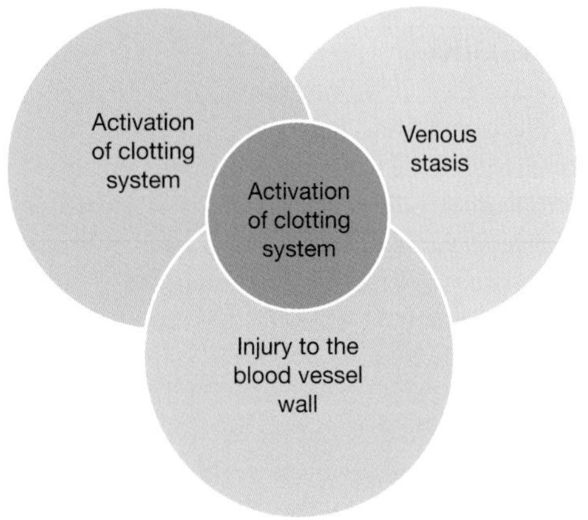
Activation
of clotting
system
Venous
stasis
Activation
of clotting
system
Injury to the
blood vessel
wall

Figure 36.2 Deep vein thrombosis

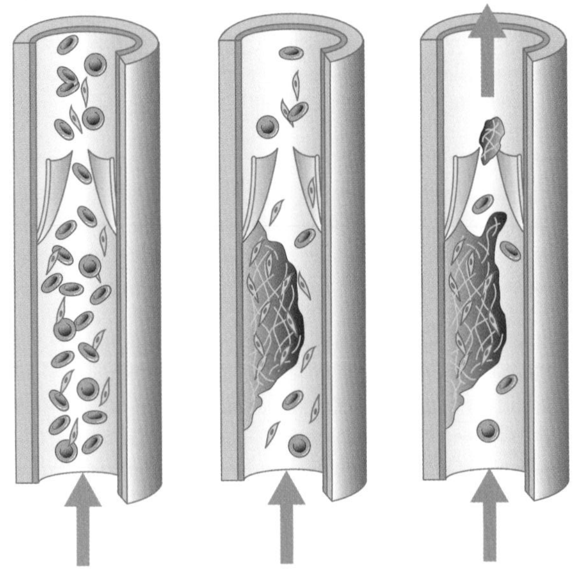
Normal blood flow
Deep vein
thrombosis
Embolus

Box 36.1 Wells' score: deep vein thrombosis
Source: Adapted from Wells PS, et al. *JAMA* 2006: 295; 199–207.

Clinical parameter score	Score
Active cancer (treatment ongoing, or within 6 months or palliative)	+1
Paralysis or recent plaster immobilisation of the lower extremities	+1
Recent bedridden for >3 days or major surgery <4 weeks	+1
Localised tenderness along the distribution of the deep venous system	+1
Entire leg swelling	+1
Calf swelling >3 cm compared with the asymptomatic leg	+1
Pitting oedema (greater in the symptomatic leg)	+1
Previous DVT documented	+1
Collateral superficial veins (non-varicose)	+1
Alternative diagnosis (as likely or greater than that of DVT)	−2
Total score	
High probability	>3
Moderate probability	1 or 2
Low probability	<0

Box 36.2 Wells' score: pulmonary embolus
Source: Wells PS, et al. *Thromb Haemost* 2000: 83; 416–20 and Kearon C, et al. *Ann Intern Med* 2006:144; 812–21.

Clinical signs and symptoms compatible with DVT	3
PE judged to be the most likely diagnosis	3
Surgery or bedridden for more than 3 days during past 4 weeks	1.5
Previous DVT or PE	1.5
Heart rate >100 min	1.5
Haemoptysis	1
Active cancer (treatment ongoing or within previous 6 months, or palliative treatment)	1
≤4: Low (or 'PE unlikely') pretest probability 4.5–6: Moderate pretest probability >6: High pretest probability	

A venous thrombus is a blood clot that forms within a vein. When a thrombus forms within a deep vein, for example in a deep calf vein, it is referred to as a deep vein thrombosis (DVT).

When a venous thrombus detaches or 'breaks off' it is called an embolus. This embolus can then travel through the venous system and form a clot within the lungs, called pulmonary embolism (PE). PE is a serious life-threatening condition requiring urgent medical attention.

What causes a thrombo-embolism?

Virchow's triad (Figure 36.1) is a good illustration of the three factors that causes blood to clot abnormally.

The first part of the triad is hypercoagulability which can be caused by congenital disorders such as factor V Leiden or protein S or C deficiency. Pregnancy and malignancy also cause hypercoagulability, with cancer patients having a seven times increased risk for venous thrombo-embolism.

Venous stasis refers to blood that is static within veins, with clots forming during periods of immobility or long haul flights.

Endothelial injury refers to damage of a blood vessel such as ligament injuries or rupture of calf muscles.

Risk factors for DVT/PE therefore include recent immobilisation, pregnancy, cancer, recent surgery, congenital thrombophilias and oral hormonal medications (i.e. hormone replacement therapy and contraceptive pills).

DVT

The symptoms of DVT are usually pain or swelling in one limb, usually described as cramping or 'bursting'. A Wells' test (Box 36.1) can be used to aid probability to assist diagnosis for DVT. The gold standard diagnostic investigation is by Doppler ultrasound which should occur within 3 days. Therapeutic low molecular weight heparin (LMWH) should be given while awaiting a scan.

Pulmonary embolus

An embolus develops when a clot or a piece of clot becomes dislodged; this then travels in the circulation. If the embolus then becomes lodged within a part of the pulmonary circulation a PE can result causing a serious complication (Figure 36.2).

The symptoms of PE are usually an abrupt onset of dyspnoea, cough and syncope. Pleuritic chest pain and haemoptysis are also key features. Large PEs will often cause haemodynamic instability and hypoxia, both fatal if left untreated. Similarly to DVT, a Wells' test can be used to aid probability (Box 36.2). The gold standard investigation is CT pulmonary angiogram or ventilation–perfusion (VQ) scan alongside therapeutic LMWH while awaiting the scan.

Treatment

Treatment of PE and DVT is conducted through anticoagulation. Colloquially known as 'thinning the blood', anticoagulant drugs do not actually affect the thickness of the blood, but alter the blood's ability to form clots. For this reason, some anticoagulants can increase the risk of bleeding or haemorrhage and patients require extensive counselling before starting these therapies.

Warfarin

A common form of anticoagulation therapy is warfarin. This vitamin K antagonist inhibits the production of active clotting factors. The effect of warfarin is shown in a blood test called International Normalised Ratio (INR) which tells how long it takes for the blood to clot. The INR of a healthy adult is usually a 1.0, and the desired goal for warfarin therapy is often between 2 and 3. Warfarin is not safe in pregnancy.

Newer anticoagulants

New oral anticoagulants have recently joined the market such as rivaroxaban and apixaban. These work by inhibiting factor Xa and affect the clotting cascade. Doses of these medications are fixed and do not require regular blood test monitoring.

Low molecular weight heparins

Usually given daily by subcutaneous injection, LMWHs such as enoxaparin predominantly inhibit factor Xa in the clotting cascade. These are useful as they are safe in pregnancy, have a rapid onset in action and short half-life. This makes this therapy safer for patients at risk of bleeding or injury (i.e. falls risk).

The length of treatment depends on whether the thrombosis was provoked alongside previous history of thrombosis. The type of treatment used depends on the patient's co-morbidities, other medications and patient preference.

Thrombolysis or embolectomy

In emergency scenarios for massive PE, treatment with thrombolysis, such as reteplase is used to disperse a clot rapidly. Severe haemorrhage can be a serious but rare complication.

Surgical removal of thrombus, embolectomy, is rarely used and is often a last resort. This can be performed using a catheter balloon technique or through surgical incision into the vessel.

Ambulatory care

There is a variation in how patients are managed for DVT and PE, with a drive to allowing patients to stay at home during the diagnostic stage.

DVT management is commonly delivered as an outpatient with a variety of models in use (Chapter 4).

Further reading

British Thoracic Society (2012) www.brit-thoracic.org.uk/guidelines-and-quality-standards/pulmonary-embolism/ (accessed 25 February 2016).

NICE (2012) Venous thromboembolic diseases: diagnosis, management and thrombophiliawww.nice.org.uk/guidance/cg144 (accessed 25 February 2016).

NICE (2015) Clinical Knowledge Summaries: Anticoagulation: oral http://cks.nice.org.uk/anticoagulation-oral (accessed 25 February 2016).

37 HIV and respiratory disease

Box 37.1 AIDS–defining clinical conditions

2008 CDC case definition for HIV infection: Aids–defining clinical conditions

- Candidiasis (trachea, bronchia or lung)
- Candidiasis (oesophageal)
- Cervical cancer (invasive)
- Coccidioidomycosis (disseminated or extrapulmonary)
- Cryptococcosis (extrapulmonary)
- Cryptosporidiosis (intestinal for longer than 1 month)
- Cytomegalovirus disease (other than liver, spleen or nodes)
- Cytomegalovirus retinitis (with loss of vision)
- Encephalopathy (HIV-related)
- Herpes simplex: chronic ulcers (present for longer than 1 month)
- Herpes simplex: bronchitis, pneumonitis or oesophagitis
- Histoplasmosis (disseminated or extrapulmonary)
- Isosporiasis (intestinal, for longer than 1 month)
- Kaposi's sarcoma
- Lymphoma, Burkitt's (or equivalent term)
- Lymphoma, immunoblastic (or equivalent)
- Lymphoma primary of brain
- *Mycobacterium avium* complex, disseminated or extrapulmonary
- *Mycobacterium kansasii*, disseminated or extrapulmonary
- *Mycobacterium tuberculosis*, any site (pulmonary or extrapulmonary)
- *Mycobacterium*, other species or unidentified species, disseminated or extrapulmonary
- *Pneumocystis carinii* pneumonia
- Recurrent pneumonia (≥2 episodes in 1-year period)
- Progressive multifocal leukoencephalopathy
- Salmonella (recurrent septicaemia)
- Toxoplasmosis (brain)
- Wasting syndrome due to HIV: >10% involuntary weight loss plus either chronic diarrhoea (≥2 stools per day for at least 30 days) or chronic weakness and documented fever (for at least 30 days) in the absence of a concurrent illness or condition other than HIV that could explain this finding

Figure 37.1 Diagnosis by chest X-ray

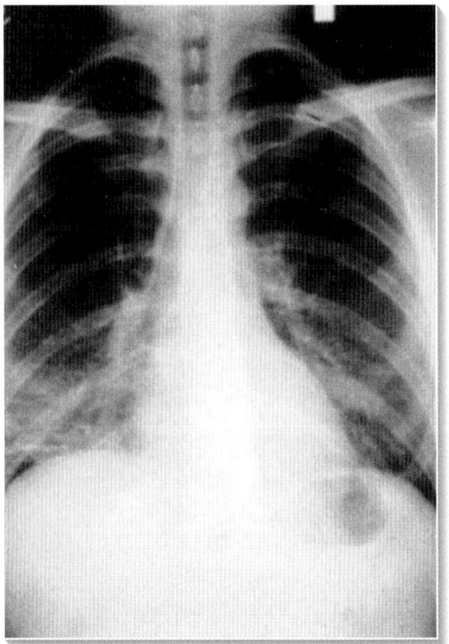

Figure 37.2 Kaposi's sarcoma
Source: Anatomy & Physiology, Connexions website, https:// commons. wikimedia. org/wiki/File:Kaposis_Sarcoma_Lesions.jpg. Used under CCA 3.0.

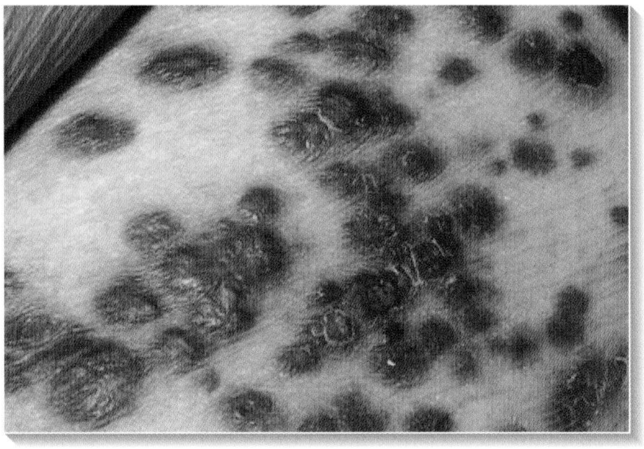

Human immunodeficiency virus (HIV) is a virus that attacks vital components of the immune system. The virus targets CD4 T-lymphocyte cells which protect the body from bacteria and other disease-causing agents. People living with HIV can have a low number of CD4 cells and are therefore immunocompromised.

Acquired immunodefiency syndrome (AIDS) is said to be present when people with HIV contract an opportunistic infection or cancer as a result of their compromised immune system. A list of these is shown in Table 37.1. People living with HIV now expect a near-normal life expectancy because of a range of medications that can help treat the virus and preserve the immune system. However, non-compliance, poor access to medications in the developing world and late diagnosis mean that HIV/AIDS is still a global health concern.

The rates of HIV in the UK continue to rise. Figures for the Health Protection Agency indicate that almost one-quarter of people infected are unaware of their diagnosis. HIV is a communicable disease that is transmitted through certain bodily fluids. The main risk factors are unprotected sex (both homosexual and heterosexual) and intravenous drug use.

HIV/AIDS and respiratory disease

Many patients with AIDS, especially during late diagnosis situations, present with respiratory disease. This is why many guidelines recommend HIV testing, especially in otherwise healthy adults presenting with tuberculosis (TB) and pneumonia. Conditions presenting with AIDS carry a high mortality rate and early testing can save lives.

A list of associated pulmonary infections with different CD4 counts is presented in Box 37.1.

Pneumocystis carinii pneumonia

Pneumocystis carinii pneumonia (PCP) is the most common first sign of illness in most persons with AIDS. The pneumonia is caused by the *Pneumocystis jiroveci* bacteria. The risk of PCP increases significantly when CD4 count falls below 200 cells/uL.

Common symptoms include respiratory distress, cough and fever. Patients will also have significantly low PAO_2 than would be expected with the presenting symptoms.

Diagnosis can be made by chest X-ray (Figure 37.1) often showing widespread pulmonary infiltrates. Specimens of sputum can be sent off for polymerase chain reaction (PCR) for specific diagnosis.

Treatment is often with atovaquone or co-trimoxazole. Steroids are often given to reduce inflammation. Prophylaxis is often given to HIV patients with low CD4 counts to help prevent PCP.

Tuberculosis

As discussed in Chapter 35, tuberculosis is a significant global health concern, HIV suppresses the immune system, opening the door for new TB disease but also reactivation of latent or dormant TB.

Disseminated *Mycobacterium avium* complex

This organism exists in the environment and rarely causes lung disease in healthy people. In immunocompromised states, it is fatal if left untreated. It can affect one part of the body such as the lungs (localised infection) but can spread and affect the bones and gastrointestinal tract (disseminated infection).

It is often diagnosed using a combination of CT scans and biopsies. It is more common in patients with CD4 counts less than 50 cells/uL.

Treatment is with anti-TB drug regimens. Prophylaxis should also be given to HIV patients with low CD4 counts with drugs such as rifabutin.

Fungal and bacterial infection

People with HIV are at risk of various viral, fungal and bacterial infections because of a reduction in host immunity. These range from candidiasis, aspergillus, herpes simplex and haemophilus influenza. The overall risk of pulmonary infection increases significantly with a lower CD4 count.

Lymphoma

Lymphoma is significantly associated with HIV/AIDS, especially Burkitt's and immunoblastic categories.

The incidence of intrathoracic manifestations of AIDS-associated lymphoma can be as high as 31%.

Lung involvement is usually seen in association with other sites of disease but occasionally it can be the initial site of the disease.

Kaposi's sarcoma

Kaposi's sarcoma is a tumour caused by infection with human herpes virus 8 (HHV8). Patients commonly present with red–purple nodules on the skin (Figure 37.2). They are typically found in the skin but can be found in the gastrointestinal or respiratory tracts.

Symptoms include haemoptysis, shortness of breath and fever. Diagnosis is made by bronchoscopy where the lesions are seen and biopsied.

Kaposi's sarcoma is not curable, but treating the cause of immunosuppression can slow or stop progression. It is commonly found in patients with CD4 counts <200 but also found in other immunosuppressed conditions, such as patients undergoing transplant. Patients with severe disease can present with large pleural effusions and alveolar haemorrhage. Chemotherapy and radiation can also be used for treatment.

Screening

The UK guidelines for national HIV testing recommend that HIV testing be offered to all patients with TB and pneumocystis. Testing should also be offered to patients with bacterial pneumonia and aspergillosis. Patients with lymphadenopathy of unknown causes and recurrent candidiasis should also be offered HIV testing.

Further reading

Fakoya A, Lamba H, Mackie N, et al. (2008) British HIV Association, BASHH and FSRH guidelines for the management of the sexual and reproductive health of people living with HIV infection. *HIV Med* 9: 681–672.

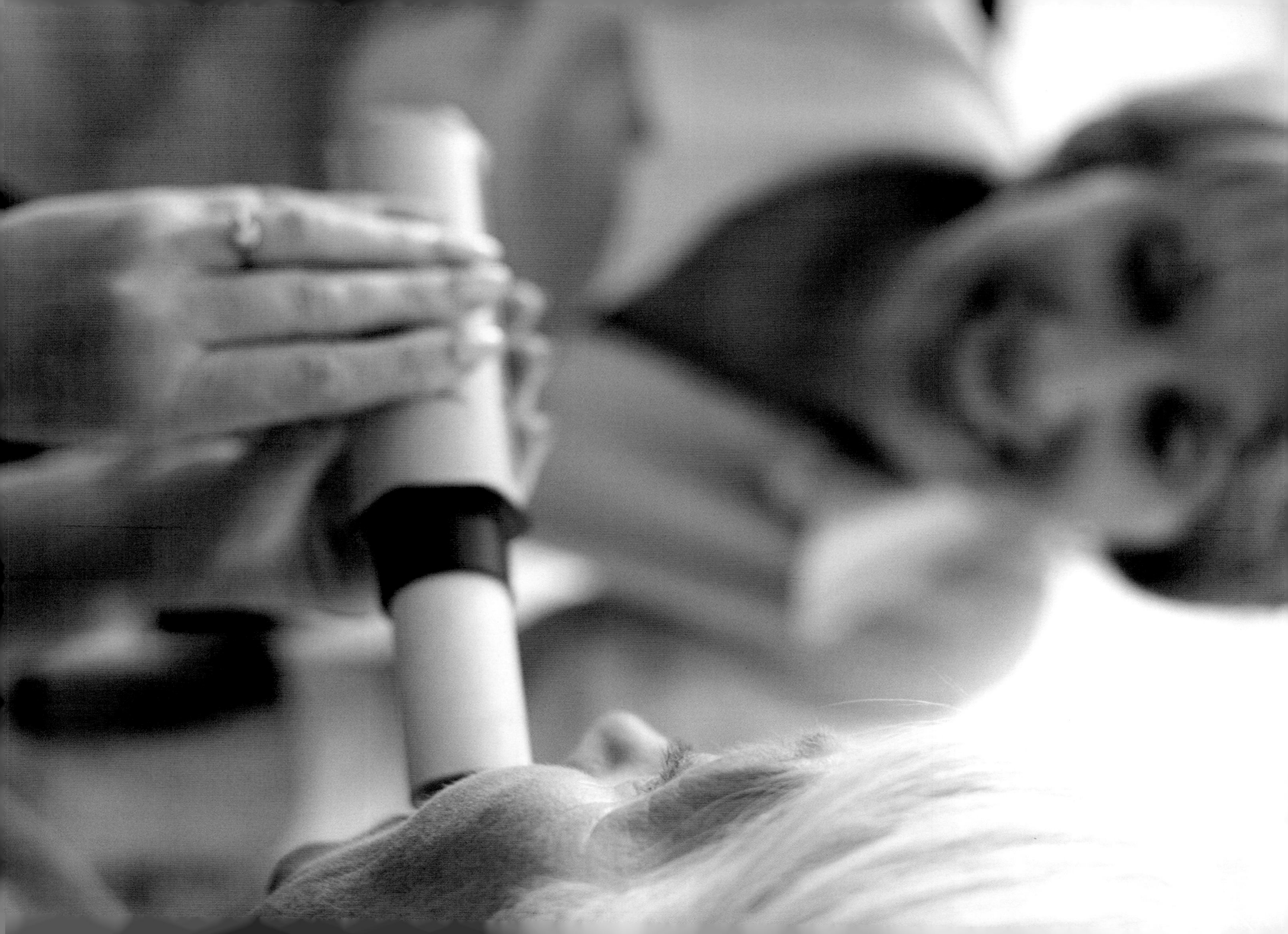

Models of care

Part 5

Chapters

Overview

Respiratory care utilises many different models of care and strategies similar to other acute and chronic disease management. Part 5 gives an overview of some models and pathways with a focus on self-management, patient education and support available.

38 Care pathways and care bundles

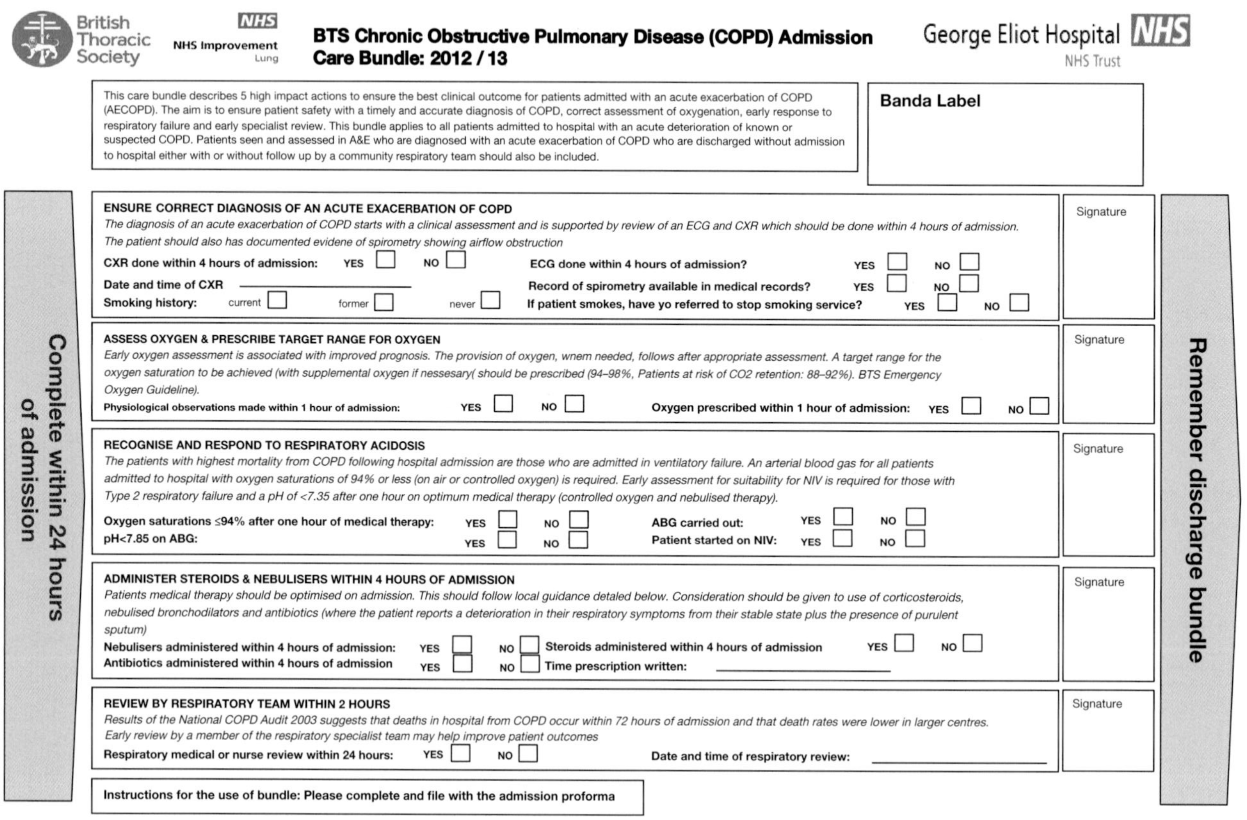
BTS Chronic Obstructive Pulmonary Disease (COPD) Admission Care Bundle: 2012 / 13

British Thoracic Society | NHS Improvement Lung | George Eliot Hospital NHS Trust

This care bundle describes 5 high impact actions to ensure the best clinical outcome for patients admitted with an acute exacerbation of COPD (AECOPD). The aim is to ensure patient safety with a timely and accurate diagnosis of COPD, correct assessment of oxygenation, early response to respiratory failure and early specialist review. This bundle applies to all patients admitted to hospital with an acute deterioration of known or suspected COPD. Patients seen and assessed in A&E who are diagnosed with an acute exacerbation of COPD who are discharged without admission to hospital either with or without follow up by a community respiratory team should also be included.

Banda Label

Complete within 24 hours of admission

ENSURE CORRECT DIAGNOSIS OF AN ACUTE EXACERBATION OF COPD

The diagnosis of an acute exacerbation of COPD starts with a clinical assessment and is supported by review of an ECG and CXR which should be done within 4 hours of admission. The patient should also has documented evidene of spirometry showing airflow obstruction

CXR done within 4 hours of admission: YES ☐ NO ☐ ECG done within 4 hours of admission? YES ☐ NO ☐

Date and time of CXR ________ Record of spirometry available in medical records? YES ☐ NO ☐

Smoking history: current ☐ former ☐ never ☐ If patient smokes, have yo referred to stop smoking service? YES ☐ NO ☐

Signature

ASSESS OXYGEN & PRESCRIBE TARGET RANGE FOR OXYGEN

Early oxygen assessment is associated with improved prognosis. The provision of oxygen, wnem needed, follows after appropriate assessment. A target range for the oxygen saturation to be achieved (with supplemental oxygen if nessesary(should be prescribed (94–98%, Patients at risk of CO2 retention: 88–92%). BTS Emergency Oxygen Guideline).

Physiological observations made within 1 hour of admission: YES ☐ NO ☐ Oxygen prescribed within 1 hour of admission: YES ☐ NO ☐

Signature

RECOGNISE AND RESPOND TO RESPIRATORY ACIDOSIS

The patients with highest mortality from COPD following hospital admission are those who are admitted in ventilatory failure. An arterial blood gas for all patients admitted to hospital with oxygen saturations of 94% or less (on air or controlled oxygen) is required. Early assessment for suitability for NIV is required for those with Type 2 respiratory failure and a pH of <7.35 after one hour on optimum medical therapy (controlled oxygen and nebulised therapy).

Oxygen saturations ≤94% after one hour of medical therapy: YES ☐ NO ☐ ABG carried out: YES ☐ NO ☐

pH<7.85 on ABG: YES ☐ NO ☐ Patient started on NIV: YES ☐ NO ☐

Signature

ADMINISTER STEROIDS & NEBULISERS WITHIN 4 HOURS OF ADMISSION

Patients medical therapy should be optimised on admission. This should follow local guidance detaled below. Consideration should be given to use of corticosteroids, nebulised bronchodilators and antibiotics (where the patient reports a deterioration in their respiratory symptoms from their stable state plus the presence of purulent sputum)

Nebulisers administered within 4 hours of admission: YES ☐ NO ☐ Steroids administered within 4 hours of admission YES ☐ NO ☐

Antibiotics administered within 4 hours of admission YES ☐ NO ☐ Time prescription written: ________

Signature

REVIEW BY RESPIRATORY TEAM WITHIN 2 HOURS

Results of the National COPD Audit 2003 suggests that deaths in hospital from COPD occur within 72 hours of admission and that death rates were lower in larger centres. Early review by a member of the respiratory specialist team may help improve patient outcomes

Respiratory medical or nurse review within 24 hours: YES ☐ NO ☐ Date and time of respiratory review: ________

Signature

Remember discharge bundle

Instructions for the use of bundle: Please complete and file with the admission proforma

Figure 38.1 COPD admission care bundle

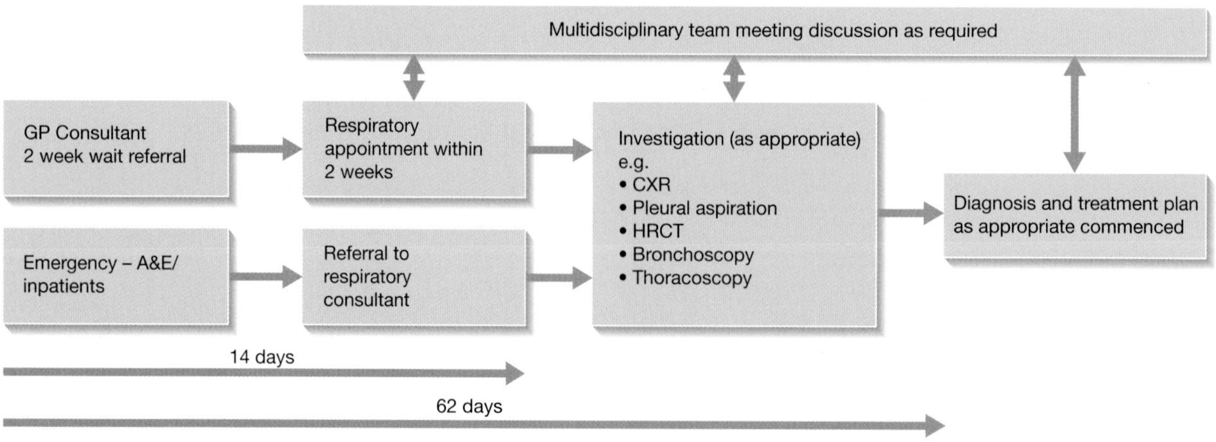
Multidisciplinary team meeting discussion as required
GP Consultant
2 week wait referral
Respiratory appointment within 2 weeks
Emergency – A&E/ inpatients
Referral to respiratory consultant
Investigation (as appropriate) e.g.
• CXR
• Pleural aspiration
• HRCT
• Bronchoscopy
• Thoracoscopy
Diagnosis and treatment plan as appropriate commenced
14 days
62 days

Figure 38.2 Lung referral and process pathway CXR, chest X-ray; HRCT, high resolution computed tomography

Background

Care bundles help identify quality of care by demonstrating evidence of the use of interventions that prevent avoidable mortality and morbidity. This approach allows for a systematic method of measuring and improving care processes and helps to ensure that all patients receive the best evidence-based care.

A care bundle combines guidelines and evidence-based research into a systematic, easy-to-follow checklist which ensures uniformity of care delivery. Care bundles are often designed for the management of specific conditions and list individual aspects that are widely accepted as good practice. They act as an aide-memoire and do not diminish the judgement or responsibilities of clinicians.

Benefits

Care bundles contribute to improvements in care delivery in several ways. First, delivering care more reliably ensures that all patients in a designated patient group receive all the aspects of care that they need. The possibility of treatment omission is therefore reduced and avoidable morbidity is also reduced. Secondly, decreasing unwarranted variation can save both time and resources.

Getting treatment right for the patient at the outset through the use of bundles helps to reduce length of stay. Care bundles are also an excellent mechanism for educating staff regarding evidence-based practice but also empowers them to implement it. Moreover, care bundles can be used as an audit to sustain and improve best practice.

The overall value of care bundles across a number of conditions has been demonstrated in the UK by Robb et al. (2010) who observed a fall of 18.5 points in their hospital standardised mortality (HSRM) following bundle implementation for 13 different diagnoses.

Examples in practice

In the context of respiratory care, common care bundles frequently used in practice are for chronic obstructive pulmonary disease (COPD) (Figure 38.1) and pneumonia.

The community-acquired pneumonia care bundle, championed by the British Thoracic Society, ensures that evidence-based care is delivered to patients presenting with pneumonia. It dictates steps that must be performed within 6 hours of admission:

1 *Diagnosis* – ensuring symptoms fit with pneumonia and diagnosis confirmed by chest X-ray
2 *Information* – CAP leaflet given to patient and/or family
3 *Oxygen* – ensure oxygen saturations are recorded and oxygen prescribed as needed (Chapter 47)
4 *CURB 65* calculated (Chapter 29)
5 *Smoking* assessment (Chapter 10)
6 *Decide* treatment according to severity.

Care pathways

A care pathway is similar to a care bundle except that it describes a much wider context rather than specific tasks that must be conducted or initiated by a specific individual. A care pathway is a tool or concept used to embed guidelines, protocols and evidence-based patient-centred care.

For example, a pathway can follow a patient from admission, through acute care, discharge and rehabilitation. These elements build together to construct a unique journey for each patient according to their needs. Holistic care requires a coordinated approach by everyone in the multi-disciplinary team to ensure quality care with the best outcomes for patients. Working to an agreed care pathway allows for process to be mapped and targets for treatment defined. The care can be given by right team members at the right time and in the right place in a manner that can be measured and compliance (outcome) recorded.

In a respiratory context, a pathway for diagnosis and management of suspected lung cancer will necessitate the steps to achieve diagnosis via diagnostic access, biopsy, oncology referral, palliative care and CNS input (Figure 38.2). It ensures a multi-disciplinary, patient-centred approach in a timely manner to meet guidelines (Chapter 27).

Further reading

Robb E, Jarman B, Suntharalingam G, et al. (2010) Using care bundles to reduce in-hospital mortality: quantitative survey. *BMJ* 340: c1234.

39 Self-management in chronic respiratory disease

Box 39.1 Impact of chronic lung disease

- Non-elective hospital admissions are increasing year on year
- 115,000 hospital admissions for those with an acute exacerbation of COPD
- More than 54,000 hospital admissions for asthma
- 16,000 die within 90 days following admission for acute exacerbation of COPD

(NHS England, 2014)

Box 39.2 Quality of life impacts

- ☐ Breathlessness
- ☐ Decreased exercise tolerance: impacting upon activities such as gardening, playing with children
- ☐ Chest tightness
- ☐ Cough
- ☐ Sputum
- ☐ Exacerbations
- ☐ Reduced appetite
- ☐ Poor sleep pattern
- ☐ Impaired ability to work
- ☐ Financial concerns
- ☐ Fearful of the future
- ☐ Anxiety
- ☐ Depression
- ☐ Hospital admissions
- ☐ Treatments: such as oxygen therapy restricting lifestyle
- ☐ Social isolation
- ☐ Relationship impacts – including sex

Box 39.3 Core components to self-management

Preparation and readiness for behaviour change
Collaborative and partnership working
Education
Practice
Empowerment
Emotional support
Motivation

Figure 39.1 Asthma management plan
Source: Reproduced with permission of Asthma UK.

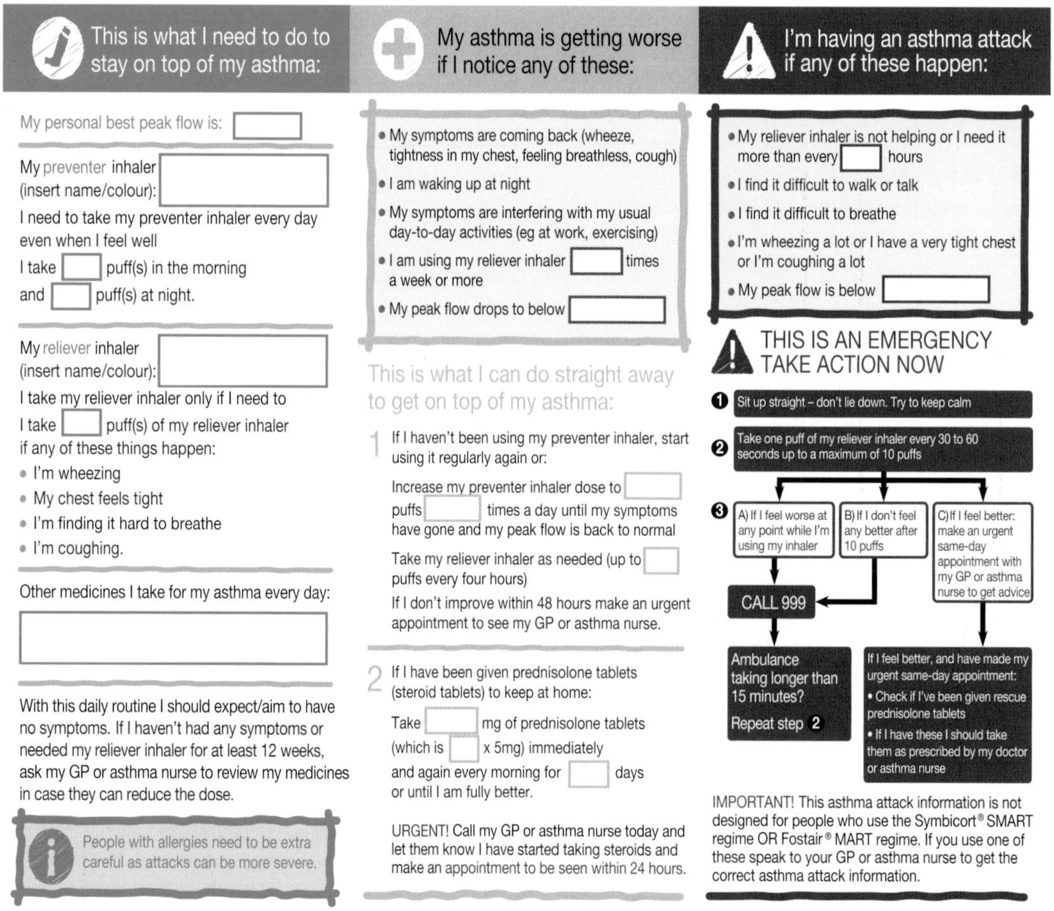

This is what I need to do to stay on top of my asthma:

My personal best peak flow is: ☐

My preventer inhaler (insert name/colour): ☐
I need to take my preventer inhaler every day even when I feel well
I take ☐ puff(s) in the morning and ☐ puff(s) at night.

My reliever inhaler (insert name/colour): ☐
I take my reliever inhaler only if I need to
I take ☐ puff(s) of my reliever inhaler if any of these things happen:
- I'm wheezing
- My chest feels tight
- I'm finding it hard to breathe
- I'm coughing.

Other medicines I take for my asthma every day: ☐

With this daily routine I should expect/aim to have no symptoms. If I haven't had any symptoms or needed my reliever inhaler for at least 12 weeks, ask my GP or asthma nurse to review my medicines in case they can reduce the dose.

People with allergies need to be extra careful as attacks can be more severe.

My asthma is getting worse if I notice any of these:

- My symptoms are coming back (wheeze, tightness in my chest, feeling breathless, cough)
- I am waking up at night
- My symptoms are interfering with my usual day-to-day activities (eg at work, exercising)
- I am using my reliever inhaler ☐ times a week or more
- My peak flow drops to below ☐

This is what I can do straight away to get on top of my asthma:

1 If I haven't been using my preventer inhaler, start using it regularly again or:
Increase my preventer inhaler dose to ☐ puffs ☐ times a day until my symptoms have gone and my peak flow is back to normal
Take my reliever inhaler as needed (up to ☐ puffs every four hours)
If I don't improve within 48 hours make an urgent appointment to see my GP or asthma nurse.

2 If I have been given prednisolone tablets (steroid tablets) to keep at home:
Take ☐ mg of prednisolone tablets (which is ☐ x 5mg) immediately and again every morning for ☐ days or until I am fully better.

URGENT! Call my GP or asthma nurse today and let them know I have started taking steroids and make an appointment to be seen within 24 hours.

I'm having an asthma attack if any of these happen:

- My reliever inhaler is not helping or I need it more than every ☐ hours
- I find it difficult to walk or talk
- I find it difficult to breathe
- I'm wheezing a lot or I have a very tight chest or I'm coughing a lot
- My peak flow is below ☐

THIS IS AN EMERGENCY TAKE ACTION NOW

1. Sit up straight – don't lie down. Try to keep calm
2. Take one puff of my reliever inhaler every 30 to 60 seconds up to a maximum of 10 puffs
3. A) If I feel worse at any point while I'm using my inhaler → CALL 999
   B) If I don't feel any better after 10 puffs → CALL 999
   C) If I feel better: make an urgent same-day appointment with my GP or asthma nurse to get advice

CALL 999 → Ambulance taking longer than 15 minutes? Repeat step 2

If I feel better, and have made my urgent same-day appointment:
- Check if I've been given rescue prednisolone tablets
- If I have these I should take them as prescribed by my doctor or asthma nurse

IMPORTANT! This asthma attack information is not designed for people who use the Symbicort® SMART regime OR Fostair® MART regime. If you use one of these speak to your GP or asthma nurse to get the correct asthma attack information.

The case for self-management in chronic respiratory disease

The term 'self-management', also termed 'self-care' has gained much publicity over recent years, particularly in association with the management of chronic respiratory diseases. Chronic diseases, such as asthma and chronic obstructive pulmonary disease (COPD) are conditions that can commonly be managed without the need for hospitalisation, but this is not being reflected in hospital admission data (Box 39.1).

Improvements in diagnosis, treatment and the increasing growth of the ageing population, highlight both current and future demands that supporting those with chronic respiratory disease places upon health and social care systems. This concern is further heightened given that 50% of patients diagnosed with COPD are currently less than 65 years of age.

Living with a chronic respiratory disease often has very disabling effects and severely impacts upon the quality of life for those affected (Box 39.2). A further significant factor for those living in the UK with chronic respiratory disease is the notably high premature mortality rate. This is considerably higher in the UK than the rest of Europe for reasons that are unclear.

High and increasing hospital admissions, premature mortality rates, multiple impacts upon patient's quality of life and a growth in the chronic respiratory disease population demonstrate that changes to current models of care are urgently needed.

Self-management

Self-management seeks to enable patient-centred care. It is a model of care that educates and supports patients to become active decision makers, empowering them to manage their own health and social care needs effectively.

Self-management has the potential to improve health outcomes and to improve patient experiences with reported benefits in increased confidence and reduced anxiety. Structured programmes have been shown to reduce unplanned hospital admissions for both asthma and COPD, with improved adherence to treatment and medications.

Current self-management education and support for patients with respiratory disease is largely delivered via pulmonary rehabilitation programmes. This specialist peer group intervention has positive effects for those with chronic respiratory disease and is particularly effective in improving mood, confidence and physical functioning (Chapter 11).

For many patients and health care workers, implementing and sustaining self-management strategies requires certain key components (Box 39.3). Incorporating these key components and tailoring personalised care improves an individual's confidence and thus ability to cope with the medical and emotional management of living with a chronic respiratory disease.

Self-management in practice

Personalised written self-management plans are recommended for all patients with asthma or COPD. A written self-management plan is formulated jointly between the patient and health professional. It is retained by patients and/or carers and utilised as a reference source, enhancing independent management of respiratory conditions. Figure 39.1 shows Asthma UK's Self-Management Plan.

As Figure 39.1 demonstrates, personalising peak flow measurements with symptom presence, guides the patient with asthma to make independent changes or to seek further health care advice and assessment. The green, amber and red sections (often referred to as a traffic light system) assist the visualisation of deteriorating respiratory signs and symptoms, which seek to enable patients to act promptly when necessary. In a similar manner, action plans for patients with COPD highlight early warning signs of an acute exacerbation and guide the patient regarding the action necessary.

Box 39.2 shows there are many quality of life impacts for those living with a chronic respiratory disease, but that many of these could be reduced through the utilisation of supported self-management strategies targeted at specific impacts, including breathing and cough techniques, exercise ability, anxiety, depression, nutritional intake, energy conservation and relaxation training.

Key considerations to effective self-management are appropriate timing of implementation and ensuring a holistic approach is taken, both of which are vital to the success of self-management in chronic respiratory disease.

Further reading

Asthma UK (2016) Written asthma action plans. https://www.asthma.org.uk/advice/resources/#action-p (accessed 23 March 2016).

British Lung Foundation (2016) COPD self-management tools for health care professionals. www.blf.org.uk/Page/Self-management-tools (accessed 26 February 2016).

Patient (2014) http://patient.info/doctor/management-of-adult-asthma (accessed 23 March 2016).

40 Telemedicine and telehealth

Figure 40.1 Telehealth and telehealthcare

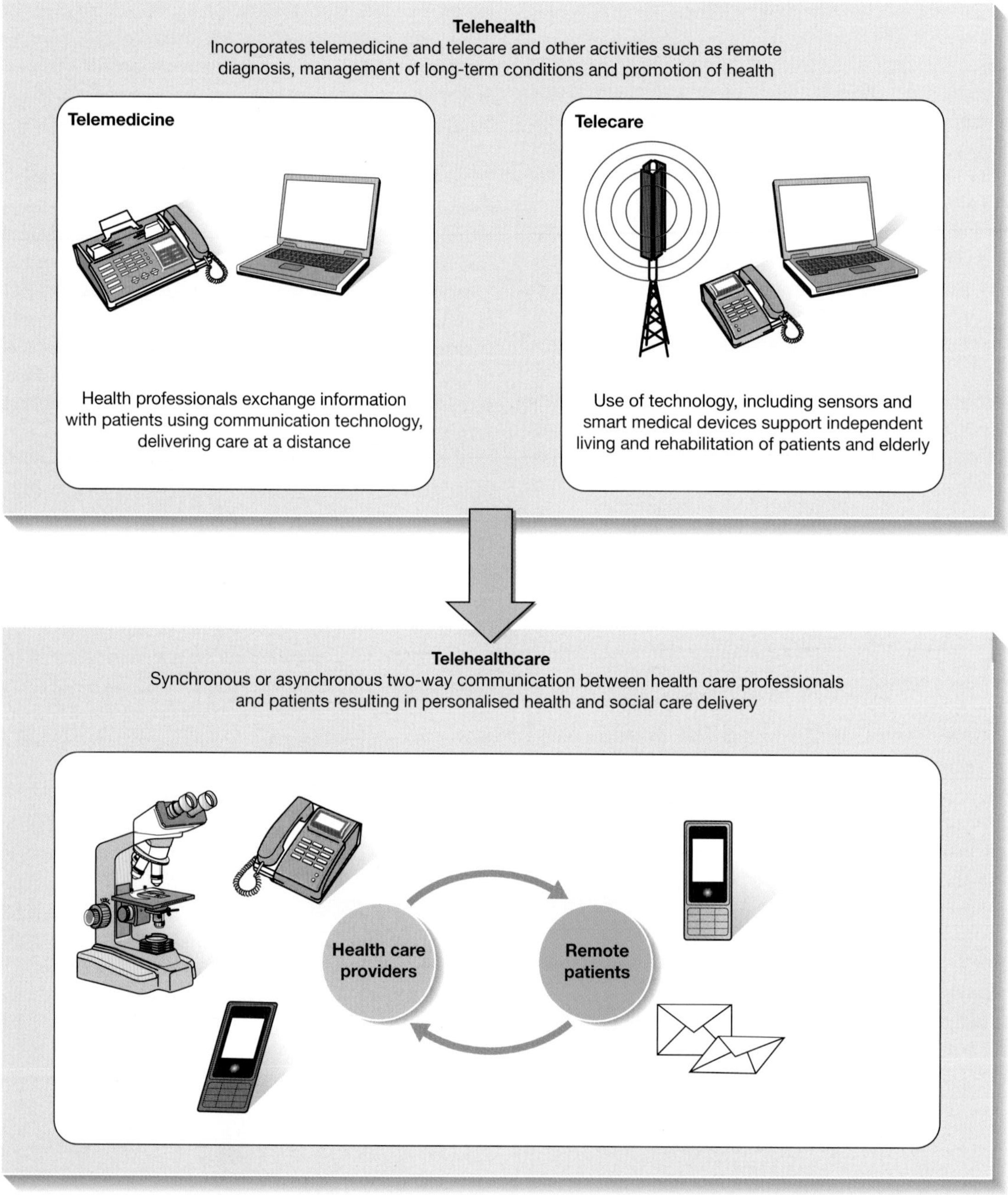
Telehealth
Incorporates telemedicine and telecare and other activities such as remote diagnosis, management of long-term conditions and promotion of health
Telemedicine
Health professionals exchange information with patients using communication technology, delivering care at a distance
Telecare
Use of technology, including sensors and smart medical devices support independent living and rehabilitation of patients and elderly
Telehealthcare
Synchronous or asynchronous two-way communication between health care professionals and patients resulting in personalised health and social care delivery
Health care providers
Remote patients

The terms telemedicine and telehealth, and more recently telehealthcare, can be used to describe a range of interventions. Telemedicine, a term that became prominent in the late 1990s, refers to the use of technology to enable the exchange of information between health professionals and patients, who usually lived in remote locations. Telehealth, however, is a term that encompasses a wider range of activities such as promotion of health (Figure 40.1). Telehealth incorporates telemedicine and telecare, and in time the term telemedicine may become redundant (Darkins and Carey, 2000).

More recently, the term telehealthcare has been used; indeed, McLean et al. (2012) use the term telehealthcare in their recent Cochrane review and meta-analysis. Telehealthcare involves obtaining information from patients, such as pulse oximetry and symptoms, but importantly it includes a health professional interpreting the information and providing individualised feedback. Crucially, telehealthcare can be synchronous (e.g. telephone), or asynchronous (e.g. email). The former permits real-time two-way communication.

Telehealthcare can be facilitated using technology that ranges from simple SMS messages through to complex computerised programs which incorporates instruments such as pulse oximeters.

Advantages of telehealthcare

At its most basic level, which is arguably SMS messaging, interactive telehealthcare can result in positive outcomes for patients with asthma, and indeed with other variables that have relevance to respiratory care such as compliance. A Cochrane review indicated that markers of asthma control can be improved by SMS interventions (De Jongh et al., 2012). These improvements included peak expiratory flow variability and a pooled symptom score comprising of cough, night symptoms, sleep quality and maximum tolerated activity.

A systematic review by Vervloet et al. (2012) concluded that general adherence is improved by SMS messages. Trials focusing on the impact of SMS interventions on asthma compliance also showed positive outcomes. A randomised controlled trial (Petrie et al., 2012) demonstrated an improvement in self-reported adherence to asthma preventer medication, and Strandbygaard et al. (2010) demonstrated a difference in mean asthma medication adherence rates at 12 weeks. Importantly, none of the reviewed SMS studies exceeded 12 months and little is known about the long-term benefits of SMS. Moreover, SMS messaging is generally used by younger people, and it may be difficult to realise the benefits of SMS interaction in older people.

The more advanced interventions tend to utilise complex interactive technology. These have also been shown to have some positive outcomes. For example, Gellis et al. (2012) performed a randomised controlled trial examining the impact of a multifaceted telehealth intervention on health, mental health and service utilisation. The patients who received the intervention were compared with people who had usual care and education. They had heart failure or COPD and tended to be house-bound. The telehealth group experienced improvements in general health and social functioning, and had reduced depression (improved depression symptom scores). They also experienced significantly fewer visits to the emergency department than the control group.

These findings are supported by a Cochrane review (McLean et al., 2012). The review concluded that telehealthcare for patients with COPD can produce statistically significant reductions in emergency department visits over 12 months, in hospitalisations at 3 months and 12 months, and a reduction in the relative risk of exacerbations. Moreover, qualitative data gave strong indications that patients are satisfied with telehealthcare provided that they could have face-to-face interaction when needed.

There is no evidence that telehealthcare can produce a difference in death rates or quality of life.

Using telehealthcare

The best evidence for telehealthcare is produced by a service that includes redesigning the care pathway. This incorporates personalised interaction which enables the delivery of feedback from a health care professional, once the patient provides their data (McLean et al., 2012). Indeed, the more interactive real-time SMS messaging provide more improved outcomes than SMS reminders alone.

It follows therefore that telehealthcare should be implemented as part of a service redesign. Without the right support, there is the potential that emergency admissions and health care utilisation might increase because of patient concerns. This is an important consideration when commissioning a service. Staff education and preparation is also crucial to the success of this intervention.

Further reading

McLean S, Nurmatov U, Liu J, et al. (2012) Telehealthcare for chronic obstructive pulmonary disease: Cochrane Review and meta-analysis. *Br J Gen Pract* 62: e738–749.

41 Patient education

Box 41.1 Benefits of patient education

- Increased understanding
- Increased concordance
- Positive engagement with healthcare
- Increased patient self-confidence
- Resource efficient – for both patient and healthcare
- Increased quality of life

Figure 41.1 Blooms' taxonomy of learning (1956)
Source: Adapted by Anderson and Krathwohl (2001).

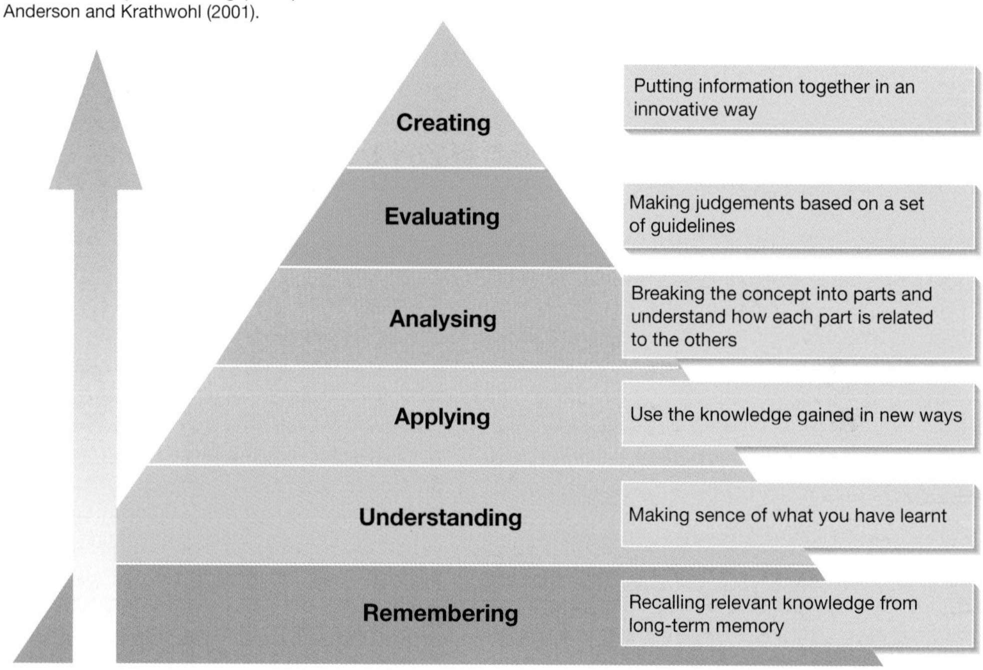
Creating
Putting information together in an innovative way
Evaluating
Making judgements based on a set of guidelines
Analysing
Breaking the concept into parts and understand how each part is related to the others
Applying
Use the knowledge gained in new ways
Understanding
Making sence of what you have learnt
Remembering
Recalling relevant knowledge from long-term memory

Box 41.2 Examples of respiratory education in action

Spirometry buses/workstations
Signage on cigarette packaging
Teaching someone how to use an inhaler
Emergency Ventolin inhalers in schools
Pulmonary rehabilitation
Smoking in cars with children ban
Banning smoking in public places
Various media platforms – internet, radio, television, leaflets

Box 41.3 Teaching resources

Placebo devices
Written personalised plans
Leaflets
'Expert' patients
Internet resources
Videos
Pictures

Education is a process that seeks to increase learning by raising another person's knowledge and awareness. In health care, the goal of patient education is that the patient will not only understand his or her current health status, but also be able to make appropriate health care decisions and make changes as necessary to reach optimal health. For this to be effective, the patient needs to be an active participant and the health care professional needs to be knowledgeable.

Imparting knowledge in order to increase patient awareness and understanding is an activity undertaken with particular frequency in health care. It is also an activity that occurs at various time points, including periods of illness and wellness, demonstrating a relationship between the constructs 'promoting health' and 'educating patients'.

Why is it important?

Educating patients and moving away from a traditional paternalistic biomedical model of health care has gradually evolved over recent years, giving rise and much focus to 'patient centred-care' and 'shared decision making'. This has many benefits for patients as well as the health and social care systems supporting them (Box 41.1).

Understanding the educational process

A critical step in applying and understanding the principles of learning is for the health professional to understand what information the patient needs and wants. This is critical because adults bring with them lifelong learning that has been acquired from a variety of sources. It is from this foundation that the health professional must begin and this signifies the importance of 'assessment'. Assessment is where individual patient needs are identified, such as does the patient have the ability to read and write? What language is most suited to the patient's needs? Does the patient have visual or hearing impairments? If so, how will the health professional adapt the educational process and are there tools and resources that will assist both parties to do this.

Blooms' taxonomy of learning (1956), adapted by Anderson and Krathwohl (2001) (Figure 41.1) is an example of an available tool that demonstrates the processes used for knowledge acquisition and application. It also serves as a helpful evaluation tool for health professionals when seeking to clarify patients' understanding. Applying this tool to the teaching of inhaler technique:

- *Remembering* – establishing patients' past experience relative to respiratory disease and the purpose of the need for the inhaler device.
- *Understanding* – patients to explain in their own words their understanding and introduction of the device.
- *Applying* – practice and application of the skill.
- *Analysing* – making sense of the task and the rationale for undertaking it.
- *Evaluating* - what works well and what does not, for example the need to exhale prior to inspiration.
- *Creating* – the final stage, empowering patients to synthesise all they have learnt and consider how will this work best for them. For example, if I leave my combination inhaler with my toothbrush I will remember to take it twice a day as prescribed and rinse my mouth after

Teaching strategies

Teaching and education relative to the respiratory field occurs (often subtly) within many local and national fields. These are often driven by individuals, communities and strategically (Box 41.2). A community that contributes to raising knowledge and awareness is charitable organisations, often offering widespread resources available for health professionals, patients and carers to utilise and share. Box 41.3 highlights some of the range of teaching resources that can be used. The utilisation of resource tools is interesting. As combining them increases interest and thus knowledge retention; take, for example, inhaler technique – practice with placebo, written instructions on how to take and watching a video that demonstrates correct technique in contrast to giving a patient written instructions alone.

Furthermore, personalising patient education through the use of simple explanations and diagrams over generic leaflet distribution also has many benefits and improves knowledge retention. Similarly, educational activities occurring within groups that have shared interests, such as pulmonary rehabilitation programmes, are particularly successful.

The role of the health professional in supporting the education of patients is very important. Understanding and then applying the fundamentals of how the learning process works is integral to its success.

Further reading

British Lung Foundation (2016) www.blf.org.uk/News/Detail/New-pilot-programme-for-patients-with-COPD (accessed 27 February 2016).

42 Voluntary organisations and patient support groups

Figure 42.1 Reducing the burden of lung disease
Source: British Lung Foundation.

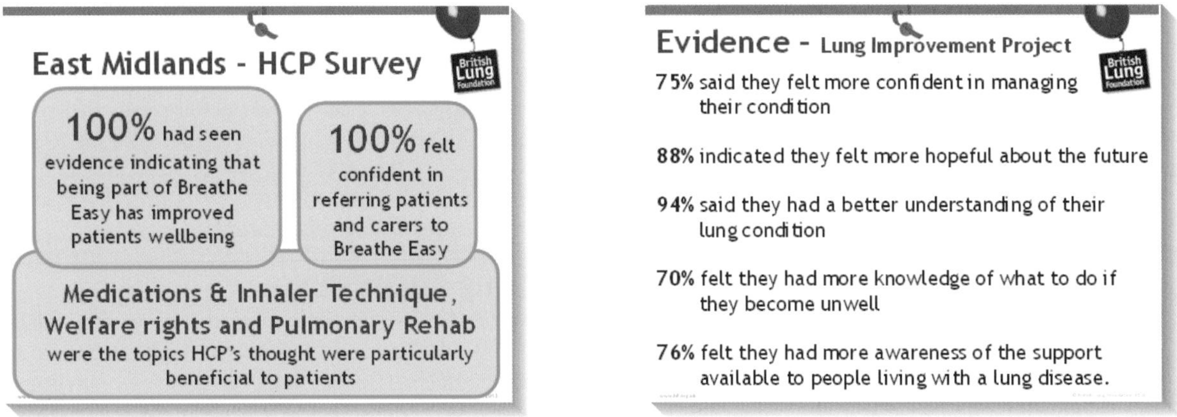
East Midlands - HCP Survey
British Lung Foundation
100% had seen evidence indicating that being part of Breathe Easy has improved patients wellbeing
100% felt confident in referring patients and carers to Breathe Easy
Medications & Inhaler Technique, Welfare rights and Pulmonary Rehab were the topics HCP's thought were particularly beneficial to patients
Evidence - Lung Improvement Project
British Lung Foundation
75% said they felt more confident in managing their condition
88% indicated they felt more hopeful about the future
94% said they had a better understanding of their lung condition
70% felt they had more knowledge of what to do if they become unwell
76% felt they had more awareness of the support available to people living with a lung disease.

Figure 42.2 An example of self-help resource from the British Lung Foundation
Source: British Lung Foundation.

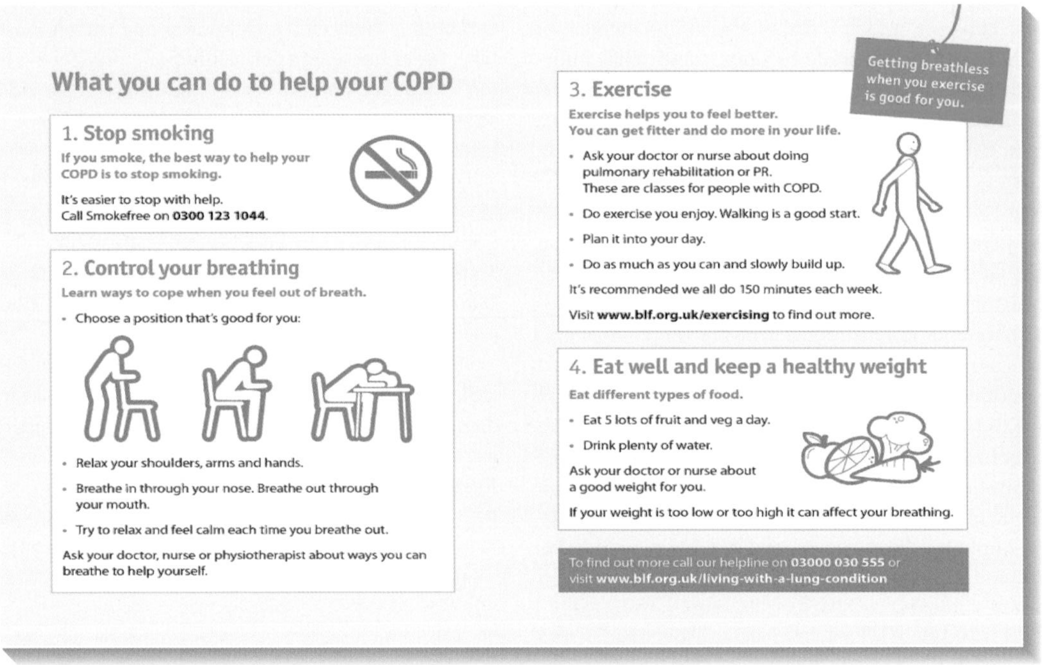
What you can do to help your COPD
1. Stop smoking
If you smoke, the best way to help your COPD is to stop smoking.
It's easier to stop with help.
Call Smokefree on 0300 123 1044.
2. Control your breathing
Learn ways to cope when you feel out of breath.
• Choose a position that's good for you:
• Relax your shoulders, arms and hands.
• Breathe in through your nose. Breathe out through your mouth.
• Try to relax and feel calm each time you breathe out.
Ask your doctor, nurse or physiotherapist about ways you can breathe to help yourself.
Getting breathless when you exercise is good for you.
3. Exercise
Exercise helps you to feel better.
You can get fitter and do more in your life.
• Ask your doctor or nurse about doing pulmonary rehabilitation or PR.
These are classes for people with COPD.
• Do exercise you enjoy. Walking is a good start.
• Plan it into your day.
• Do as much as you can and slowly build up.
It's recommended we all do 150 minutes each week.
Visit www.blf.org.uk/exercising to find out more.
4. Eat well and keep a healthy weight
Eat different types of food.
• Eat 5 lots of fruit and veg a day.
• Drink plenty of water.
Ask your doctor or nurse about a good weight for you.
If your weight is too low or too high it can affect your breathing.
To find out more call our helpline on 03000 030 555 or visit www.blf.org.uk/living-with-a-lung-condition

Figure 42.3 Singing for Breathing Group

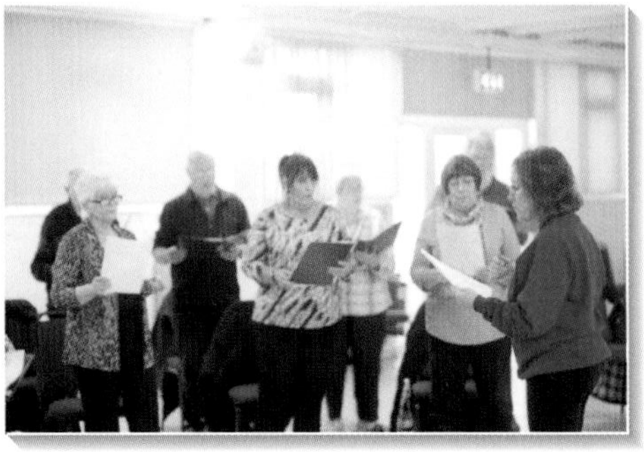

Essential to the aspiration of providing person-centred care is supporting patient self-management and improving information and patient understanding. In essence these are the factors that support shared decision making and promote prevention. Patient support groups have a key role in terms of improving supported self-management and therefore ultimately making the aspiration of effective person-centred care nearer to a reality.

Patient support groups such as the network of British Lung Foundation's (BLF) Breathe Easy groups work with professionals, patients and carers to promote better self-management and improve patient well-being. In our experience these groups work best when health care professionals, clinical commissioners and the BLF work collaboratively to ensure the support group is properly integrated into the local respiratory care pathway. The aim, where this happens, is to reduce the burden of lung disease on both the individual and the local health economy (Figure 42.1).

Activities at Breathe Easy support group meetings aim to ensure:
- Peer learning, where members share experience and knowledge
- Peer support, where patients find ways to support each other
- Education and instruction from the BLF and from a variety of health care professionals (Figure 42.2)
- Signposting to other local relevant support services
- Patients are supported to use their voice to review and improve local services.

The outcomes for patients include:
- Better understanding of their lung condition
- Increased medicine management and compliance
- Increased opportunities for social contact (reduced isolation), increased confidence
- Better understanding of health services
- Plus confidence to self-manage/self-care.

For the local health economy there is potential to achieve:
- Reduced call upon GP services
- Reduced risk of unnecessary hospital admissions.

It has been found that the scope of activities at support group meetings diversifies as patient numbers grow and individual member confidence increases. The opportunities for maintenance exercise sessions following completion of a pulmonary rehabilitation programme are increasing with 30% of groups now offering some form of exercise session in addition to their traditional activities. Walking groups and group singing activities are also growing (5% and 11%, respectively) indicating a desire amongst patients to try a menu of activities with an emphasis on improved self-care.

There has been little in the way of research on the effectiveness of patient support groups to support better self-management. However, what is clear is that if people want to improve their health they need support to do so. A survey commissioned by the Department of Health reported that:
- 75% of patients said that if they had guidance and support from a peer or a health care professional they would feel more confident about taking care of their own health
- 90% were interested in being more active self-carers
- 82% of patients said they have an active role in their care but would like to do more.

So the evidence of patient need and desire for support is there and in terms of patient outcomes the BLF has commissioned the University of Kent to conduct an independent study looking at evidence of outcomes for patients attending Breathe Easy groups. This study is due to report in 2016.

In terms of the benefits of support groups for health care professionals a study (for the Department of Health) reported that attendance of a professional at support group meetings highlighted how many concerns patients have and their reluctance to approach or voice those concerns in ordinary consultations. It found that patients are more likely to raise concerns in an informal environment than a formal consultation and this may highlight service wide issues relating to clinical provision elsewhere.

Figure 42.1 also shows more qualitative evidence. Conducted amongst a limited number of health care professionals involved in integrated Breath Easy groups in the East Midlands, this and much wider anecdotal evidence, provides a basis to support the premise that health care professionals gain significant benefit from attendance at patient support group meetings.

Summary and further resources

Voluntary organisations and patient support groups are an important resource for many patients and professionals. There are several respiratory charities supporting such groups:
- British Lung Foundation – details of local Breathe Easy groups can be found at www.blf.org.uk/BreatheEasy
- Asthma UK – resources and support for health care professionals and patients can be found at http://www.asthma.org.uk/
- Cystic Fibrosis Trust UK – information for patients and health care professionals can be found at www.cysticfibrosis.org.uk

However, it has to be accepted that joining support groups is not for everyone and so charities like the BLF offer a range of patient support opportunities, including:
- Helplines – for example, BLF Helpline free advice, information and support available from respiratory nurse specialists and specialist welfare benefits advisers (03000 030 555)
- Web communities – BLF on-line forum with over 10,500 members
- Singing groups and exercise classes (Figure 42.3)
- Patient information and literature free to order online: http://www.asthma.org.uk/sites/healthcare-professionals
- www.blf.org.uk/page/conditions
- Web site and social media feeds: www.blf.org.uk @lunguk or https://www.facebook.com/britishlungfoundation @asthmauk
- Self-management products for patients and professionals: http://www.asthma.org.uk/advice-asthma-action-plan and www.blf.org.uk/Page/Stay-in-control-of-your-lung-condition

Further reading

National Voices (2015) Prioritising person centred care: summarising evidence from systematic reviews. BLF Breathe Easy patient survey.

MORI, commissioned by Department of Health (2005) *Public Attitudes to Self-Care: Baseline Survey*. MORI.

NHS Improvement Lung (2011) Managing COPD as a long term condition: emerging learning from national improvement projects. http://www.slideshare.net/NHSImprovement/managing-copd-as-a-long-term-condition-emerging-learning-from-the-national-improvement-projects (accessed 1 March 2016).

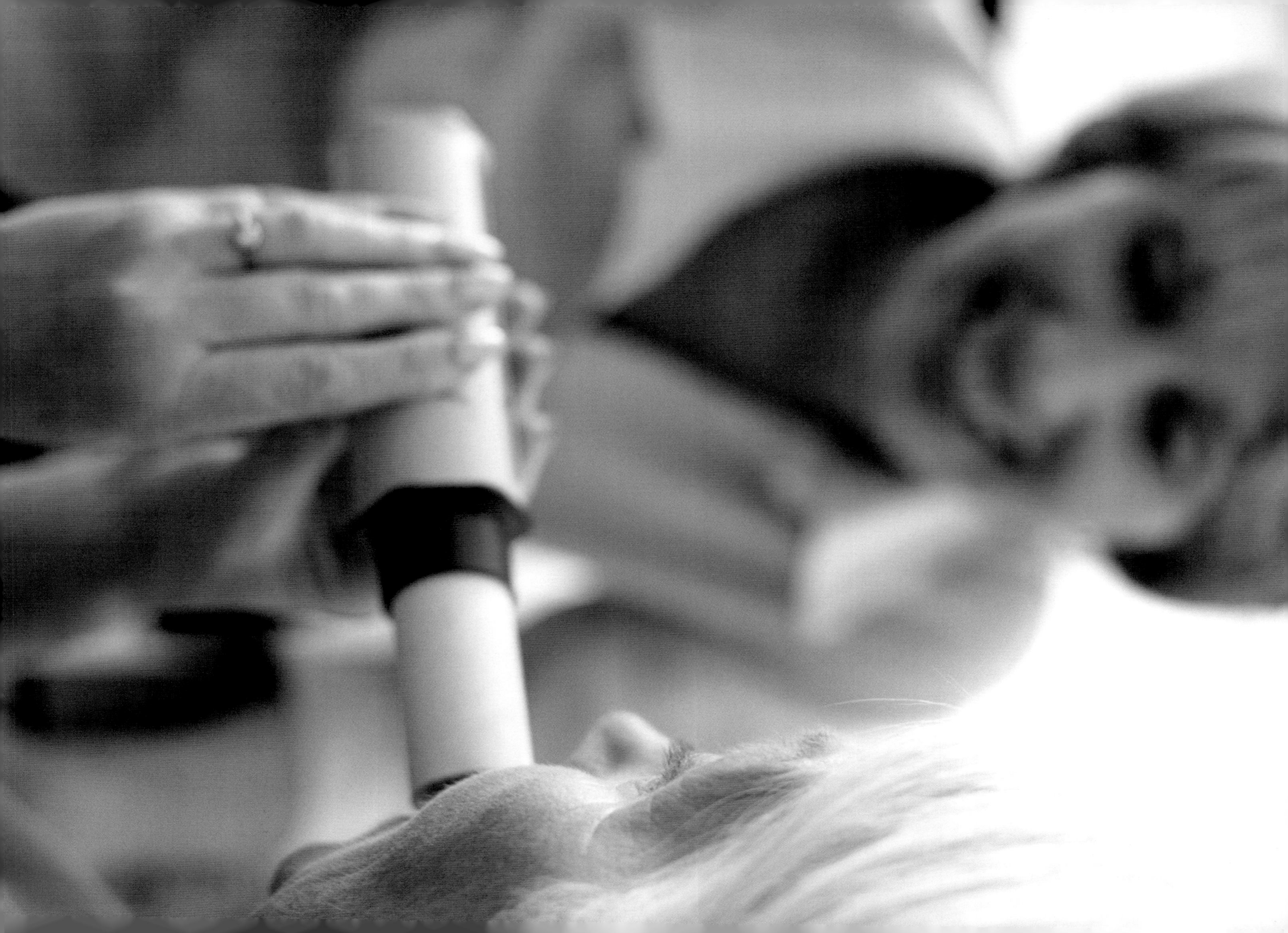

Respiratory medication

Part 6

Chapters

Overview

Pharmacology related to respiratory medicine focused on the role of the nurse is explored in Part 6. The different administration routes are briefly covered with a focus on oxygen therapy. The importance of achieving adherence and concordance to optimise patient outcomes is summarised.

43 Pharmacology and prescribing

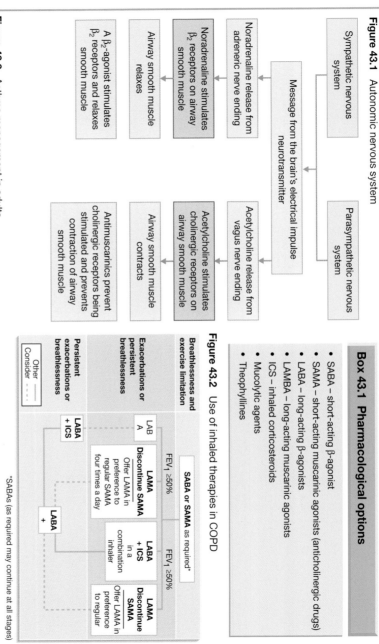

Figure 43.1 Autonomic nervous system

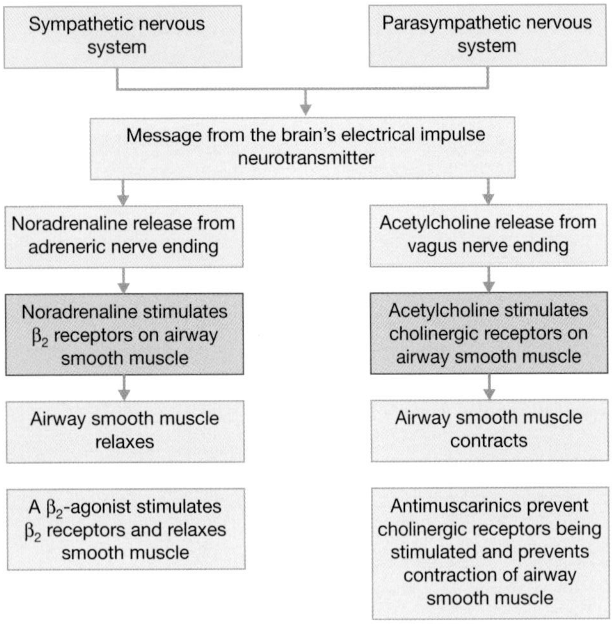
Sympathetic nervous system
Parasympathetic nervous system
Message from the brain's electrical impulse neurotransmitter
Noradrenaline release from adreneric nerve ending
Acetylcholine release from vagus nerve ending
Noradrenaline stimulates β2 receptors on airway smooth muscle
Acetylcholine stimulates cholinergic receptors on airway smooth muscle
Airway smooth muscle relaxes
Airway smooth muscle contracts
A β2-agonist stimulates β2 receptors and relaxes smooth muscle
Antimuscarinics prevent cholinergic receptors being stimulated and prevents contraction of airway smooth muscle

Box 43.1 Pharmacological options

- SABA – short-acting β-agonist
- SAMA – short-acting muscarinic agonists (anticholinergic drugs)
- LABA – long-acting β-agonists
- LAMBA – long-acting muscarinic agonists
- ICS – inhaled corticosteroids
- Mucolytic agents
- Theophyllines

Figure 43.2 Use of inhaled therapies in COPD

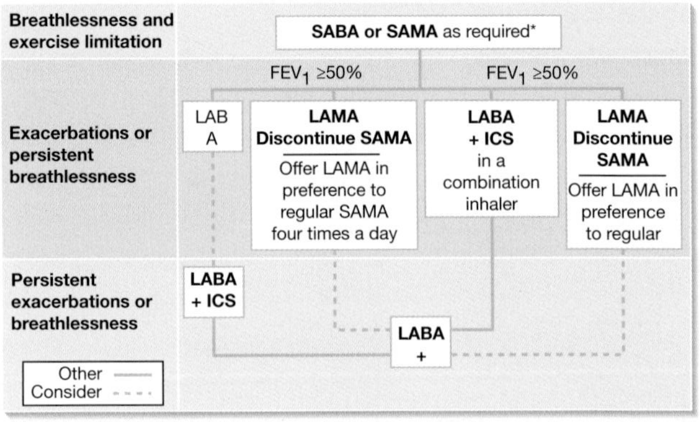
Breathlessness and exercise limitation
SABA or SAMA as required*
FEV1 ≥50%
FEV1 ≥50%
Exacerbations or persistent breathlessness
LABA
LAMA Discontinue SAMA
Offer LAMA in preference to regular SAMA four times a day
LABA + ICS in a combination inhaler
LAMA Discontinue SAMA
Offer LAMA in preference to regular
Persistent exacerbations or breathlessness
LABA + ICS
LABA +
Other
Consider

*SABAs (as required may continue at all stages)

Figure 43.3 Asthma management in adults
Source: BTS SIGN. (2014) *Thorax* 69: i1-i192. Reproduced with permission of BMJ Publishing Ltd.

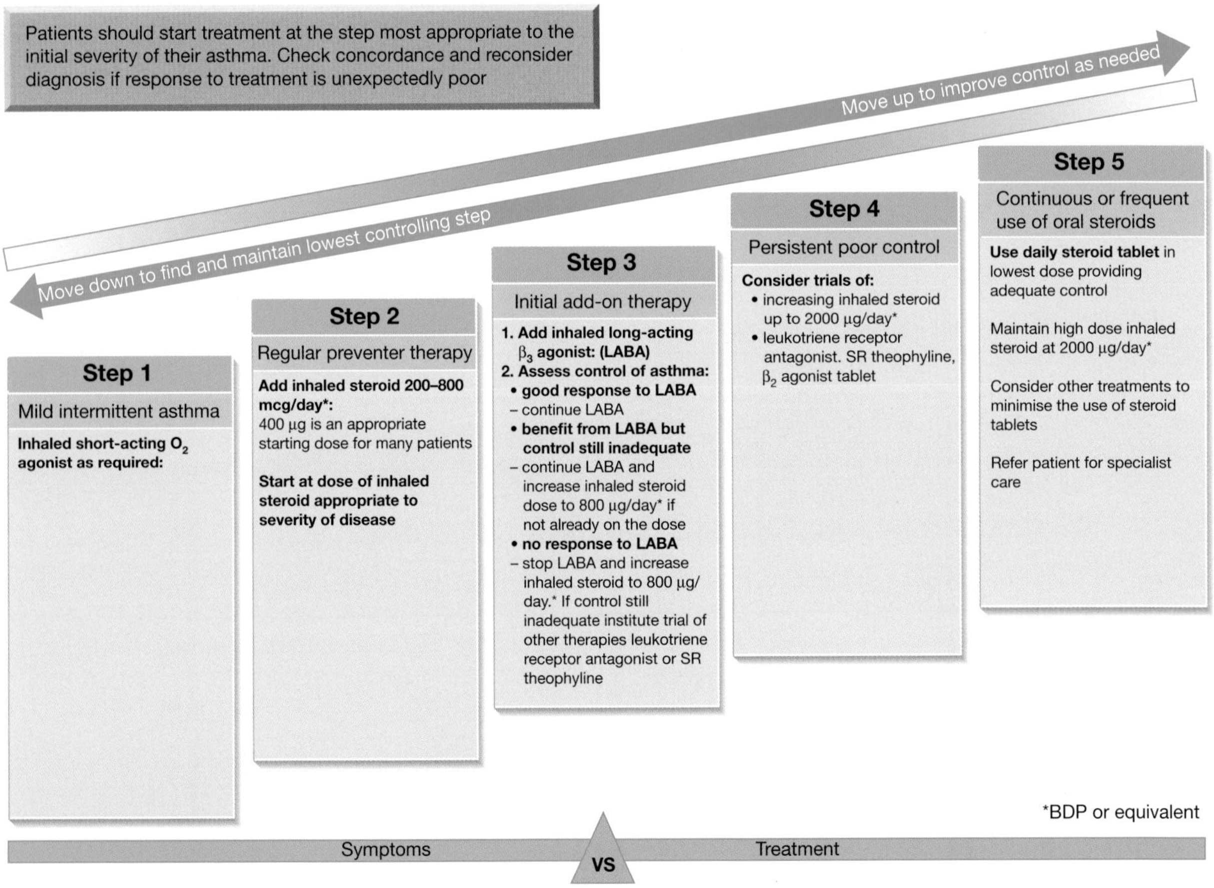
Patients should start treatment at the step most appropriate to the initial severity of their asthma. Check concordance and reconsider diagnosis if response to treatment is unexpectedly poor
Move up to improve control as needed
Move down to find and maintain lowest controlling step
Step 1
Mild intermittent asthma
Inhaled short-acting O2 agonist as required:
Step 2
Regular preventer therapy
Add inhaled steroid 200–800 mcg/day*:
400 μg is an appropriate starting dose for many patients
Start at dose of inhaled steroid appropriate to severity of disease
Step 3
Initial add-on therapy
1. Add inhaled long-acting β3 agonist: (LABA)
2. Assess control of asthma:
• good response to LABA
– continue LABA
• benefit from LABA but control still inadequate
– continue LABA and increase inhaled steroid dose to 800 μg/day* if not already on the dose
• no response to LABA
– stop LABA and increase inhaled steroid to 800 μg/day.* If control still inadequate institute trial of other therapies leukotriene receptor antagonist or SR theophyline
Step 4
Persistent poor control
Consider trials of:
• increasing inhaled steroid up to 2000 μg/day*
• leukotriene receptor antagonist. SR theophyline, β2 agonist tablet
Step 5
Continuous or frequent use of oral steroids
Use daily steroid tablet in lowest dose providing adequate control
Maintain high dose inhaled steroid at 2000 μg/day*
Consider other treatments to minimise the use of steroid tablets
Refer patient for specialist care
*BDP or equivalent
Symptoms
VS
Treatment

Pharmacology is the study of the actions, mechanisms, uses and adverse effects of a drug. In order to decide on appropriate pharmacological therapy it is important to understand the pharmacokinetics and pharmacodynamics of the therapies used.

Pharmacokinetics considers how drugs are absorbed, distributed within the body, metabolised and excreted. Factors that can influence the pharmacokinetics include the dose of the drug given, the patient's condition, dosing schedule of the drug and the route of administration.

Pharmacodynamics considers the effect the drug will have on the cells that it reaches. Once the drug reaches the site of action it will either have a specific mechanism, affecting the way the cell works, or a non-specific mechanism, causing changes to the cellular environment. Adverse drug reactions (ADRs) also need to be considered and are classified into common predictable ADRs and rare unpredictable ADRs. ADRs should be reported via the Yellow Card system.

Bronchodilators

The main action of these drugs is to relieve symptoms by opening up the airways.

Short and long-acting inhaled β_2 agonists

Inhaled β_2 agonists act on the β_2 receptors of the sympathetic nervous system (Figure 43.1). When these receptors are stimulated they relax bronchial smooth muscle and dilate the bronchi. They also inhibit the release of mediators from mast cells.

Side effects of β_2 agonists include tremor, tachycardia, headaches and muscle cramps; interactions can occur with digoxin and hypokalaemia can result when used with corticosteroids, diuretics or theophyllines.

Short-acting β_2 agonists

Short-acting β_2 agonists (e.g. salbutamol, terbutaline) work within 5–15 minutes and last for approximately 4 hours. They are recommended for use as required for wheeze, cough, breathlessness and chest tightness. Asthmatics should not need to use short-acting bronchodilators routinely, and increased use in asthma is an indicator of poor control or exacerbation. Patients with chronic obstructive pulmonary disease (COPD) may need to use their β_2 agonists more frequently as their disease progresses.

Long-acting β_2 agonists

Long-acting β_2 agonists have a longer duration of action (12–24 hours) and are used to treat moderate to severe persistent asthma as an add-on therapy to inhaled corticosteroids. For patients with COPD they are used for symptomatic relief of breathlessness in those requiring more that just short-acting therapy.

Antimuscarinic (anticholinergic) bronchodilators

These drugs act on the parasympathetic nervous system by inhibiting the vagal control of bronchial smooth muscle tone in response to irritants and thus reduce bronchoconstriction (Figure 43.1). They also reduce production of excess mucus in the airways.

Side effects are rare but include dry mouth, nausea, constipation, urinary retention and headache.

Short-acting antimuscarinics

Short-acting antimuscarinics (e.g. ipratropium bromide) work within 30–60 minutes and last for 3–6 hours. They are only used as add-on therapy for patients with asthma during a severe exacerbation. They can be used for patients with COPD as an alternative to salbutamol for rapid relief of symptoms.

Long-acting antimuscarinics

Long-acting antimuscarinics have more specific and therefore more effective action than the short-acting variety. There are a number of these available which work for between 12 and 36 hours, depending on therapy. They are used for symptomatic control of breathlessness in patients with COPD and also have an effect on reducing the frequency of exacerbations. The British National Formulary provides information for available products and licensing.

Methylxanthines

These drugs have been used for patients with asthma and COPD for over 50 years and appear to work by preventing the breakdown of cyclic adenosine monophosphate (cAMP), thus increasing the amount of cAMP in smooth muscle causing bronchodilatation in the same way as β_2 agonists. They should be prescribed by brand because of varying absorption rates.

Common side effects include nausea, vomiting and restlessness. High plasma concentrations can lead to convulsions, arrhythmias and hypotension. Blood plasma levels should be monitored (Chapter 48).

Inhaled corticosteroids

Corticosteroids are anti-inflamatory agents. Inhaled corticosteroids reduce eosinophils, T cells and mast cells in the airways. They inhibit late bronchoconstrictor response caused by allergen exposure and suppress inflammatory cell infiltration of the airways, also reducing mucus hyper-secretion and can reverse epithelial damage.

They are the cornerstone of treatment for all but the mildest asthma. Their role in COPD is less clear and current research aims to identify the likelihood of patients having a response to corticosteroids. They are used in patients with a history of exacerbation with severe to very severe COPD.

Inhaled bronchodilator and corticosteroid therapies are available in a variety of combination products for use in appropriate patients with asthma and COPD. With all inhaled therapy, ensuring the patient has good inhaler technique is crucial to ensuring optimal effect from the therapy.

Guidelines

National, international and local guidelines aid decision making when prescribing – knowledge of all of the guidelines will enable the clinician to make an appropriate choice for the patient (Box 43.1; Figure 43.2 and Figure 43.3).

Nurse prescribing

Non-medical prescribing is a useful skill for respiratory nurses to acquire. It improves holistic patient care and autonomy.

Further reading

Beckwith S, Franklin P. (eds.) (2011) *Oxford Handbook of Prescribing for Nurses and Allied Health Professionals.* Oxford University Press, Oxford.

Simmons M. (2012) *Pharmacology: An Illustrated Review.* Thieme, New York.

44 Inhaler technique

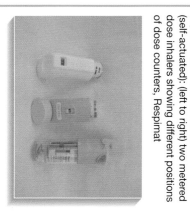

Figure 44.1 Aerosol inhalers (self-actuated): (left to right) two metered dose inhalers showing different positions of dose counters, Respimat

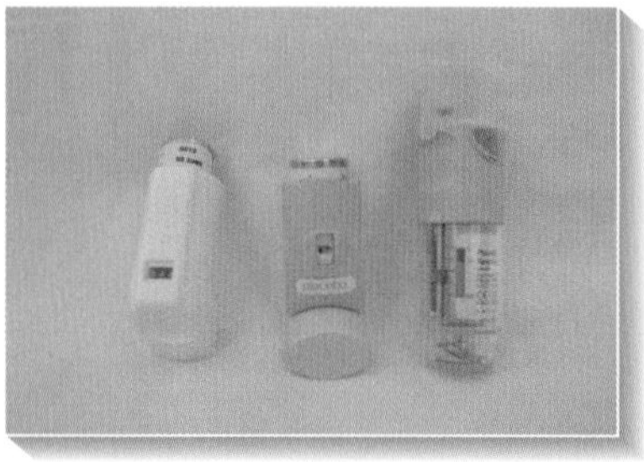

Figure 44.2 Aerosol inhalers (breath-actuated): Autodialler and Easi-breathe

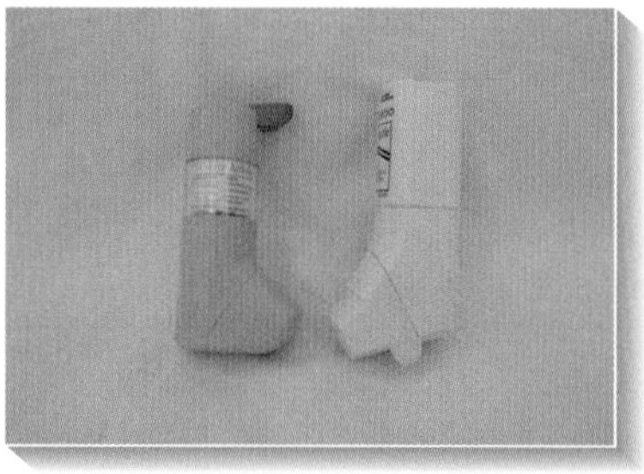

Figure 44.3 Inhaler aids: Haleraid 200 and 120 for MDI; twishgrip for Tubohaler (right)

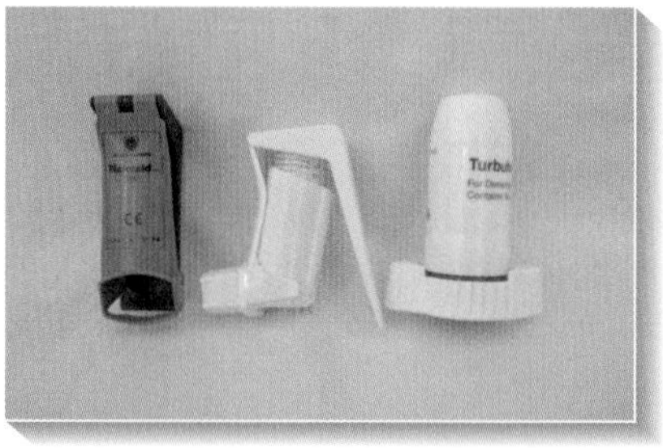

Figure 44.4 Spacers: (left to right) paediatric Aerochamber, adult Aerochamber and Volumatic

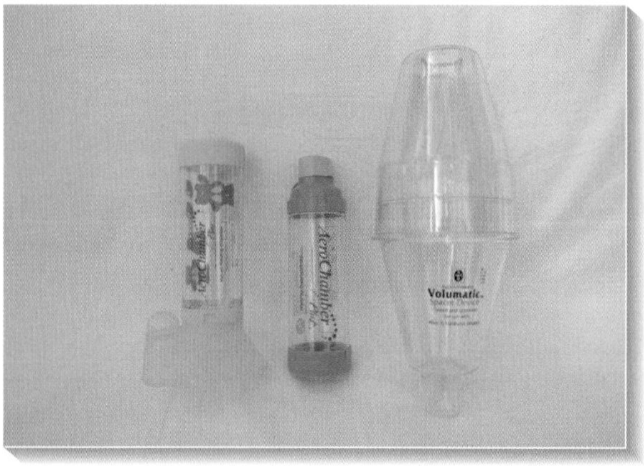
Volumatic

Figure 44.5 Dry power inhalers (capsule): HandiHaler and Breezhaler

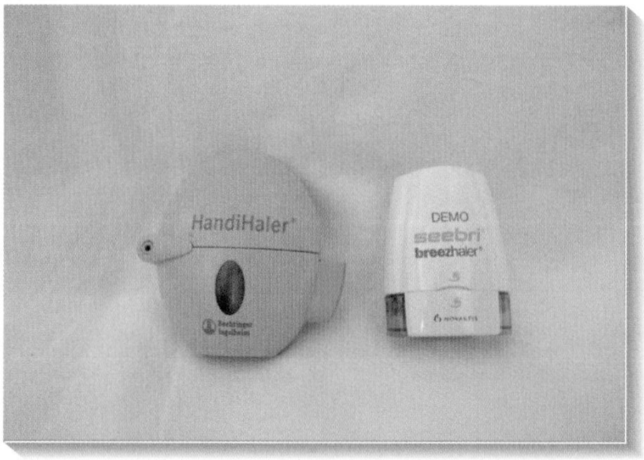
HandiHaler
DEMO
seebri
breezhaler

Figure 44.6 Dry power inhalers (multi-dose): (top row left to right) Accuhaler, Easyhaler, Ellipa; (bottom row left to right) Genuair, Turbohaler, Nexthaler, Spiromax

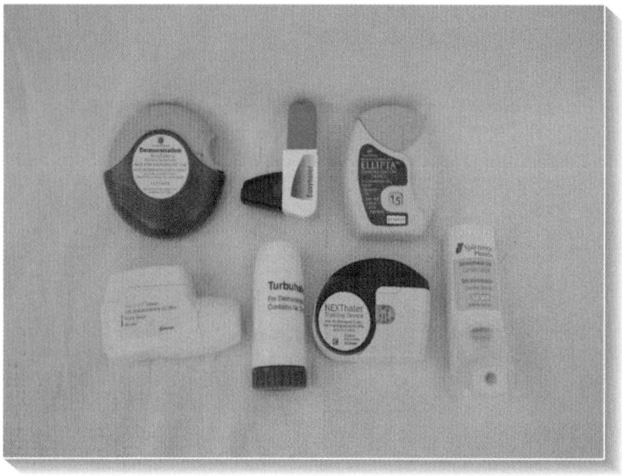
ELLIPTA
NEXThaler

Figure 44.7 Inspiratory flow training aids: (top row, left to right) inspiratory flow whistles for Accuhaler, Ellipa, Turbohaler; (bottom row) In-Check inspiratory flow meter

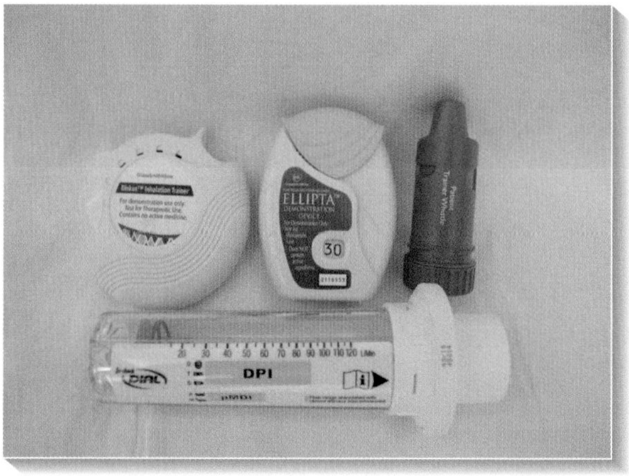
ELLIPTA
30
DPI

Inhaled therapy is the mainstay of treatment for people with asthma and COPD. Drugs are delivered directly to the airways where they are needed, work quickly and effectively. Lower doses can be used, and usually there are fewer side effects than with oral drugs.

Inhaled therapy requires a delivery device to be able to hold the drug, and to deliver it to the airway at the required moment. Correct inhaler technique is essential, and it is vital that health care professionals receive appropriate training and education to support correct use of devices by patients.

Inhaler technique should be checked when first prescribing the device, and at least once a year as part of a regular review. More frequent checks should be made if the patient shows poor control, or after attack or exacerbation.

Choosing the correct device should be led by the health care professional, and agreed by the patient. Sometimes the choice of device is determined by the choice of drug. The best device is the one the patient will use, and is able to use correctly.

In the UK there is a National Inhaler Group which aims to ensure there is consistency of education for health care professionals.

Bronchodilators and anti-inflammatories are delivered via either aerosol or dry powder inhalers (DPI). These two device types require different techniques to ensure drugs are delivered safely to the airways.

Manufacturers' instruction leaflets, which accompany each device, contain useful information about breath-hold, cleaning, storing and problem solving. Patients should be encouraged to read these wherever possible.

Aerosol inhalers

The drug is stored as liquid, contained inside a pressurised canister (Figure 44.1). In most cases the canister includes a propellant as well, with the exception of the Respimat, which uses a spring to expel the contents and produce a 'soft mist' of drug. When the device is activated, the drug is released under pressure. It passes through a 'venturi' or narrowing, becoming atomised as a gas, before leaving the inhaler. Good technique requires a slow and long inspiratory breath, which must coincide with activation of the device. One of the more common mistakes with aerosol inhalers is breathing in too quickly or too hard.

Metered dose inhaler

Instructions for using a metered dose inhaler (MDI):

1 Shake the inhaler to mix the drug and propellant
2 Remove the cap
3 Breathe out, away from the inhaler
4 Secure a good seal with the lips around the mouthpiece
5 Commence a slow breath in
6 Compress the canister to activate, and continue to breathe in slowly and deeply
7. Hold the breath for about 5–10 seconds.

Breath actuated MDI (e.g. Easi-Breathe, Autohaler)

The technique for using a Breath-Actuated MDI is similar to an MDI. The main difference is that the device will fire automatically without compressing the top of the canister (Figure 44.2).

Spacers

Use of a spacer with an MDI is recommended to increase lung deposition (Figure 44.4). Spacers also reduce risks of failing to synchronise inhalation and activation of the MDI.

Large volume spacers (e.g. Volumatic) have been shown to be comparable to a nebuliser in an emergency. Small volume spacers may be less efficient, but are more portable.

Instructions for using a spacer:

1 Shake the inhaler to mix the drug and propellant
2 Remove the cap
3 Place the MDI into the aperture of the spacer
4 Squeeze the canister to activate
5 Secure a good seal with the lips around the mouthpiece of the spacer
6 Take four or five deep breaths.

Dry powder inhalers

The drug is stored as powder, contained either within a capsule or within the inhaler itself (Figures 44.5 and 44.6). The drug leaves the device only when the patient inhales sufficiently. A good technique involves a strong, forceful inspiratory breath. This is the opposite of the technique used for aerosol inhalers.

Capsule DPIs (e.g. Handihaler, Breezhaler)

Instructions for use of a dry powder inhaler (DPI):

1 Remove a capsule from the foil blister packaging, observing the manufacturer's instructions
2 Open the inhaler, and place the capsule inside the chamber
3 Close the inhaler
4 Pierce the capsule by squeezing the button on the side of the inhaler
5 Secure a good seal with the lips around the mouthpiece
6 Inhale as hard as possible
7 Hold the breath for 5–10 seconds
8 If any powder is left, repeat steps 5–6.

Multi-dose DPIs (e.g. Turbohaler, Accuhaler, Easyhaler, Genuair, Ellipta, Nexthaler, Spiromax)

This represents the most diverse group of inhalers. While the technique is broadly similar, each device has its own specific priming mechanism. The technique is similar to capsule DPIs, but rather than inserting a capsule, the device is primed by opening the cover, sliding a lever, pushing a button or twisting the base.

Some DPIs leave no taste, and it is important to forewarn patients especially if they are changing from an aerosol inhaler, which can have a very different taste and feel in the mouth.

Inhaler aids

Inspiratory flow whistles obtained from some manufacturers whistle if the patient has sufficient inspiratory flow to inhale powder from the device. Similarly, the Flo-Tone Trainer can help assess MDI technique. The In-Check DIAL meter can also be used to assess inspiratory flow in a range of devices. There are devices available to help patients with dexterity issues (Figure 44.3).

A full table of drugs and devices can be downloaded from the ARNS website: http://arns.co.uk/inhaler-device-summary-resource/

45 Nebuliser therapy

Figure 45.1 Particle deposition in the airways and lungs

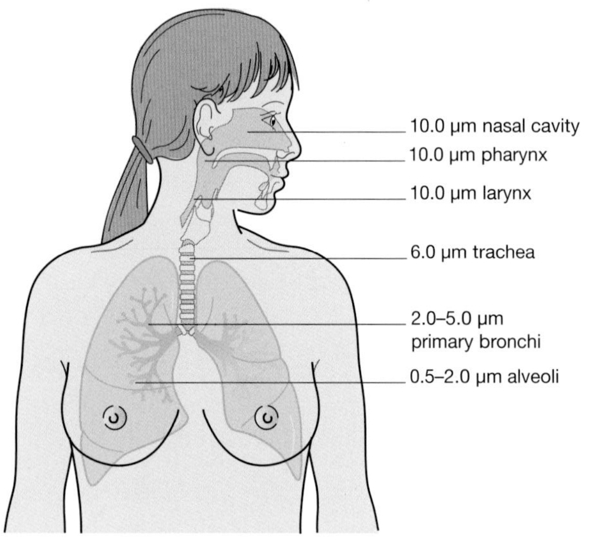

10.0 μm nasal cavity
10.0 μm pharynx
10.0 μm larynx
6.0 μm trachea
2.0–5.0 μm primary bronchi
0.5–2.0 μm alveoli

Figure 45.2 Nebulisation equipment

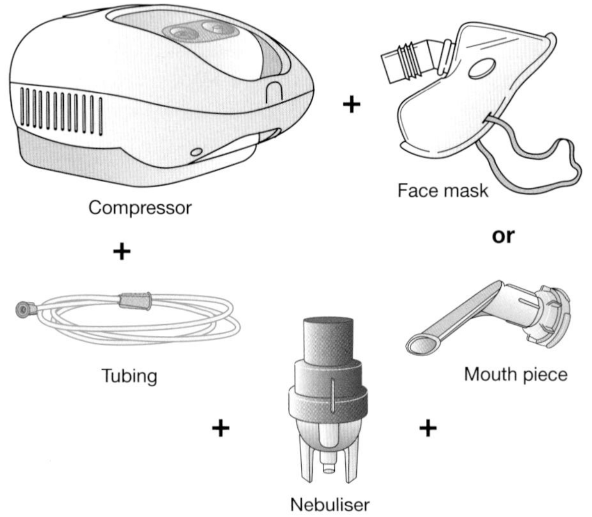

Compressor
+
Face mask
or
Tubing
Mouth piece
+
Nebuliser
+

Figure 45.3 How a nebuliser works: (a) jet nebuliiser; (b) ultrasonic nebuliser

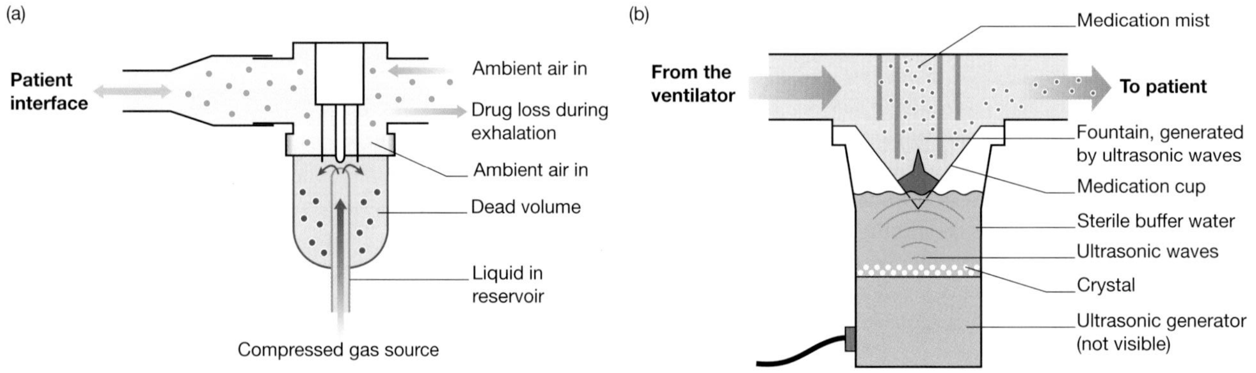

(a)
Patient interface
Ambient air in
Drug loss during exhalation
Ambient air in
Dead volume
Liquid in reservoir
Compressed gas source
(b)
Medication mist
From the ventilator
To patient
Fountain, generated by ultrasonic waves
Medication cup
Sterile buffer water
Ultrasonic waves
Crystal
Ultrasonic generator (not visible)

Figure 45.4 (a) Mask; (b) mouthpiece

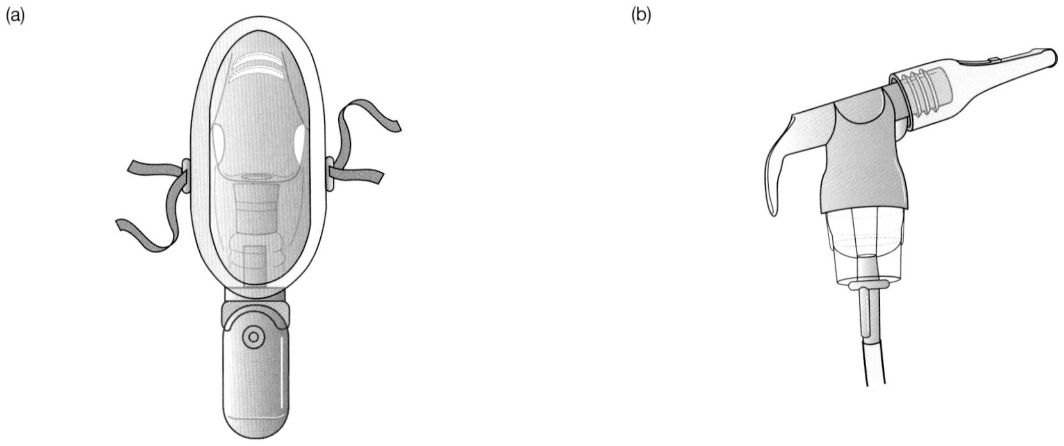

(a)
(b)

A nebuliser is a device that converts a liquid into an aerosol suitable for inhalation. In respiratory medicine this allows drugs, usually at higher doses than standard inhalers, to be converted to an aerosol that can be delivered to the lungs. Administration via this route increases speed of effect, requires lower doses of drug than if given systemically and therefore usually causes fewer side effects. The amount of deposition of the drug is dependent on the condition of the lungs, the pattern of breathing and the particle size of the medication. In order to reach the airways the particle size needs to be 1–5 μm in diameter; for alveolar deposition a diameter of 1–2 μm is necessary. Deposition of the medication varies and around 10% of the particles reach the necessary part of the airway (Figure 45.1). The remaining solution is left in the chamber as residual volume, in the tubing or mouthpiece (Bourke and Burns, 2015).

Use of nebulisers

It is widely regarded that most bronchodilator and corticosteroid therapy is best administered via a hand-held inhaler device, often with a spacer. However, for some patients with severe illness or poor manual dexterity a trial of nebulised therapy can be considered.

There are a variety of medications that can be used in a nebuliser. β_2 agonists and antimuscarinics are bronchodilators, corticosteroids can be used to reduce airway inflammation, antibiotics to treat infection locally and mucolytics facilitate expectoration by reducing the viscosity of sputum. In some cases the drug is available only in a nebulised preparation, such as dornase alpha (rhDNase), a synthetic enzyme that reduces viscosity and aids sputum expectoration.

Nebuliser drivers and equipment

The main nebuliser system is made up of a driver, nebuliser/medication pot and delivery device (mouthpiece/mask; Figure 45.2).

To enable a nebuliser to create an aerosol for inhalation there is a need for driver; this is often mistaken as the nebuliser. Jet-driven nebulisers (Figure 45.3a) are the most commonly used and rely on compressed gas to drive the nebuliser, either piped air or oxygen, at a flow rate of at least 6–8 L/minute or with an electric compressor. It is important to note that during an exacerbation of asthma the preferred gas is oxygen. However, in patients with COPD who are at risk of hypercapnia, air should be used to drive the nebuliser with supplemental oxygen via nasal cannula if required to manage hypoxia. Ultrasonic nebulisers are becoming more common; they tend to be smaller, quieter and more portable, relying on a vibrating piezoelectric crystal to drive the nebuliser (Figure 45.3b). Nebulisers produce a steady stream of aerosolized droplets. However, in some devices this can be moderated by breath actuated mechanisms. It is essential that the nebulised chamber is matched to the type of driver.

Nebulised medication can be delivered either by a mask or a mouthpiece (Figure 45.4a,b). Patient preference must be taken into consideration; however, an important factor that needs to be taken into account is the drug being delivered. A mouthpiece may be preferable to a mask when using antimuscarinic drugs to avoid any risk of glaucoma (caused by close proximity of the vapour to the eyes). Equally, when nebulising antibiotics or steroids a facemask should be avoided to prevent contact of the drug with the skin and eyes. If the user is unable to use a mouthpiece and a mask is necessary, then it should be very well fitting and eye protection should be considered in order to reduce risk. When nebulising antibiotics, a filter or hosing system will be necessary to protect other people from unnecessary exposure.

Education of user

It has been demonstrated that patients' understanding of the principles of nebulised therapy and the equipment is poor (Boyter and Carter, 2005). It is therefore essential that if a person is to use nebulised therapy at home that they, or their carer, are coached regarding assembly of the equipment and installation of the medication; how to use the medication and when the administration is complete; how to clean the equipment, maintenance, service and what to do should the equipment fail. This should be supported with written instructions.

Use

While nebulisers vary, the fill volume is usually between 2.5 and 5 mL. It is important not to exceed this otherwise performance will be affected and nebulisation time prolonged. A characteristic 'splutter' signifies when the nebuliser has stopped working. At this point any residual fluid should be discarded before the next nebulisation.

Cleaning

The mask or mouthpiece and chamber of the nebuliser should be cleaned daily by washing in warm water and detergent, then left to air dry overnight. The tubing should not be washed in water. Once reassembled the nebuliser should be run for a few seconds to clear the tubing.

Maintenance

With the jet nebuliser the mask or mouthpiece, nebuliser chamber and tubing needs to be changed as per the manufacturer's instructions; this can vary between 3 months and 1 year depending on the type of nebuliser. Nebulisers are for single patient use; some are for single use only – these are commonly used in emergency and pre-hospital settings. Attention also needs to be paid to the compressor where disposable parts such as the filter will need to be changed dependent on usage and the manufacturer's instructions. Compressors require servicing again as per manufacturer's instructions.

Breakdown

In the event of a breakdown, the user should have clear instructions regarding what to do. This advice should include which medication to substitute for the 'missed' nebulised dose if possible and who to contact to arrange a substitution/replacement and repair.

Further reading

Nebulisers and nebulised medication. (2014) www.lothianrespiratorymcn.scot.nhs.uk/wp-content/uploads/2014/09/nebuliser-professional-advice-v2-0.pdf (accessed 27 February 2016).

46 Emergency oxygen therapy

Box 46.1 Indications for oxygen therapy in acute illness

- Cardiac/respiratory arrest or peri-arrest
- Hypoxaemia
- Shock, sepsis, major trauma, anaphylaxis
- Carbon monoxide poisoning

Figure 46.1 Titrating oxygen dose: a stepwise approach to adjusting dose up or down (BTS 2008)

Titrating oxygen up or down	
Venturi 24% 2.4 L/min (blue)	Nasal cannulae 1 L/min
Venturi 28% 4–6 L/min (white)	Nasal cannulae 2 L/min
Venturi 35% 8–10 L/min (yellow)	Nasal cannulae 4–6 L/min
Venturi 40% 10–12 L/min (red)	Simple face mask 5–6 L/min
Venturi 60% 12–15 L/min (green)	Simple face mask 7–10 L/min
Reservoir mask at 15 L/min	

Figure 46.3 Simple face mask ('low flow' mask)

- For short-term use e.g. post-operative recovery
- Oxygen at flow rates 2–10 L/min is supplemented with air drawn into the mask during breathing, FiO_2 achieved cannot be predicted – depends on the rate and depth of breathing
- At flow rates of <5 L/min exhaled CO_2 may build up in the mask, resulting in rebreathing. Should not be used tor patients at risk of hypercapnic failure

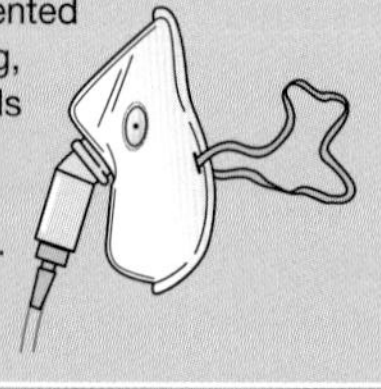

Box 46.2 Potential risks of inappropriate administration of oxygen

- CO_2 retention in patients at risk of hypercapnic respiratory failure
- Rebound hypoxaemia – occurs if oxygen is withdrawn abruptly in patients with acute hypercapnic respiratory failure
- Vasoconstriction in non-hypoxaemic stroke and acute coronary syndromes
- Alveolar membrane damage with prolonged exposure to FiO_2 >60% leading to widespread pulmonary inflammation and fibrosis
- Fire–oxygen supports burning and serious burns can occur when oils, alcohol gels or naked flames are used in an oxygen enriched environment

Figure 46.2 Reservoir mask (non-rebreathing mask)

- At high risk (10–15L/min) flow rate delivers oxygen at >60%
- Recommended for short-term use in patients who are critically ill
- Reservoir bag must be filled with oxygen before use and ensure a close fit on the patient's face. One-way valve prevents exhaled air entering the bag

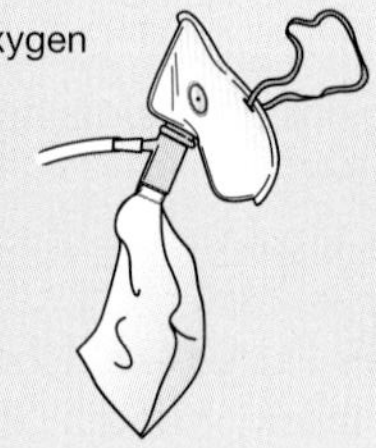

Figure 46.4 Nasal cannulae

- Comfortable and well tolerated by most patients
- Do not interfere with coughing, talking or eating
- Oxygen is inhaled even when mouth breathing
- Flow rates >4 L/min can cause drying of nasal mucosa and are more uncomfortable
- FiO_2 varies with rate and depth of breathing; not recommended for acute use in patients with unstable hypercapnic failure, other than during meals or to provide supplemental oxygen during air driven nebulised therapy

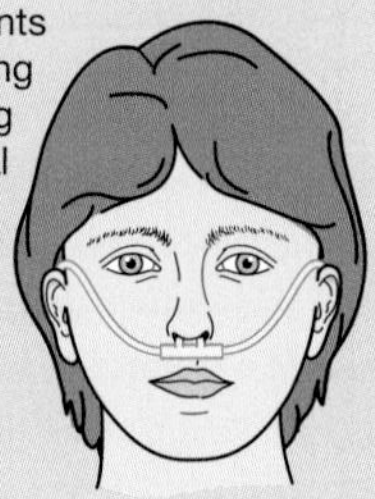

Figure 46.5 Fixed performance devices (controlled oxygen deliverey systems)

Deliver accurate percentage of oxygen independent of patient's breathing rate or volumes by entraining or precise proportion of air with fixed oxygen flow rate. Recommended for use in unstable patients and those at risk of hypercapnic respiratory failure

Venturi valves are colour coded to denote the fixed percentage of oxygen delivered, from 24% (blue) to 60% (green) provided that the minimum oxygen flow rate on the barrel of the device is given. Minimum oxygen flow rate required is noted on the device (varies between manufacturers). Increasing the oxygen flow rate by 50% (e.g. 2 L/min to 3 L/min) increases the gas flow into the mask without increasing the percentage of oxygen delivered and may be more comfortable

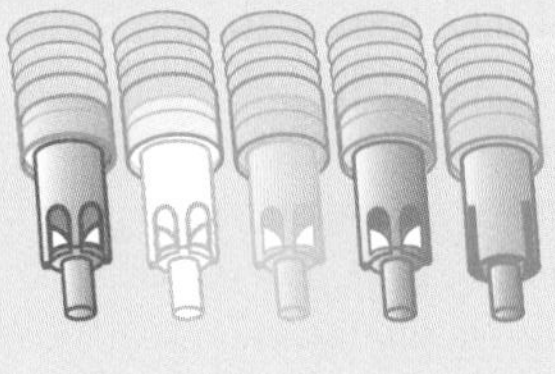

Oxygen is required by all tissues to support cell metabolism; in acute illness, low tissue oxygenation (hypoxia) can occur because of a failure in any of the systems that deliver and circulate oxygen. Box 46.1 lists indications for oxygen therapy.

Oxygen therapy can be life-saving but given without appropriate assessment and ongoing evaluation it can also be detrimental (Box 46.2). The British Thoracic Society (BTS) 2008 Emergency Oxygen Guideline recommends the administration of oxygen to treat hypoxaemia (low blood oxygen levels) and the use of a target oxygen saturation range to guide therapeutic treatment. Oxygen does not treat breathlessness in the absence of hypoxaemia.

In an emergency situation, immediate assessment of airway patency, breathing and circulation (e.g. A–E approach) is essential and in critical illness, such as peri-arrest, high concentration oxygen should be commenced via reservoir mask at 10–15 L/min until the patient is stable and appropriate target range can be prescribed (Resuscitation Council UK, 2015).

Target saturation range is prescribed according to risk of type 2 (hypercapnic/CO_2 retention) respiratory failure pending arterial blood gas measurement. For most patients a target of 94–98% is appropriate; for those at risk of CO_2 retention (hypercapnia) a target of 88–92% ensures safe levels of oxygenation and minimises risk of initiating or worsening respiratory acidosis. Those at risk include patients with moderate or severe chronic obstructive pulmonary disease (COPD)/emphysema, severe bronchiectasis, neuromuscular disease, cystic fibrosis, neuromuscular and chest wall disorders and morbid obesity.

Pulse oximetry measures tissue hypoxia and must be available in all settings where emergency oxygen is used. It is essential that the fraction of inspired oxygen (FiO_2) and delivery device is recorded alongside oxygen saturations and that the effect of any changes to FiO_2 is monitored and documented.

Commencing oxygen therapy in acutely ill patients

Baseline observations should be recorded in order to determine response to treatment, including saturations, respiratory rate, blood pressure and pulse. It is also important to note colour, respiratory effort and level of consciousness.

Oxygen is a drug and, with the exception of the peri-arrest situation, must be given with a prescription. Where there is no known risk of CO_2 retention, a target range of 94–98% is prescribed and oxygen therapy commenced via reservoir mask at 10–15 L/min. Where there is a risk of CO_2 retention, a target of 88–92% is prescribed and oxygen therapy commenced via 28% Venturi device and mask. The mask is placed on the patient's face and the nose clip and elastic straps adjusted to ensure a close fit. Patients often require reassurance; being breathless is very frightening and an oxygen mask can feel very claustrophobic. Venturi masks can be substituted with nasal cannulae at low flow rates (1–2 L/min) to achieve the same target range once the patient has stabilised.

Response to oxygen therapy is monitored and compared with baseline – oxygen saturations should be reviewed 5 minutes after each adjustment to oxygen dose and the FiO_2 titrated accordingly to maintain saturations within the prescribed target range. All adjustments to oxygen dose must be documented alongside saturations.

Patients should be nursed in an upright position to maximise ventilation unless contraindicated by underlying clinical problems (e.g. spinal or skeletal trauma).

Ongoing care of patients requiring oxygen therapy in the acute setting

Oxygen saturations should be recorded at least four times a day, more often if clinically indicated. Saturations are recorded at rest and should be documented alongside FiO_2 *in situ* at the time. Oxygen dose is titrated to keep saturations within prescribed range (Figure 46.1). Patients requiring increasing doses of oxygen or with signs of respiratory deterioration (increasing respiratory rate, drowsiness, headache, tremor, increasing early warning score) require prompt medical review and further assessment including arterial blood gas monitoring.

Choice of oxygen delivery device will be determined by the cause of hypoxia and underlying medical condition (Figures 46.2–46.5). Fixed performance devices deliver a fixed proportion of air and oxygen via a Venturi valve, ensuring an accurate concentration of oxygen is delivered regardless of the patient's rate and depth of breathing. Fixed performance devices are recommended for patients at risk of CO_2 retention. Stable patients may be more comfortable with nasal cannulae but it is important to be aware that FiO_2 will vary with rate and depth of breathing. Patients requiring air driven nebulised therapy may require supplemental oxygen via nasal cannulae at low flow rates for the duration of the treatment.

Humidification is not required for the delivery of low-flow oxygen or for the short-term use of high-flow oxygen. It is not therefore required in pre-hospital care. However, oxygen has a drying effect on oral and nasopharyngeal mucosa, particularly at high flow rates. It is reasonable therefore to use humidified oxygen for patients who require high-flow oxygen systems for more than 24 hours or who report upper airway discomfort resulting from dryness.

Discontinuation of oxygen therapy can be considered once the patient is stable and saturations are within target range on at least two consecutive recordings. Saturations should be monitored for 5 minutes after stopping oxygen and rechecked after 1 hour.

Further reading

O'Driscoll R, Howard LS, Davison AG; British Thoracic Society (2008) Guideline for emergency oxygen use in adult patients. *Thorax* 63(Suppl 6): 1–68.

Resuscitation Council (UK) (2015) Resuscitation guidelines. https://www.resus.org.uk/resuscitation-guidelines/ (accessed 23 March 2016).

47 Domiciliary oxygen therapy

Figure 47.1 Oxygen concentrator

The concentration filter room air and stores the concentrated oxygen in a small reservoir for delivery via up to 15 metres of tubing. It may be installed as a 'free line' to enable use while mobilising around the home or as a 'fixed install' to reduce risk of trips and falls

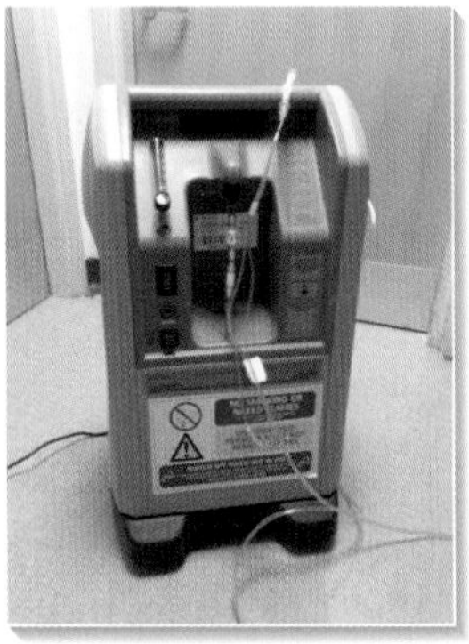

Figure 47.2 Standard ambulatory cylinder

Weighs approximately 3.5 kg and can deliver flow rates of 1–15 l/min. Approximate duration of 31/2 hours from full at 2 l/min

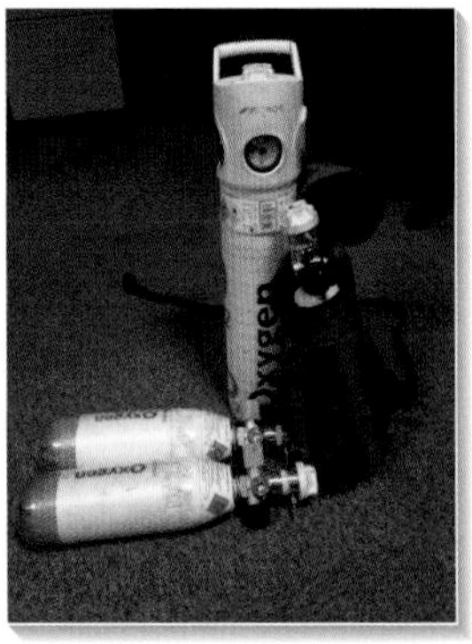

Figure 47.3 Standard ambulatory cylinder

Smaller than standard cylinder and weighing approximately 2.7 kg. Delivers flow rates of 0.1–15 l/min, with duration of approximately 2 hours at 2 l/min

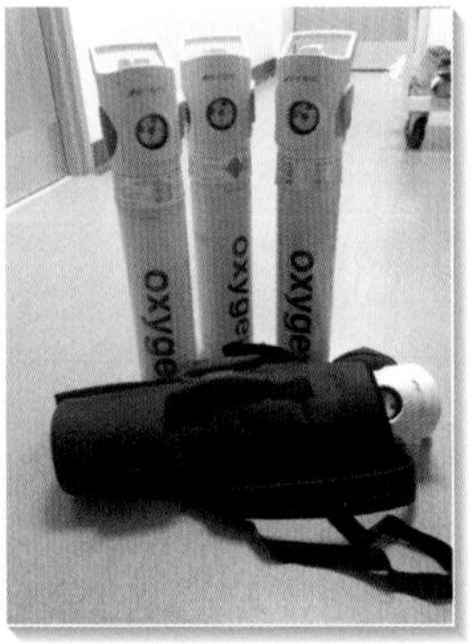

Liquid-oxygen: Liquid units provide more flexibility for patients, enabling them to refill the portable unit as and when needed. They do require reasonable manual dexterity to refill and safe external storage. Duration of use is variable as there can be considerable evaporation from the unit but typically will last about 6–7 hours at 2 l/min

Breathlessness is a common symptom in chronic cardiorespiratory conditions, and can be distressing and disabling. Supplementary oxygen therapy is often recommended but the evidence for its effectiveness to palliate the symptom of breathlessness is largely unknown (Uronis et al., 2015). However, home oxygen is widely used and is associated with significant potential costs both to the individual patient, in terms of quality of life and to the wider health care economy.

Domiciliary oxygen therapy is categorised according to intended usage; the British Thoracic Society (BTS) guidelines (Hardinge et al., 2015) provide evidence-based guidance on the assessment and use of each category of oxygen in the home setting (Hardinge et al., 2015). Prior to considering home oxygen, patients should have a definite diagnosis and optimal medical management. Assessment for oxygen should be undertaken in a specialist oxygen service, with appropriate clinical expertise and access to equipment that will be used in the home (Hardinge et al., 2015).

Long-term oxygen therapy

Long-term oxygen therapy (LTOT) is defined as supplemental oxygen used for at least 15 hours/day including overnight (Hardinge et al., 2015). Two landmark trials in the early 1980s assessed the use of oxygen in patients with chronic obstructive pulmonary disease (COPD) and severe resting hypoxaemia (arterial oxygen (PaO_2) ≤7.3 kPa). Both NOTT (1980) and MRC (1981) trials demonstrated a survival benefit in those receiving oxygen for more than 15 hours/day. The evidence that LTOT confers a mortality benefit in non-COPD respiratory failure is lacking (Zielinski, 2000; Ringbaek, 2005) but it is generally accepted in clinical practice that the same arterial blood gas criteria should be applied. LTOT appears to offer variable effects on health-related quality of life, with some studies suggesting minor improvements but others demonstrating no benefit (Eaton et al., 2004; Hardinge et al., 2015).

Pulse oximetry is used to screen patients for referral for LTOT assessment; those with resting oxygen saturation of ≤92% on air should be referred for arterial blood gas assessment. Patients should be stable, at least 8 weeks after an acute exacerbation (Hardinge et al., 2015). Those with clinical evidence of peripheral oedema, polycythaemia or pulmonary hypertension can be considered for earlier referral for assessment for LTOT.

The need for LTOT is confirmed by undertaking arterial blood gas (ABG) sampling on two occasions, at least 3 weeks apart, to confirm chronic hypoxaemia (Chapter 20). LTOT is indicated if PaO_2 ≤7.3 kPa (or ≤8 kPa in presence of signs of cor pulmonale or polycythaemia). Gorecka et al. (1997) found no survival benefit in patients with COPD and moderate hypoxaemia (7.4–8.7 kPa). ABG should be reassessed on oxygen to ensure adequate correction of oxygenation is achieved without causing or worsening hypercapnia (CO_2 retention). Ear lobe capillary blood gas (CBG) sampling gives an accurate estimate of pH and $paCO_2$ and may be used as an alternative to ABG during oxygen titration (Hardinge et al., 2015).

LTOT is delivered via an oxygen concentrator (Figure 47.1), a motor driven machine that plugs into an electrical supply and filters room air through a series of internal chemical filters, venting nitrogen as a 'waste' gas. The concentrated oxygen is stored in a small reservoir and delivered to the patient via standard oxygen delivery devices, usually nasal cannulae. Patients are supplied with large back-up cylinders in case of machine or power failure.

Commencing LTOT has significant implications for patients and their carers. It is important that there is adequate follow-up and support by a specialist home oxygen team to improve compliance with therapy, determine continued need and provide appropriate education and risk assessment.

It is not known whether patients who continue to smoke derive the same survival benefit potential from LTOT (Hardinge et al., 2015). Continuing to smoke is associated with an increased risk of accelerated decline in lung function and increased mortality in COPD and it is possible that the negative effects of smoking offset any benefit from LTOT. Patients who continue to smoke should be counselled that the potential for clinical benefit might be limited (Hardinge et al., 2015). Additionally, there are significant risks of fire and injury related to home oxygen use and smoking. Oxygen is not explosive but will support vigorous burning in the presence of a heat source; lighting a cigarette is the most common cause of injury (Hardinge et al., 2015) with burns sustained to the face, hands and inhalation injury from oxygen flare fires. An additional risk has been identified of fires associated with e-cigarettes and their chargers. Both clinicians prescribing home oxygen and home oxygen suppliers have a responsibility to undertake risk assessments prior to installation and it may be necessary to withhold oxygen therapy if safety is significantly compromised. All patients and families should be made aware of the dangers of using home oxygen in the vicinity of naked flames and smoking cessation should be discussed at each review if patients continue to smoke (Chapter 10).

Ambulatory oxygen therapy

Breathlessness, in chronic respiratory disease, is often exacerbated by progressive inactivity and muscle deconditioning. Some patients who are not hypoxaemic at rest but desaturate significantly on exertion can benefit from ambulatory oxygen therapy (AOT) during activity. AOT does not confer a survival benefit but enables some patients to tolerate more prolonged levels of activity and can increase hours for those on LTOT who are regularly out of the home (Hardinge et al., 2015).

Patients should undergo formal AOT assessment with oximetry during an exercise test. AOT should only be recommended if there is objective evidence of increased exercise capacity and a reduction in symptoms of breathlessness. Patients should be reviewed regularly to determine benefit, usage and ongoing requirement for oxygen.

AOT is delivered by portable oxygen systems, most commonly cylinders (Figure 47.2), but many patients find these difficult to manage as a result of their weight and size. The burden of AOT can outweigh any perceived symptom benefit and AOT has not been shown to improve quality of life or exercise capacity in the long term (Hardinge et al., 2015; Uronis et al., 2015). Smaller delivery systems, such as lightweight cylinders (Figure 47.3) and liquid oxygen can be more manageable for some patients and should be assessed on an individual basis. Patients with high respiratory rates (e.g. interstitial lung disease) can derive more benefit from AOT delivered at a high flow via Venturi mask.

Palliative oxygen therapy

Oxygen therapy is often considered for patients with advanced disease resulting in intractable breathlessness. However, in the absence of hypoxaemia there is little evidence that breathlessness is relieved by oxygen (Abernethy et al., 2010). Alternative strategies for managing breathlessness, such as fan therapy, breathlessness management techniques or opioids can be more effective (Davidson and Johnson, 2011; Kamal et al., 2012). Patients should be assessed individually to determine effect of palliative oxygen therapy (POT) on reducing symptom burden and improving quality of life (Hardinge et al., 2015).

Short burst oxygen therapy

Short burst oxygen therapy is described as intermittent use of oxygen for short periods and has traditionally been offered to patients for relief of breathlessness pre or post-exertion. It is usually provided via large static cylinders. There is no evidence that it improves quality of life or exercise capacity in respiratory disease used in this way and is not recommended (Hardinge et al., 2015).

Further reading

Hardinge M, Annandale J, Bourne S, et al. (2015) British Thoracic Society guidelines for home oxygen use in adults. *Thorax* 70: 1–143.

48 Other routes of administration

Currently inhaled medicines are the core treatment options for managing respiratory conditions as they are used to prevent and maintain symptoms primarily caused by the drug being delivered directly to the site of action (the airways). In some instances there can be a need to administer medicines via alternative routes such as intravenous, intradermal and intramuscular to provide a systemic advantage to managing the patient's respiratory condition.

Antibiotics

Oral antimicrobial agents are promoted particularly for general practice and parenteral antimicrobial agents for hospital practice. Antibiotics delivered directly to the airways by nebulisation have been shown to be very effective in managing pulmonary complications. Inhaled antibiotics are related to the local delivery of the drug to the lung resulting in much higher sputum concentrations than those of intravenous or oral agents. In addition, nebulised antibiotics seem to have a lower side effect profile and toxicity.

Patients with a pulmonary exacerbation or with persisting low grade symptoms particularly in cystic fibrosis (CF), that are unresponsive to oral antibiotics should receive intravenous antibiotics through specialist hospital advice. For organisms other than *Pseudomonas aeruginosa* a single agent may be appropriate. For *P. aeruginosa*, a combination of two antibiotics with a different mechanisms of action should be used for intravenous treatment in specific respiratory patients. Ceftazidime and tobramycin are commonly used but meropenem and colistin is a suitable alternative combination. A once daily aminoglycoside regimen may be more convenient for most patients, though some find the use of a 30-minute infusion difficult. Once daily tobramycin is associated with less acute nephrotoxicity in children with CF.

In CF, tobramycin is the aminoglycoside of choice and gentamicin should be avoided. Co-administration of other nephrotoxic drugs should be avoided. Plasma creatinine should be measured before the first dose of tobramycin and again before the eighth dose. Trough and peak serum aminoglycoside levels should be measured depending upon the dosing regimen used. In patients receiving repeated courses of nephrotoxic antibiotics, glomerular filtration rate should be measured or estimated annually, along with plasma magnesium as a measure of renal tubular function. In order to reduce cochlear and vestibular toxicity the use of an aminoglycoside should be restricted to alternate courses of intravenous antibiotics, where the patient's clinical condition permits. Drug allergy should be managed with an appropriate desensitisation regimen. Antibiotics use should be ideally initiated following specialist input from the microbiology department to ensure appropriate and effective use to minimise inappropriate resistance.

Vaccinations

Pneumococcal vaccinations are provided annually for all respiratory diseases (Chapter 6). The inactivated influenza vaccines given by intramuscular injection should be given preferably into the upper arm (or anterolateral thigh in infants). However, individuals with a bleeding disorder should be given vaccine by deep subcutaneous injection to reduce the risk of bleeding.

Intravenous bronchodilators

Parenteral β agonists should be reserved for those patients who cannot reliably use inhaled therapy. This approach is predominately used in a specialist setting to ensure appropriate management and monitoring. The regular use of β_2 agonists by the subcutaneous route is not recommended because the evidence of benefit is uncertain and it may be difficult to withdraw such treatment once started. β_2 agonists can also be given by intramuscular injection.

Methylxanthines

Theophylline has a narrow therapeutic range of 55–110 μmol/L (10–20 mg/L); blood levels should be within this range for maximum bronchodilatation and minimum side effects. The pharmacokinetics of methylxanthines are complex and can be influenced by many factors.

Plasma clearance of therapy is reduced in patients with severe congestive heart failure, cor pulmonale, pulmonary oedema, severe liver disease and hypoxaemic state. The dose may need to be lowered in these patients.

Theophylline clearance is increased in smokers, with macrolide and quinolone antibiotics, calcium channel blockers, and cimetidine. In addition, plasma theopylline levels may be reduced by rifampacin, lithium, phenytoin and carbamazapine (see current BNF for complete listing).

Signs of toxicity: nausea, vomiting, diarrhea, tremor, epigastric headache, insomnia, hypotension, cardiac arrhythmias and convulsions.

Magnesium sulfate

A single dose of magnesium sulfate injection (unlicensed indication) 1.2–2 g (equivalent to approx. 4.8–8 mmol Mg^{2+}) by intravenous infusion over 20 minutes can be used for patients with severe acute asthma, but evidence of benefit is limited.

Leukotriene receptor agonists

Cysteinyl leukotrienes are mediators involved in the inflammatory process of asthma. Anti-leukotriene medication is used in asthma and allergic rhinitis to block leukotriene receptor sites and inhibit both early and late response to allergens.

Mucolytics

These are mucus controlling agents that work by altering the molecular composition of mucus, making it less thick and sticky and easier to expectorate. They are used in COPD and bronchiectasis when patients have difficulty expectorating despite being well hydrated and using optimal chest clearance techniques.

Anti-IgE monoclonal antibodies

These are used in IgE-mediated asthma when guideline therapy has failed to control symptoms. They block IgE from binding to the mast cells and thus decrease the allergic response. They are only prescribed from specialist centres under consultant management.

Further reading

Simmons M. (2012) *Pharmacology: An Illustrated Review*. Thieme, New York.

49 Adherence and concordance

An important part of the management of long-term conditions such as asthma and chronic obstructive pulmonary disease (COPD) is to encourage active management on the patient's part. This is important given that many patients may only encounter clinicians once a year. It has been recognised for a long time, however, that adherence to treatment regimens is suboptimal in many cases, and indeed may be so even where treatment periods are short, as in the case of antibiotics. This chapter describes how poor adherence can be classified, offers specific examples related to respiratory care and discusses ways in which adherence can be optimised.

Classifying adherence

The easiest way is to consider this as either *intentional* or *non-intentional*. In intentional non-adherence, patients make conscious decisions not to adhere to advice or prescriptions. Reasons for this vary, but common ones include the following:

- Fear of side effects from a drug. Steroids are often cited as inducing anxiety in patients. Almost two-thirds of patients in one study expressed fear regarding side effects of inhaled corticosteroids (Boulet, 1998).
- Misunderstanding. For example, patients with poorly controlled asthma who are prescribed a long-acting β_2 agonist (LABA) as add-on therapy may think the LABA replaces the inhaled corticosteroid (ICS) they are already taking – hence the need to prescribe combination inhalers in these circumstances.
- Perceived lack of efficacy. ICS will take a number of days to produce noticeable improvements in asthma and patients may not be aware of this. Patients with COPD receiving long-term oxygen therapy may not appreciate the rationale for the therapy and expect marked improvements in their breathing.
- Cost can be an issue for some people who do not qualify for free prescriptions.

Unintentional non-adherence implies that the patient is willing to follow advice, but has, for example, forgotten some elements of that advice, or perhaps lacks technical skill in some way. Common examples here include the following:

- Confusion of dosing schedules – for instance in asthma, the patient may be taking a reliever medication regularly and a preventer medication on a PRN basis.
- Simply forgetting to take regularly prescribed medication for asthma or COPD.
- In respiratory care, poor inhaler technique is a common, important and avoidable example of unintentional non-adherence (Lavorini et al,. 2008).

Other areas of poor adherence in respiratory care include failure to adhere to, or fabrication of, peak flow recordings; underuse of home-based non-invasive ventilation; overuse of bronchodilator drugs; and continued smoking in the presence of established respiratory disease.

Optimising adherence

Arguably, good communication, teaching and demonstration where appropriate will resolve many issues. However, it is well recognised that many patients have quite complex health beliefs which may clash with advice given by clinicians. On a simple level, any of the following could be considered as basic issues in improving adherence:

- Discuss diagnosis and treatment with patients; explain how treatments work, timescales, what sort of improvements might be expected.
- Ask about concerns, for instance, side effects of treatments. Many of these may be exaggerated concerns, and can be easily dealt with.
- Try to be concise – keep things simple.
- Some evidence indicates that summarising a consultation or discussion into 4–5 main areas can enhance patients' recall of a consultation.
- Avoid overloading patients with information – this is easily done and can lead to dissatisfaction – both of these issues individually can decrease adherence, as they can in combination.
- For inhaler technique, demonstration of technique using a placebo device (even if it is the clinician using it) is superior to simply describing how to use it to the patient (Chapter 44).
- Use of written information is useful but care should be taken as poor leaflet design (including use of language, size of type, presentation of the information and other issues) can be counter-productive.
- In relation to the above, a specific example is the use of written care/action plans. There is an abundance of evidence for these in asthma (e.g. Gibson and Powell, 2004), and a smaller body for COPD (e.g. Bucknall et al., 2012; Walters et al. 2010). See Chapter 39 for further information on self-management.

Further reading

Lavorini F, Magnan A, Dubus C, et al. (2008) Effect of incorrect use of dry powder inhalers on management of patients with asthma and COPD. *Respir Med* 102: 593–564.

Walters J, Turnock A, Walters E, Wood-Baker R. (2010) Action plans with limited patient education only for exacerbations of chronic obstructive pulmonary disease. *Cochrane Database Syst Rev* 5: CD005074.

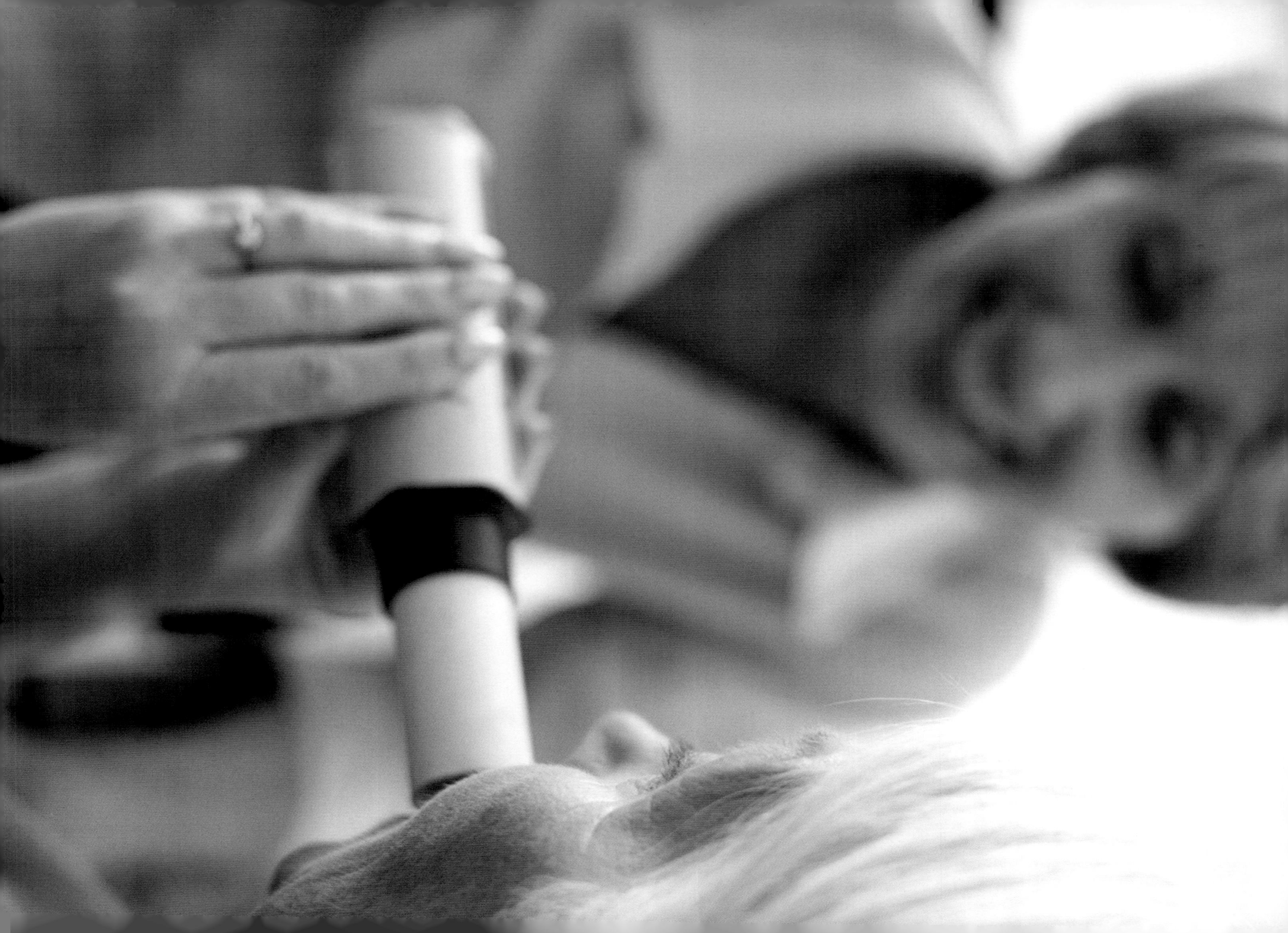

Acute care of the respiratory patient

Part 7

Chapters

Overview

Part 7 gives an overview of some aspects of caring for the acutely ill respiratory patient. While it is not possible to include all presentations here some of the more common ones are discussed and the main management strategies outlined. Non-invasive ventilation, tracheostomy care and pleural procedures are summarised.

50 Respiratory failure

Table 50.1 Conditions causing respiratory failure

Type	Examples	Part of lungs
Conditions that affects the blood flow and cause damage	Pulmonary embolism	Pulmonary artery
Conditions that affect the nerves and muscles	Muscular dystrophy Amyotrophic lateral sclerosis (ALS) Spinal cord injuries	Diaphragm
Conditions that affect the brain	Stroke Drugs/alcohol overdose	Brain
Conditions that affect the flow of air into and out of the lungs	COPD Cystic fibrosis	Lungs
Conditions that affect the gas exchange in the alveoli (air sacs)	Acute respiratory distress syndrome (ARDS) Pneumonia	Alveoli (air sacs)

Box 50.1 Types of respiratory failure

Type 1 Hypoxaemic

PaO_2 <60 mmHg/8.0 kPa
$PaCO_2$ (low or normal)

Type 2 Hypercapnic

PaO_2 <60 mmHg/8.0 kPa
$PaCO_2$ >45 mmHg/6.0 kPa

Common causes of respiratory failure

Type I respiratory failure	Type II respiratory failure
Asthma	COPD
Pneumonia	Drugs overdose
COPD	Cystic fibrosis
Pulmonary oedema	Sleep apnoea
Pulmonary embolism	Chronic neuromuscular disorders
	Chest wall disorders
	Morbid obesity

Please note: Type I respiratory failure may deteriorate to type II respiratory failure

Figure 50.1 Demonstrating the action of the mechanical pump during respiration

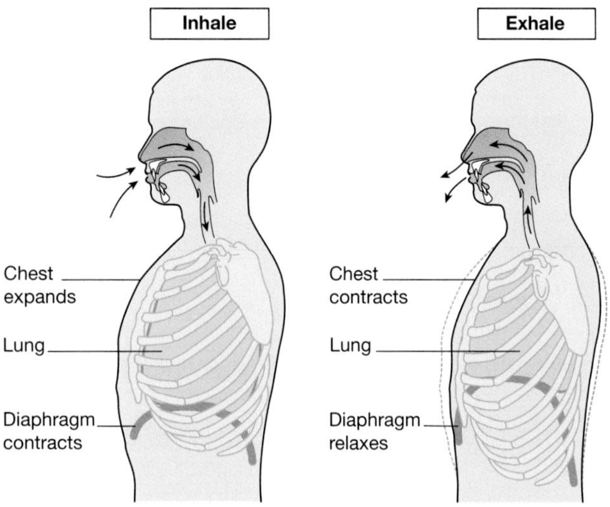
Inhale
Exhale
Chest expands
Lung
Diaphragm contracts
Chest contracts
Lung
Diaphragm relaxes

Figure 50.2 Demonstrating a pulmonary shunt
Note underventilating alveoli unable to pick up deoxygenated blood

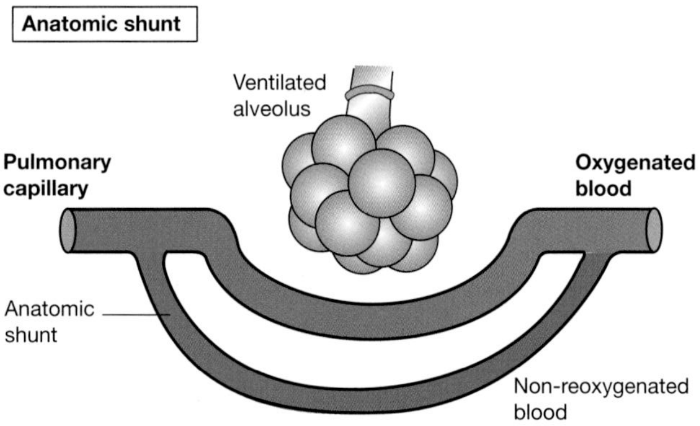
Anatomic shunt
Ventilated alveolus
Pulmonary capillary
Oxygenated blood
Anatomic shunt
Non-reoxygenated blood

Figure 50.3 Symptoms of respiratory acidosis

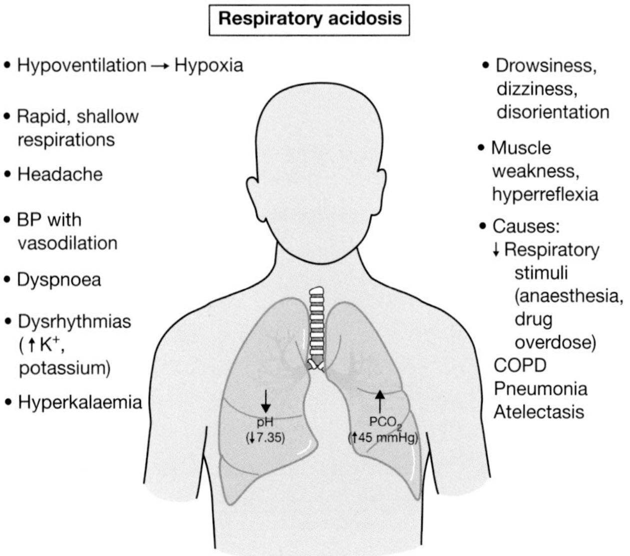
Respiratory acidosis
• Hypoventilation → Hypoxia
• Rapid, shallow respirations
• Headache
• BP with vasodilation
• Dyspnoea
• Dysrhythmias (↑K+, potassium)
• Hyperkalaemia
• Drowsiness, dizziness, disorientation
• Muscle weakness, hyperreflexia
• Causes: ↓Respiratory stimuli (anaesthesia, drug overdose) COPD Pneumonia Atelectasis
pH (↓7.35)
PCO2 (↑45 mmHg)

What is respiratory failure?

Respiratory failure falls into two categories and two subtypes. First, the failure of gases to exchange effectively to maintain the internal equilibrium of the body. Secondly, the piston/pump mechanism fails to produce enough mechanical force to ventilate alveoli resulting in decreased gas exchange which can in time result in an acid–base imbalance and hypoxia.

The subtypes are type 1 respiratory failure (hypoxia), which is often linked to an acute episode, and type 2 respiratory failure (hypercapnia) which is linked to an acute, chronic or acute on chronic respiratory failure, where underlying CO_2 retention already occurs and an acute episode exacerbates the retention. Depending on which category and cause for respiratory failure occurs, the results and treatments vary.

Failure of gas exchange

Oxygenation

As already seen in Chapter 20, the ability to exchange gases effectively is paramount for the body to function to its maximum capacity. To oxygenate effectively the lungs require:

1 An adequate supply of oxygen and the ability to expel CO_2
2 A toned and well-tuned mechanical pump to create enough pressure to inflate alveoli to allow gas exchange to occur with little or no resistance.

When failure occurs because of conditions affecting the brain (e.g. cerebrovascular accident) the flow of oxygen into and out of the lungs (e.g. chronic obstructive pulmonary disease), blockages limiting or preventing the flow of oxygen and carbon dioxide in and out of the pulmonary system (e.g. pulmonary embolism) and conditions affecting the nerve and muscle supply which assist the mechanical pump system to inflate and deflate the lungs as seen in Figure 50.1 is required. As a result, the respiratory system attempts to modify the impact of the failure by adjusting mechanisms that monitor acid–base balance (Chapter 20). When the body becomes overwhelmed by prolonged management or an acute change with no time to react, the result is failure to maintain internal equilibrium and external treatment is required to optimise patient outcome.

The mechanical pump

The function of contracting chest muscles and the diaphragm is to create a negative pressure within the thorax to draw air into the airways and down the peripheries of the pulmonary system (alveoli) to facilitate gas exchange (Tortora et al., 1993). As the diaphragm relaxes, the air flows out of the lungs and rises into a dome shape which rises into the thorax. When the diaphragm contracts it pulls downwards causing a negative pressure within the thorax which pulls air into the lungs (Figure 50.1). The effectiveness of this cycle is dependent on the pleura, the tone and effectiveness of the intercostal muscles, the elasticity of connective tissue and an undisturbed flow of neurones from the respiratory centre found in the medulla oblongata.

Types of respiratory failure

Type 1 respiratory failure

Hypoxia denotes low levels of oxygen. Despite low levels of oxygen, the carbon dioxide levels remain normal or low. Research suggests that the main contributing factors for this are V/Q mismatch and shunt (Kaynar, 2015). Ventilation/perfusion (V/Q) mismatch is the lungs' inability to oxygenate because of damage to the lung tissue. The remaining lung is still able to excrete CO_2 because less functioning tissue is required for CO_2 excretion. Bronchial spasm, pulmonary oedema, pulmonary emboli, lung injury or inhalation of a foreign object, consolidation and acute respiratory distress syndrome are all precursors for type 1 respiratory failure as they all affect how oxygen travels from the alveoli to the circulatory system (Box 50.1).

Inter-pulmonary shunting relates to well-perfused alveoli but the inability for the oxygen to diffuse across into circulatory system which results in deoxygenated blood recirculating and not being able to offload already utilised oxygen and pick up oxygen ready to recirculate, resulting in hypoxaemia.

Type 2 respiratory failure

Known as hypercapnic ventilatory failure, this occurs when alveolar ventilation is inefficient which affects the transport out of the lungs of carbon dioxide. Alveolar ventilation pressure is reduced when the piston/pump mechanism becomes ineffective. The chemo-receptors of the medulla oblongata and the peripheral nervous system respond to changes in blood gas tensions and determine how fast and deep we breathe to eliminate CO_2 and take in more O_2. When ventilation is inefficient, an accumulation of CO_2 occurs and over a short or long period of time the CNS becomes overwhelmed and an increase in CO_2 occurs (Chapter 20) resulting in type 2 respiratory failure – $>CO_2$, $<pH$ – hypercapnia with respiratory acidosis. Causes of type 2 respiratory failure are shown in Figure 50.2.

Treatment options

Treatment options depend on the severity of respiratory failure and a full review of the patient's clinical condition.

Type 1 respiratory failure

Supplemental oxygen is given either by a facemask or continuous positive airway pressure (CPAP), control of secretions (physiotherapy), antibiotics to treat infection and bronchodilators. If the failure is life-threatening the patient may need to be invasively ventilated to reduce the load on the respiratory muscles.

Type 2 respiratory failure

As for the type 1 failure, treatment with controlled oxygen and regular blood gas analysis is advocated (BTS, 2016). However, if the hypercapnia is impacting on the patient's CNS then the treatment options will focus on non-invasive ventilation which may provide respite to allow other therapies to work and thus avoid endotracheal intubation (BTS, 2016).

Further reading

British Thoracic Society (BTS). (2016) Ventilatory management of acute hypercapnic respiratory failure guideline. https://www.brit-thoracic.org.uk/guidelines-and-quality-standards/ventilatory-management-of-acute-hypercapnic-respiratory-failure-guideline/ (accessed 24 March 2016).

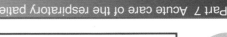

51 Pre-hospital care

Figure 51.1 The Manchester triage model
Source: ALSG (2014) Emergency Triage, 3rd edn. Reproduced with permission of John Wiley & Sons Ltd.

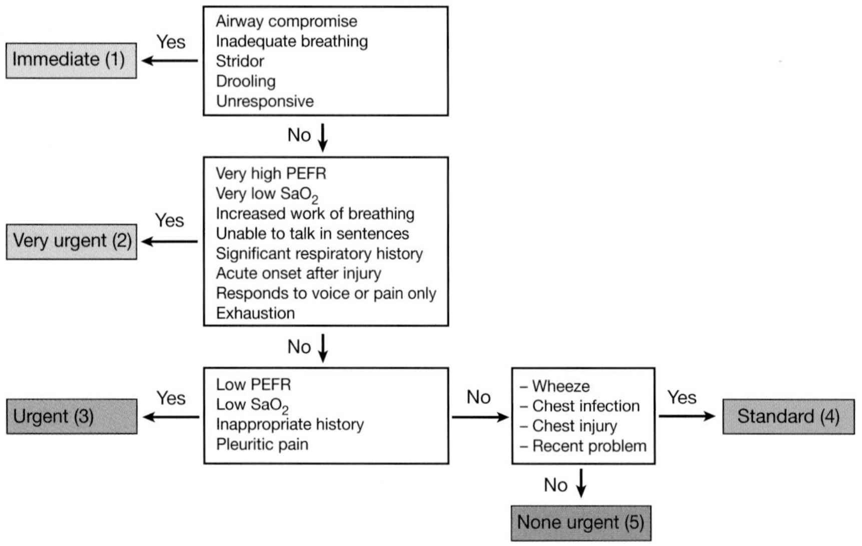
Airway compromise
Inadequate breathing
Stridor
Drooling
Unresponsive
Yes
Immediate (1)
No
Very high PEFR
Very low SaO_2
Increased work of breathing
Unable to talk in sentences
Significant respiratory history
Acute onset after injury
Responds to voice or pain only
Exhaustion
Yes
Very urgent (2)
No
Low PEFR
Low SaO_2
Inappropriate history
Pleuritic pain
Yes
Urgent (3)
No
– Wheeze
– Chest infection
– Chest injury
– Recent problem
Yes
Standard (4)
No
None urgent (5)

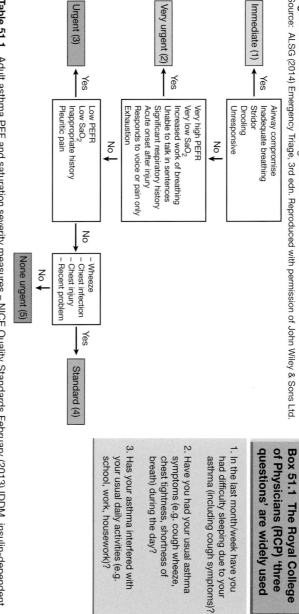

Box 51.1 The Royal College of Physicians (RCP) 'three questions' are widely used

1. In the last month/week have you had difficulty sleeping due to your asthma (including cough symptoms)?
2. Have you had your usual asthma symptoms (e.g. cough wheeze, chest tightness, shortness of breath) during the day?
3. Has your asthma interfered with your usual daily activities (e.g. school, work, housework)?

Table 51.1 Adult asthma PEF and saturation severity measures – NICE Quality Standards February (2013) IDDM, insulin-dependent diabetes mellitus; LTOT, long-term oxygen therapy

Factor	Treat at home	Treat at hospital
Able to cope at home	Yes	No
Breathlessness	Mild	Severe
General condition	Good	Poor/deteriorating
Level of activity	Good	Poor/confined to bed
Cyanosis	No	Yes
Worsening peripheral oedema	No	Yes
Level of consciousness	Normal	Impaired
Already on LTOT	No	Yes
Social circumstances	Good	Alone/not coping
Acute confusion	No	Yes
Rapid onset	No	Yes
Significant co-morbidity (particularly cardiac and IDDM)	No	Yes
SaO_2 <90%	No	Yes
Changes in chest radiograph	No	Present
Arterial pH level	≥7.35	<7.35
Arterial PaO_2	≥7 kPa	<7 kPa

Table 51.2 Adult asthma peak expiratory flow (PEF) and saturation severity measures

Measure peak expiratory flow (PEF) and arterial saturation		
PEF >50–75% best or predicted	PEF 33–60% best predicted	PEF 33% best predicted
Moderate asthma	**Acute severe asthma**	**Life-threatening asthma**
SpO_2 ≥0.2% PEF >50–75% best or predicted No features of acute severe asthma	Features of severe asthma • PEF <50% best predicted • Respiration ≥25/minute • SpO_2 ≥92% • Pulse ≥110 breaths/minute • Cannot complete sentence in 1 breath	• SpO_2 <92% • Silent chest, cyanosis, poor respiratory effort • Arrhythmia, hypotension • Exhaustion, altered consciousness

Table 51.3 Dyspnoea, obstruction, smoking and exacerbation (DOSE) frequency >4 is associated with admission or respiratory failure

	DOSE index points			
	0	**1**	**2**	**3**
MRC dyspnoea scale score	0–1	2	3	4
Obstructive FEV_1 % predicted	>50	30–49	<30	
Smoking status	Non-smoker	Smoker		
Exacerbations per year	0–1	2–3	<3	

Pre-hospital care involves a multi-disciplinary approach, and is delivered in many different settings such as the GP surgery, clinic, the patient's own home and pharmacy. The aim of pre-hospital care is to aid symptom control, optimise treatment and prevent hospital admissions and re-admissions. This chapter covers exacerbation management in the pre-hospital setting (community), discuss factors to consider when deciding to admit a patient or continue treating in the home or elsewhere. Before reading this chapter please ensure you have referred to the chapters on respiratory assessment, examination, respiratory medications and investigations.

Triaging a respiratory patient

Triage helps the clinician to decide on the urgency and order of treatment needed. The word comes from the French verb *tier*, to separate. Originally a battlefield system for assessing wounds, the NHS has adapted various models. However, triage has its limitations as using one tool for all situations can cause problems as some factors are not taken into account within these models (e.g. age, morbidities, pregnancy or obesity). Many triage models are aimed at acute hospital care. For example, the Manchester triage system has limitations in that it lacks specific observation parameters to follow so may be open to interpretation (Figure 51.1). There can be limitations for triage in the community which result from a lack of access to information regarding the patient. Additionally, access to certain types of diagnostic and blood tests may not be available. Telephone triage is often adopted in GP surgeries as a way of treating patients who cannot get an appointment or are housebound. However, the patient cannot be examined and it must be acknowledged that treatment decisions are based on patient-reported symptoms only, so this may not be suitable for some patients. As triage involves consultation, patient safety is a consideration especially if carried out remotely and should conclude with safety netting, whereby there are clear instructions in case of emergency.

Managing an acute exacerbation pre-hospital

If the patient has been triaged and a decision has been made that the best place to continue care is in the home, and it is safe to do so, available treatment options will need to be considered. Some areas have access to respiratory specialist teams in the community; many areas have local treatment guidelines and formularies which are easily accessible via the internet or NHS organisations. A face-to-face assessment with an experienced clinician can be more appropriate for acute severe illness than a telephone review. Community clinicians have access to a variety of investigations to aid the decision to treat at home such as chest X-ray and blood results including point of care blood gas analysis or C-reactive protein (CRP).

NICE COPD (2010) and BTS asthma (2014) guidance recommend individualised management plans, so that patients and practitioners recognise and treat infection and exacerbation early. There are many types of plans available on the internet which are symptom-based, or rely on set parameters such as peak flow. The plan should be discussed with the patient to see which fits best and will be more successful.

Management plans for patients with chronic obstructive pulmonary disease (COPD) include oral corticosteroids for increased breathlessness and antibiotics for purulent sputum. Management plans should direct patient decision making by providing rescue packs of antibiotics and steroids. This can help to reduce future treatment delays in appropriate patients. However, plans should advise the patient to make contact with their health care professional if they fail to improve, and adapting or reviewing the plan may be indicated.

Ongoing review should be agreed with the patient when the plan is initiated to provide monitoring and action needed. This can include sign-posting to other clinical teams and adjustment of therapies, dependent on the severity, control and type of respiratory disease, as well as response to treatment which dictates how often review will be required.

Scoring and decision tools

There are condition-specific tools such as the COPD Decision to Admit tool (NICE 2010). This guides admission to hospital or staying at home (NICE, 2010, Table 51.1). However, this type of tool relies on clinical judgement and access to blood testing to aid decision making which may not available, so it may need to be adapted. Other tools that can be found online include: dyspnoea scoring tools, Medical Respiratory Council (MRC), Royal College of Physicians (RCGP) 3 questions for asthma (Box 51.1), peak expiratory flow (PEF) and saturation severity measures (Table 51.2), early warning scoring, CURB-65 for pneumonia, BODE and DOSE index (Table 51.3). Factors such as health care consumption or mortality risk can be determined by the score or number of triggers identified when using these tools. For example, Jones et al. (2009) found DOSE scores over 4 increased the risk of admission, GP visits, accident and emergency attendances and bed days. Not all of these will be needed and individually they can be used to direct care, for example an MRC of 3 or above would be an indication to offer pulmonary rehabilitation for patients with COPD, reduced peak flows without exacerbation in patients with asthma, and can indicate a lack of control requiring treatment adjustments or referral to a specialist.

It is important to involve the patient in the decision making process but sometimes the patient may not agree (e.g. when a hospital admission is indicated). Refusal to accept care decisions must be documented and discussion with other professionals and family members are sometimes indicated.

Further reading

Jones RC, Donaldson GC, Chavannes NH, et al. (2009) Derivation and validation of a composite index of severity in chronic obstructive pulmonary disease: the DOSE Index. *Am J Respir Crit Care Med* 180: 1189–1195.

52 Non-invasive and invasive ventilation

Box 52.1 Ceiling of care decisions, to be made and documented by an experienced doctor (second year specialist trainee or above) early in the treatment

1. Immediate intubation
2. Suitable for NIV but escalation to intubation if NIV fails
3. Suitable for NIV but not for intubation
4. For full active medical treatment but not NIV
5. For palliative care

Box 52.2 Contraindications to using non-invasive ventilation (NIV)

- Need for immediate intubation e.g. respiratory arrest
- Acute asthma
- Undrained pneumothorax
- Uncontrolled vomiting
- Fixed upper airway obstruction
- Facial trauma, burns or surgery making it impossible to apply a mask or worsen the 'wound' significantly

Table 52.1 Settings for safe delivery of NIV

Level 1 (e.g. respiratory ward or admissions unit)	Level 2/3 (e.g. high dependency unit)
• pH 7.25–7.35	• pH <7.25
• Single organ failure	• Multiple organ failure
• Adequate numbers of competent staff	

Box 52.3 Treatment aims

- Improve pH >7.35 by reducing pCO2
- Maintain adequate oxygenation, SpO_2 88–92%

Table 52.2 Troubleshooting

Problem	Possible solution
Failure to increase or normalise pH	• Check mask/circuit for leak • Ensure no patient ventilator asynchrony • Increase pressure support by increasing IPAP
Failure to reduce pCO_2	• Increase pressure support by increasing IPAP • Check exhalation port patency • Check for excessive mask leak or patient/ventilator asynchrony
Low SpO_2 or pO_2	• Increase FiO_2 by entraining oxygen or more oxygen into the circuit • Increase EPAP (increasing IPAP by equal amount to maintain the same pressure support)
Excessive mask leak	• Take off and refit mask, ensuring equal pressure through all straps • Change angle of mask if possible so pressure greater at point of leak (e.g. adjust forehead support) • Check mask sizing – replace if too big or small • Mask fitted too tight – uncomfortable and can cause pressure sores • Try alternative mask • Shave a beard • Put well fitting dentures in
Patient ventilator asynchrony	• Check and correct any excessive mask leak • Adjust ventilator triggers • Back up rate set too high

Figure 52.1 Nasal mask

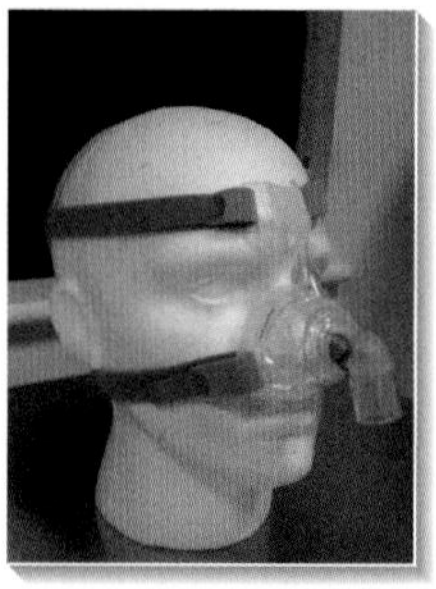

Figure 52.2 Full face mask

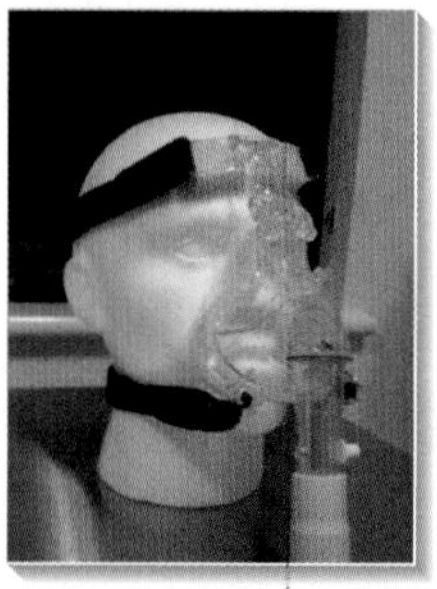

Figure 52.3 Total face mask

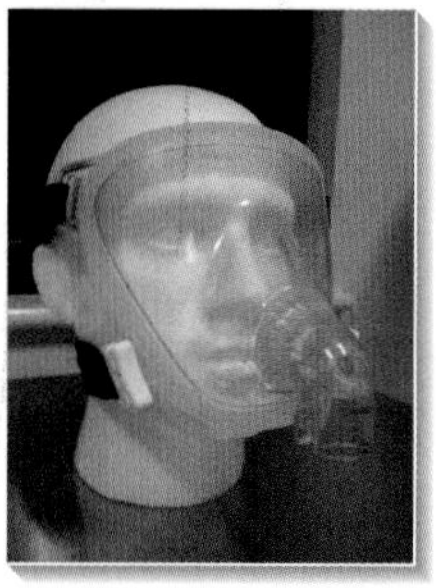

Box 52.4 Factors that can increase failure rates and reduce threshold for intubation during trial of NIV

- Pneumonia
- Life-threatening hypoxaemia
- Haemodynamic instability
- Severe co-morbidities
- Copius secretions
- Confused/agitation
- Inability to protect airway

Non-invasive ventilation

Non-invasive ventilation (NIV) is a first line treatment in the management of a respiratory acidosis secondary to an acute hypercapnic respiratory failure (type 2 respiratory failure). The severity of the acidosis reflects the severity of the condition and provides a guide to prognosis. This form of assisted bi-level ventilation is delivered by the provision of positive pressure through a well-fitting mask.

The benefits of NIV are reductions in mortality, need for intubation, length of hospital stay and hospital costs. Patients are able to have breaks to eat, drink, communicate, cough and expectorate sputum as well as to have treatments such as nebulisers and physiotherapy. Although the main body of evidence is in chronic onstructive pulmonary disease (COPD), it can also be used for patients with obesity hypoventilation, neuromuscular disease, decompensated obstructive sleep apnoea, chest wall disease (e.g. kyphoscoliosis) and cardiogenic pulmonary oedema unresponsive to continuous positive airway pressure (CPAP).

Prior to initiating NIV

A diagnosis should be established and any reversible causes treated including maintaining the SpO_2 88–92% to ensure treatment of hypoxaemia and excessive oxygen is not contributing to the hypercapnia and acidosis. A decision on the ceiling of treatment should be established before initiating NIV (Box 52.1), involving the patient and family. Early initiation will result in better outcomes, although contraindications will need excluding (Box 52.2). Informed consent should be obtained and the patient made aware of the importance and effectiveness of this treatment. For those receiving NIV but whose ceiling of care is intubation, early liaison with critical care staff facilitates a smooth transfer of care should NIV fail and could also influence the setting in which NIV is delivered (Table 52.1).

Ventilator modes and settings

A spontaneous/timed (S/T) or pressure support (PS) mode allows the patient to trigger the breaths and synchronise with the ventilator. The back-up rate will ensure the ventilator delivers a breath should the patient's respiratory rate fall or if he or she develops apnoea.

The ventilator delivers two levels of pressure: the inspiratory positive airway pressure (IPAP) and an expiratory positive airway pressure (EPAP), with the difference between the two being the pressure support (PS). The IPAP and PS deliver the pressure to inflate the alveoli; this increases the tidal volume (breath size) which results in the patient exhaling excess carbon dioxide (CO_2). The EPAP help splint open any collapsed small airways to recruit more alveoli or larger airways that collapse (e.g. in obstructive sleep apnoea), and helps improve oxygenation. Healthy lungs (e.g. neuromuscular conditions) need lower levels of EPAP. Conditions such as COPD can require moderate amounts of EPAP (6 cmH_2O). Overweight patients can require higher levels of EPAP (8–10 cmH_2O). EPAP can help to alleviate pulmonary oedema.

Pressure support should be optimised in response to the blood gas results until resolution of the acidosis (Box 52.3). It can also help to reduce tachypnoea (high respiratory rate). The increase in tidal volume for each breath can reduce the need to breathe so fast.

Interfaces

Mask selection and sizing is crucial to ensure effective ventilation by minimising leak and optimising patient comfort. Masks covering the nose and mouth are preferable as patients tend to mouth breath making nasal masks ineffective (Figure 52.1, Figure 52.2 and Figure 52.3). Most ventilators will compensate for a small mask leak so avoid over-tightening as this is uncomfortable and can cause pressure sores. If non-vented masks are used then breathing circuits must have an exhalation port to allow CO_2 excretion and improved hypercapnia. Oxygen can be entrained into the circuit at a flow rate to maintain SpO_2 88–92%.

Monitoring

Patients require close monitoring including continuous saturation checks and intermittent physiological measurements of respiratory rate, heart rate (ECG for first 12 hours), blood pressure and consciousness. Monitor for significant mask leak and patient ventilator synchrony (Table 52.2). Blood gas assessment is crucial to establish if the acidosis has resolved, at a minimum recorded at 1, 4 and 12 hours following initiation or after an hour of increased pressures. The frequency and discomfort of this may require the placement of arterial lines. Assess patient comfort with encouragement and reassurance as it is important to optimise adherence as approximately 20% will not be able to tolerate NIV or fail treatment (Box 52.4).

Breaks and weaning

NIV should be encourages as much as possible in the first 24 hours but short breaks are acceptable provided the patient's condition allows. Oxygen can be given during these periods to maintain SpO_2 88–92%. Treatment will usually continue for 48–72 hours and weaning takes place by reducing the time on NIV and not reducing the PS. Time should be reduced in the day before stopping the treatment at night. A small number of patients require treatment to continue at home (Chapter 60).

Training, competency and audit

All health care professionals involved in the care of patients receiving NIV should have the appropriate training and competency assessment. Refresher training is also important to maintain these skills and competency. Having experienced staff with local protocols are central to a successful service. Regular audit can ensure an effective service and identify areas for improvement.

Invasive mechanical ventilation

Invasive mechanical ventilation (IMV) differs from NIV in that it requires the insertion of an artificial airway in the form of an endotracheal or tracheostomy tube and has considerable risks (e.g. trauma, infection). IMV should be considered when:

- It has been decided it is an appropriate ceiling of care
- Respiratory arrest or peri-arrest on NIV with no clinical improvement despite treatment
- Unable to obtain a satisfactory mask fit on NIV
- IMV likely to give a better patient outcome
- pH <7.15 despite optimal therapy, or pH <7.25 despite optimal NIV therapy
- Significant clinical deterioration despite optimal NIV therapy.

NIV can be used successfully to support the weaning process from IMV. Its benefits include a reduction in mortality, length of stay, complications, it can accelerate extubation and a reduction in the need for re-intubation.

Further reading

BTS/RCP London/Intensive Care Society (2008) The use of non-invasive ventilation in the management of patients with chronic obstructive pulmonary disease admitted to hospital with acute type II respiratory failure. https://www.brit-thoracic.org.uk/guidelines-and-quality-standards/non-invasive-ventilation-(niv)/ (accessed 29 February 2016).

53 Pleural procedures and management

Figure 53.1 Rocket® pleural aspiration kit
Source: Inset image reproduced with permission of Rocket Medical plc.

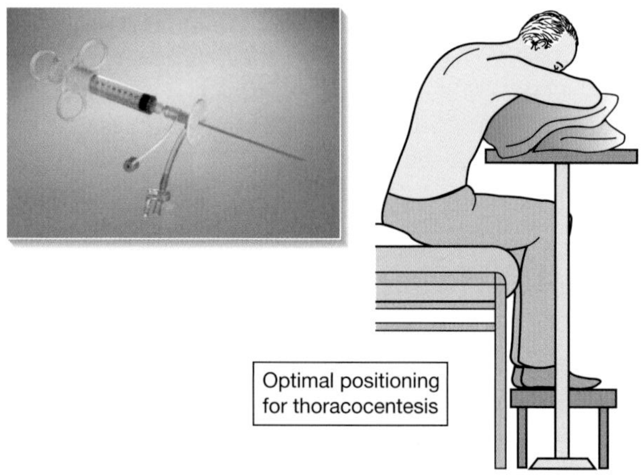
Optimal positioning
for thoracocentesis

Figure 53.2 Safe triangle

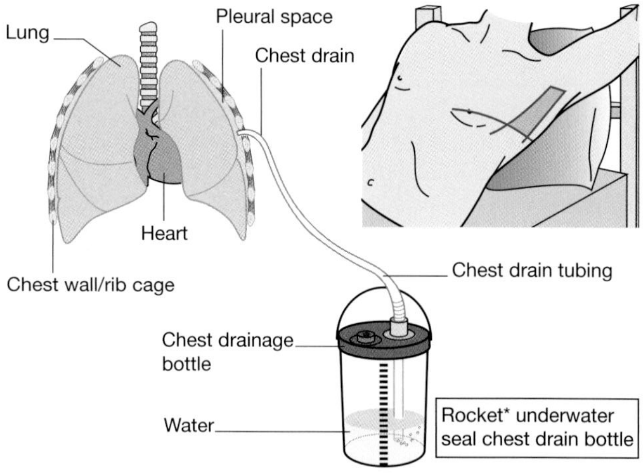
Lung
Pleural space
Chest drain
Heart
Chest wall/rib cage
Chest drain tubing
Chest drainage bottle
Water
Rocket* underwater seal chest drain bottle

Figure 53.3 Rocket® IPC dressing pack and bottle
Source: Image reproduced with permission of Rocket Medical plc.

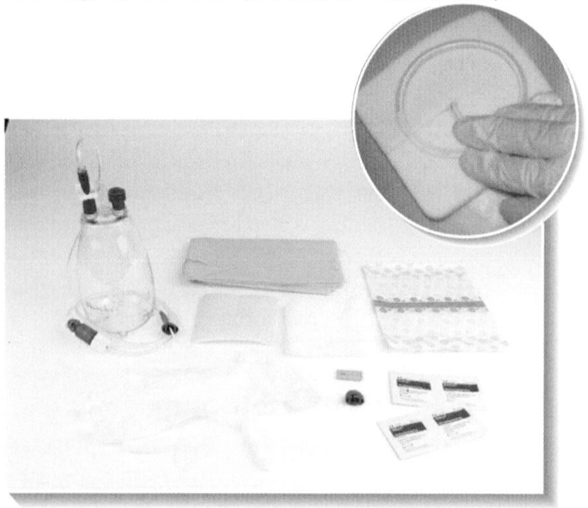

Figure 53.4 Medical thoracoscopy

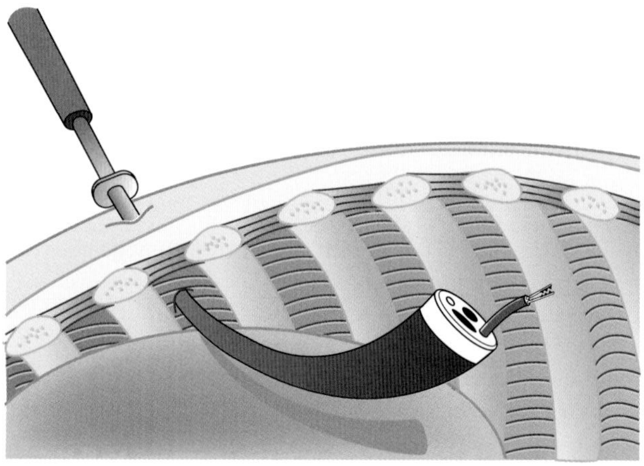

Figure 53.5 Instillation of talc via three-way tap on chest drain

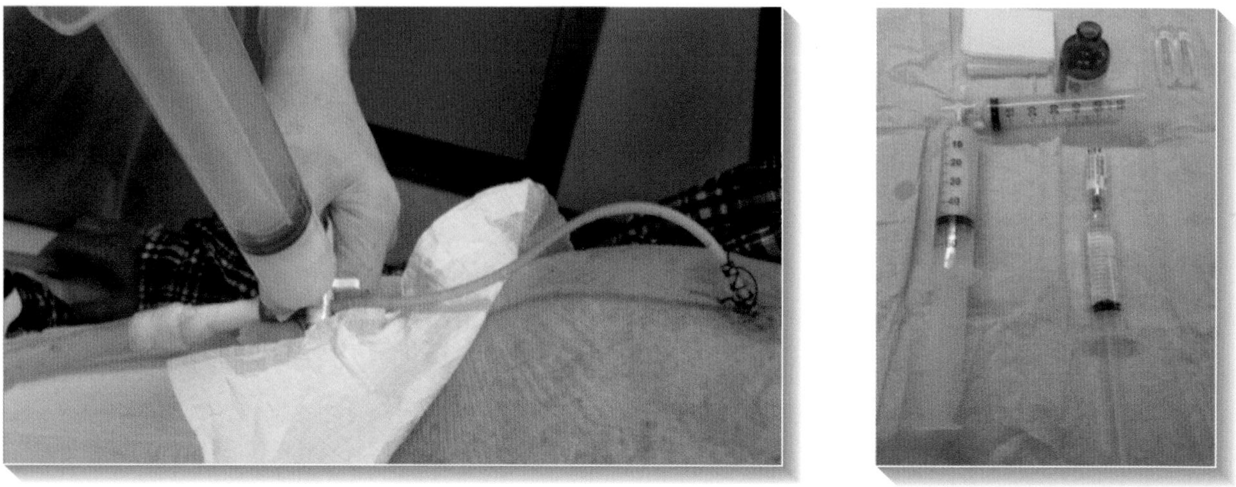

Pleural aspiration or thoracocentesis is a method used for sampling and/or draining fluid from the pleural space. It is performed to aid diagnosis in new cases of pleural effusion and for symptomatic relief in larger effusions.

The procedure is undertaken under local anaesthetic. The British Thoracic Society (BTS) strongly recommend the use of ultrasound guidance to reduce the risk of complications and improve the success rate. A diagnostic sample is aspirated with a fine bore (21G) needle and a 50-mL syringe. A purpose-made therapeutic aspiration kit (Figure 53.1) comprising a 6 French flexible fenestrated catheter and a large volume collection bag can be used to drain up to 1500 mL fluid; draining more than this puts the patient at risk of re-expansion pulmonary oedema. For diagnostic purposes fluid is sent for biochemistry, cytology and microbiological analysis. After the procedure a chest X-ray should be performed and the patient observed to monitor for any complications.

Risks associated with the procedure include pneumothorax, visceral injury, pain, bleeding, bruising and infection.

Intercostal drains

A chest drain is a hollow flexible tube inserted through the chest wall between the ribs and into the pleural cavity to allow drainage of air (pneumothorax), blood (haemothorax), fluid (pleural effusion) or pus (empyema) from the pleural space. Effective drainage requires an adequately positioned drain connected securely to a system with unidirectional flow, usually an underwater seal bottle.

Any coagulopathy defects are corrected prior to drain insertion to avoid bleeding. Other risks of the procedure include infection, pain and visceral injury. The drain should ideally be inserted in the 'safe triangle', which is delineated by the lateral border of the pectoralis major, the anterior border of the latissimus dorsi and a line horizontal with the nipple (Figure 53.2).

The drain is inserted aseptically under local anaesthetic and with ultrasound guidance to identify a safe insertion site. It is secured to the skin by a strong suture (i.e. '0' silk). Small drains (8–12 French) are inserted to minimise patient discomfort; larger drains require a wound closing suture to be tied post drain removal.

A chest X-ray ensures satisfactory position of the drain. Large pleural effusion drainage is controlled in order to prevent re-expansion pulmonary oedema by clamping the tube for 1–2 hours after draining up to 1.5 L. There is no need to clamp drains for pneumothoraces.

Chest tubes are removed when the original indication for placement is no longer present or the tube becomes non-functional. It is removed on deep expiratory breath hold or with the patient performing a valsalva manoeuvre, and the site covered with a dry occlusive dressing.

Indwelling pleural catheters

An indwelling pleural catheter (IPC) is a semi-permanent tunnelled catheter designed to drain recurrent pleural effusions (Figure 53.3). They are used predominantly in patients with malignant effusions re-accumulating rapidly, thereby minimising the need for repeated procedures so as to improve quality of life.

The IPC can be inserted during a day-case admission and is carried out under local anaesthetic. On occasion a once-only dose of prophylactic antibiotic is administered.

Initially, the catheter is secured with sutures which are generally removed after 14 days. A cuff on the catheter which sits in a subcutaneous tunnel secures its position from then on. The catheter can be managed at home by district nurses, carers or by patients themselves after suitable training has been given. Kits containing pre-vacuumed bottles and other items needed for drainage are available, making the task simple to manage.

Frequency of drainage is determined by the rate of accumulation of the effusion and by symptomatic evaluation. Frequent drainage and keeping the space dry can encourage auto-pleurodesis.

Risks involved with IPC insertion are pain, infection, bleeding and visceral injury. Ongoing risks include infection and loculated pleural space which may interfere with the efficacy of the drain, but these are infrequent. The drain can remain in situ as long as required and can be removed during a day-case admission under local anaesthetic if no longer needed.

Medical thoracoscopy

Medical thoracoscopy is a minimally invasive procedure that allows complete visualisation of the hemi-thorax and access to the pleural space using a combination of viewing and working instruments (Figure 53.4). It also allows for basic diagnostic (undiagnosed pleural fluid or pleural thickening) and therapeutic procedures (pleurodesis) to be performed safely. Lack of a pleural space, uncorrected coagulopathy and haemodynamic instability are contraindications to the procedure. Complications of medical thoracoscopy are uncommon. They include bleeding, infection of the pleural space and injury to intrathoracic organs.

This procedure is performed under local anaesthesia with or without conscious sedation with the patient positioned in lateral decubitus position with the affected hemi-thorax uppermost.

The thorascope is inserted via a trocar between the ribs into the pleural space. Fluid is evacuated using a suction catheter and the pleural cavity is inspected with the thorascope. Pleural biopsies are obtained from suspicious areas under direct vision. If indicated talc poudrage (pleurodesis) can be performed. Once the examination and procedures are completed, the scope is withdrawn, a chest drain is placed and the pneumothorax is evacuated.

Pleurodesis

Talc pleurodesis is a procedure that involves instilling sterile talc into the pleural space to prevent accumulation of air or fluid (Figure 53.5). The talc acts as an irritant, encouraging inflammation of the pleura and subsequent adherence of the lung to the chest wall. Pleurodesis is effective in 70–80% of cases.

Talc can be administered via chest drain once air or fluid has been drained and a chest X-ray shows good apposition of parietal and visceral pleura. Prior to pleurodesis, an appropriate oral analgesic is given and lidocaine is instilled into the pleural space to minimise discomfort.

When instilling talc via a chest drain for management of effusion, fluid output should be less than 200 mL per 24 hours for optimal results. The talc is diluted with normal saline and injected via a three-way tap which is then closed for up to 2 hours and then re-opened to allow drainage of any residual fluid. The drain is removed once drainage ceases.

Pleurodesis (talc poudrage) can also be performed during therapeutic medical thoracoscopy after the effusion is drained. The talc is introduced via the thoracic trocar using an atomiser.

Minor complications associated with talc pleurodesis include pain, fever, breathlessness and infection. More serious complications include acute respiratory distress syndrome (ARDS), but this is extremely rare.

Further reading

BTS (2016) www.brit-thoracic.org.uk/guidelines-and-quality-standards/pleural-disease-guideline/ (accessed 29 February 2016).

54 Tracheostomy care and management

Figure 54.1 Cuffed tracheostomy tube

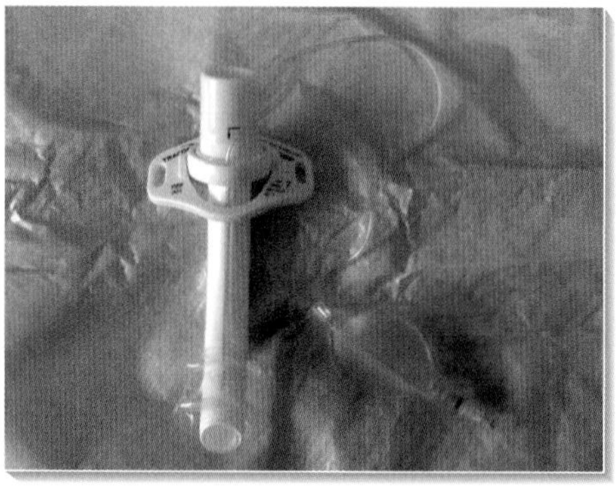

Figure 54.2 Uncuffed tracheostomy tube

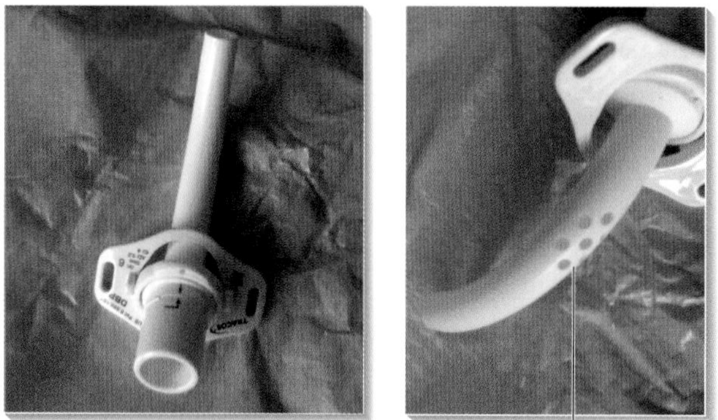
Fenestrated

Figure 54.3 Inner tubes

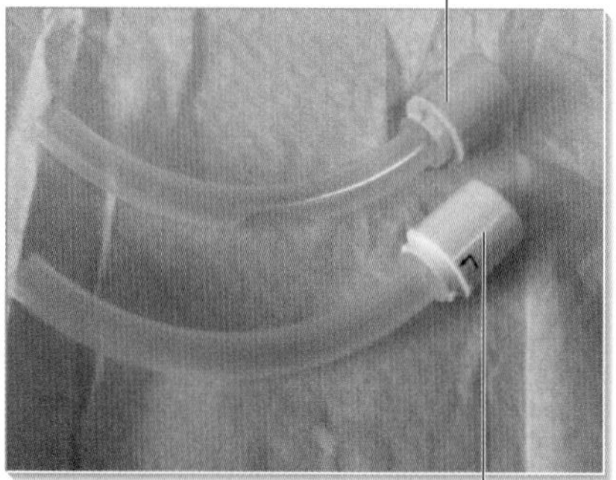
Inner tube with fenestration (blue top)
Non-fenestration inner tube (White top)

Figure 54.4 A secured tracheostomy tube and humidification system

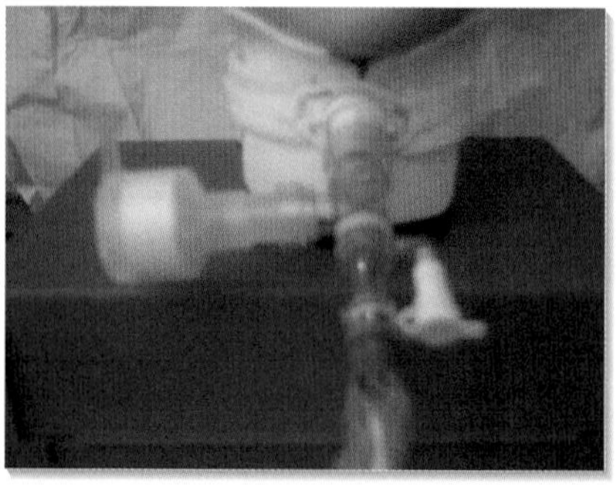

Figure 54.5 Speaking valve

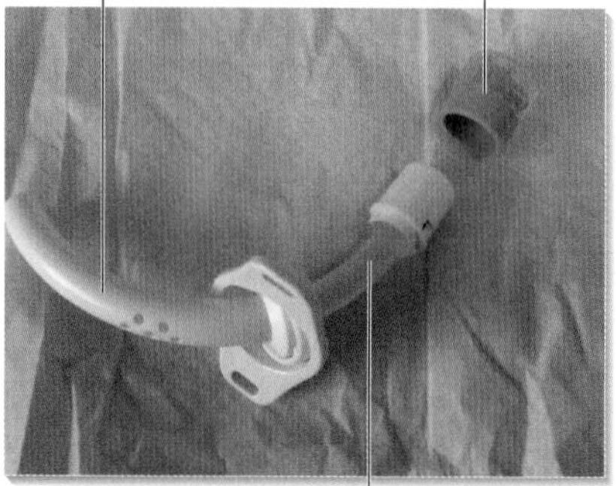
Uncuffed tracheostomy tube
Speaking valve
Fenestrated inner tube

Box 54.1 Clinical signs of tracheostomy tube obstruction

Early (tube becoming blocked):

- Clammy
- Pallor
- Panic
- Noisy respirations
- Seesaw respirations

Late (tube totally blocked):

- Absent breath sounds
- No chest expansion
- Central cyanosis
- Decreased level of consciousness

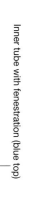

A tracheostomy is a surgical opening in the anterior wall of the trachea to facilitate breathing and the removal of secretions. It can be temporary or permanent and required for a variety of causes and circumstances.

Types of tracheostomy tube

Cuffed tubes are used when:

- There is a strong risk of aspiration
- To provide ventilation with a bag/valve system during resuscitation.

Patients with a tube that has the cuff inflated are unable to vocalise, as air does not pass over the vocal cords (Figure 54.1). Uncuffed tubes are used when there is a minimal risk of aspiration.

Both cuffed and uncuffed tubes have a removable non-fenestrated inner tube. The uncuffed tube also has a fenestrated inner tube (Figure 54.2).

Tracheostomy tubes can usually remain in situ for 30 days before changing but long-term tubes may stay in longer (see manufacturer's advice).

Unplanned removal of tracheostomy tube

Tracheostomy tubes can accidentally fall out or may be deliberately removed by the patient. By the time a patient has been transferred from ITU to a ward or home the stoma site is usually well established and a spare tracheostomy tube should be provided.

Care of inner tube

Tracheostomy inner tubes reduce the risk of occlusion and the need for frequent tube changes (Figure 54.3). They need to be kept clean, as a coating of secretions will reduce the size of the inner lumen and increase the work of breathing. Signs that the patient requires inner cannula change include:

- The patient is experiencing difficulty in breathing
- Secretions in the cannula that cannot be removed by tracheal suction/coughing
- The patient requests inner tube change
- The patient exhibits noisy breathing
- The patient stops breathing.

Securing the tube and wound care

The tracheostomy tube needs to remain in the correct position to maintain the patient's airway. Tube displacement occurs when a tube partially or completely comes out of the trachea and can lead to respiratory arrest if it is not possible to re-establish an airway.

A tracheostomy stoma is a full-thickness wound, which is susceptible to chemical and mechanical injury. Secretions can ooze out of the stoma site allowing the area to be persistently wet and can result in skin irritation and excoriation. The increased moisture can prevent the stoma site from healing and may act as a medium for bacterial growth.

Humidification

A tracheostomy bypasses the body's natural ability to warm, humidify and filter inspired air. The delivery of dry gases will slow the mucociliary elevator allowing secretion accumulation, mucosal crusting, increased airway resistance and a susceptibility to bronchial infection. The presence of a tracheostomy impedes the patient's ability to cough and clear secretions. These secretions then thicken and prove difficult to clear and in turn block the tracheostomy. It is essential to provide adequate humidification and hydration as failing to do this can be potentially fatal (Figure 54.4).

Suction

Tracheal suction is a necessary procedure but there are detrimental effects:

- Hypoxia
- Bradycardia
- Infection
- Mucosal damage
- Discomfort.

The frequency with which suction is required varies widely between patients. Some require hourly suction; others with a long-term tracheostomy seldom require suction. Each patient must be individually assessed.

Indications that the patient requires suctioning:

- Noisy or moist respirations
- Increased use of intercostals muscles
- Reduced oxygen saturation levels
- Increased or ineffective coughing
- Patient request.

Obstruction of a tracheostomy tube causes:

- Sputum plug
- Blood
- Foreign body
- Tube misplacement
- Kinking of the tube
- Over-inflation of the cuff
- Cuff herniation.

This can be recognised by:

- Unable to pass a suction catheter
- Clinical signs (Box 54.1).

Speaking valves

These can be used to help the patient vocalise. They should not be used if the patient develops copious secretions and requires frequent suction (Figure 54.5).

Nursing care

Patients must be cared for by nursing staff who have the knowledge and skills to provide tracheostomy care. Some useful care elements are as follow:

- Patients with tracheostomies when in hospital need to be cared for in an area where they are visible to nursing staff at all times. Call bells must be answered immediately as the patient may be having difficulty breathing.
- The tracheostomy tube should be correctly positioned at all times and only specifically designed dressings used (to prevent loose fibres entering the airway).
- Infection control is paramount and usually two practitioners are required during care to reduce the risk of the tube becoming dislodged.
- Patients with a tracheostomy can take diet and fluid, as appropriate. It is essential that the patient stays well hydrated.
- An awake and cooperative patient should be encouraged to cough up secretions, thereby reducing excessive secretions.
- A patient with a laryngectomy does not have a patent upper airway. Airway access is only via the stoma and any supplementary oxygen or assisted breathing must be via the stoma.

Further reading

NCEPOD On the right trach? (2014) http://www.ncepod.org.uk/2014tctoolkit.html (accessed 24 March 2016).

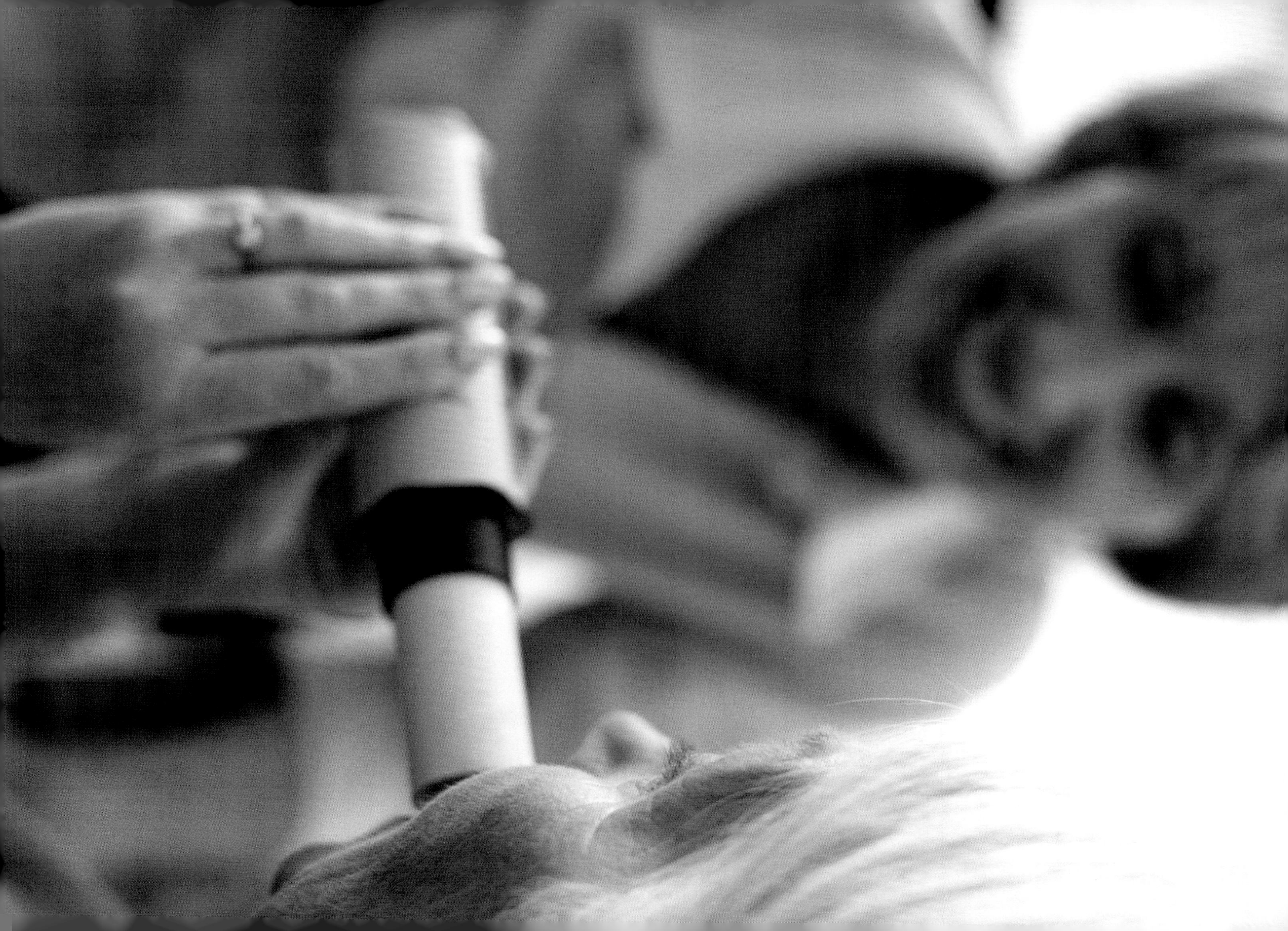

Supportive and palliative care

Part 8

Chapters

Overview

Part 8 focuses on supportive and palliative care. Communication, especially regarding end-of-life care, and planning is discussed with a chapter dedicated to support for families and carers. Psychological issues are explored and strategies to manage anxiety and other symptoms, including domiciliary non-invasive ventilation.

55 Communication

Box 55.1 SAGE and Thyme: a model for dealing with distress

- **Setting** If you notice concerns – create some privacy – sit down
- **Ask** 'Can I ask what you are concerned about?'
- **Gather** Gather all of the concerns–not just the few
- **Empathy** Respond sensitively – 'You have a lot on your mind'

and

- **Talk** 'Who do you have to talk to or support you?'
- **Help** 'How do they help?'
- **You** 'What do you think would help?'
- **Me** 'Is there something you would like me to do?'
- **End** Summarise and close – 'Can we leave it there?'

Source: University Hospital of South Manchester NHS Foundation Trust (2015). Reproduced with permission from University Hospital of South Manchester NHS Foundation Trust.

Figure 55.1 SPIKES: a model for communicating bad news

S	Setting
P	Perception
I	Invitation
K	Knowledge
E	Empathy/emotions
S	Summary/strategy

Box 55.2 Suggested approach to end-of-life care conversations in chronic obstructive pulmonary disease
Source: Momen et al. (2012) *Thorax* 67: 77–780. Reproduced with permission of BMJ Publishing Ltd.

Respect autonomy
Allow the patient to decide whether to have an end-of-life care conversation, when and with whom

Patient centred
Content, timing and pace set by the patient

Multiple opportunities
For the patient to explore issues if they wish

Maintain balance
Combine realistic hope with practical planning

Honest information
Including acknowledgement of uncertainty

Document discussion
Enable other health care professionals to be aware of the patient's preferences for care

Most people can cope with most things in life ... because they have to

... but they need to know what they are up against!

Annette Duck (2015)

According to the National End of Life Care Intelligence Network (2011), 14% of all deaths in England between 2007 and 2009 were from respiratory diseases. This proportion increased to 20% when lung cancer deaths were included. The proportion of all deaths in England with a mention of respiratory disease on the death certificate, for the same period, was 34%, illustrating the full extent of respiratory diseases.

I would like to question how many of those patients were prepared for death and what proportion had the opportunity to talk about their illness and end-of-life care before they finally passed away?

Why it is important?

Giving information about disease, medication, prognosis and impending death are an important part of everyday practice, but how do we know that patients understand what we have told them? How do we know that we have done it well? How can we expect patients to follow self-management plans if we do not talk to them in a language they understand? Communicating to patients is probably one of the most important skills a clinician needs and yet how many of us have had training on how to do it? In today's multi-cultural health care system it has become even more imperative that we communicate to patients in a language they understand and this is particularly important when talking about prognosis and giving bad news.

What do we know?

We know that patients have a high level of information needs throughout their illness and that those needs change over time. We know that the way information is conveyed can affect the way patients adjust to their illness and future relationships with health care practitioners. We know that patients prefer a known trusted health care practitioner who delivers the information sensitively, balancing realism with hope, showing empathy and encouraging questions. We know that carers' information needs differ from those of patients and we know that some patients want to talk about their prognosis and make plans for the future and some do not (Parker et al., 2007). We know from Ekington et al. (2005) that compared with cancer, end-of-life discussions are not taking place with patients with chronic obstructive pulmonary disease (COPD), despite the NICE COPD guidelines (2010) stating that patients with COPD should be offered the full range of palliative care services. Murray et al. (2005) postulate that although clinicians think that these discussions should be taking place, they are unsure when and who should be initiating these discussions. How do we work out which patients want to talk about the future and which do not? Fortunately, as this is dangerous ground for clinicians, tried and tested communication models can help to navigate this dangerous territory.

SAGE & THYME®

SAGE & THYME is a nine-step mnemonic model for dealing with the emotional concerns of patients (Box 55.1). The model was developed by a multi-specialty team, including a patient with cancer, to enable staff of all grades and roles to fulfil the role of providing psychological care to patients as recommended by NICE (2004) Improving Supportive and Palliative Care for Adults with Cancer. The model is based on the evidence relating to emotional support and communication skills. The model enables patients to describe their concerns and emotions if they wish; allows health care staff to respect those concerns; helps patients identify their own support structures; and explores the patients' own ideas and solutions before offering advice or information (Connolly et al., 2010). Information on the 3-hour foundation-level communication skills course is available from: http://www.sageandthymetraining.org.uk/.

Breaking bad news

Momen et al. (2012) suggest that clinicians need adequate training in order to feel confident about opening end-of-life discussions with their patients. Approaches that might help clinicians include respecting autonomy and allowing the patient to decide whether to have an end-of-life care conversation, when and with whom. These conversations should be patient centred as regards their content, timing and, importantly, the pace is set by the patient. The patient should be given multiple opportunities to explore issues if they wish.

There should be realistic hope but combined with this practical planning. Information needs to be honest including acknowledging any uncertainty. All discussions should be documented to enable other health care professionals to be aware of the patient's preferences for care.

It is important to listen for any cues a patient might give that they might want to talk about the future. This can often be a 'throw away' remark like 'I thought I'd had it that time' when referring to a recent hospitalisation or 'Sometimes I get so breathless, I think I am going to die.' Using cues like this and repeating back what was just said '"Had it that time" or "I think I am going to die" Is that something you have thought about? Or are worried about?' Patients who might want to talk about it will often respond to a question like this.

Using a model such as SPIKES (Baile et al., 2000) (Figure 55.1) to help clinicians through a breaking bad news conversation can be very helpful. SPIKES is a six-step pneumonic model developed by oncologists for breaking bad news.

- *Setting:* is now and here the right place and time to have this discussion? Ask the patient.
- *Perception:* what is the patient's perception of how things are? Do they realise how bad things are? Where is my starting point for giving this information? Ask the patient.
- *Invitation:* do they want to hear this? Is this the right time for telling them? Ask the patient.
- *Knowledge:* always give a 'warning shot' before giving bad news: 'I am afraid that I have bad news … on the tests.' 'I am afraid this is not the news you were hoping to hear.' It is important to pause and wait so that patients have time to prepare themselves for whatever you have to say. This may seem like a long time, but it is important not to go on until the patient gives you the prompt to continue. Follow with the information slowly and with pauses so that you allow the patient time to assimilate what you are saying. Watch how the patient is taking your news and ask whether they want you to continue. Some patients cannot take all the news at once.
- *Empathy:* make sure you acknowledge any emotion sensitively with comforting words like 'I can see you are upset by what I have just said.' 'I am sorry that I have had to tell you this.' Maybe a gesture and responding to crying by providing tissues is a comfort to patients.
- *Strategy:* finally, providing contact telephone numbers or following up on what is going to happen next will bring the conversation to a close.

Further reading

Momen N, Hadfield P, Kuhn I, Smith E, Barclay S. (2012) Discussing an uncertain future: end-of-life care conversations in chronic obstructive pulmonary disease: a systematic literature review and narrative synthesis. *Thorax* 67: 777–780.

56 Psychosocial impact of respiratory disease

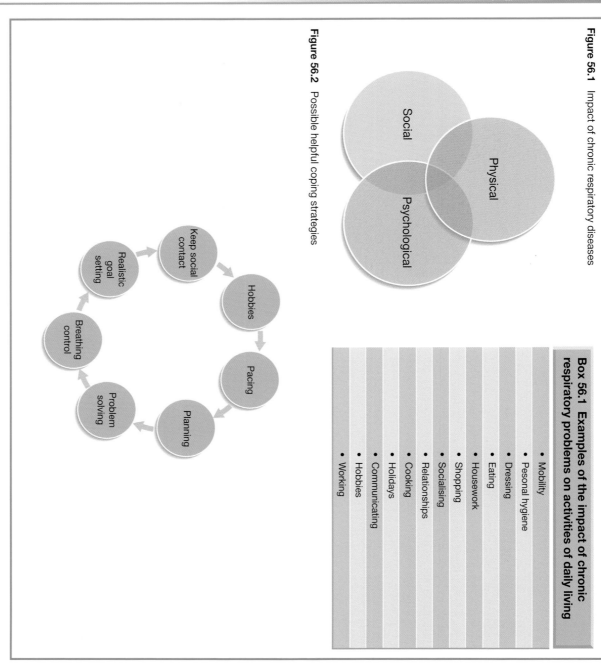

Figure 56.1 Impact of chronic respiratory diseases

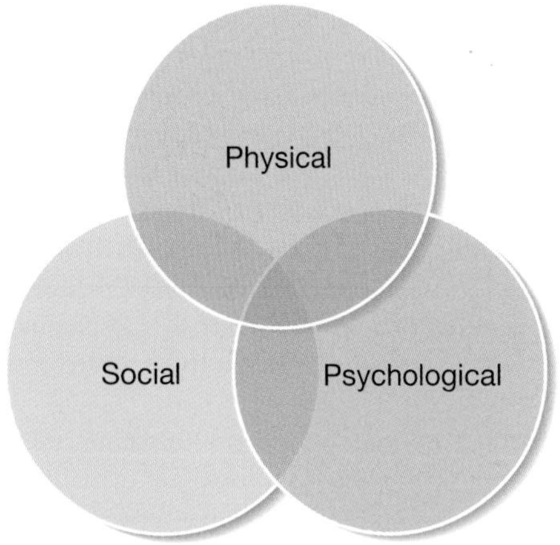
Physical
Social
Psychological

Box 56.1 Examples of the impact of chronic respiratory problems on activities of daily living

- Mobility
- Pesonal hygiene
- Dressing
- Eating
- Housework
- Shopping
- Socialising
- Relationships
- Cooking
- Holidays
- Communicating
- Hobbies
- Working

Figure 56.2 Possible helpful coping strategies

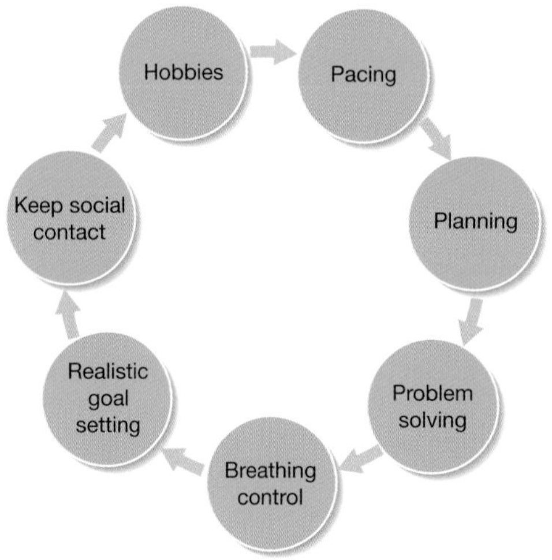
Hobbies
Pacing
Planning
Problem solving
Breathing control
Realistic goal setting
Keep social contact

Patients with chronic respiratory disease face the prospect of coping with physical decline and disabling symptoms. A term used to describe ill-health or disease burden is disability adjusted life years (DALYs). DALYs reflect the number of years lost due to ill health, disability or early death (World Health Organization, 2008). The UK has poor rankings in terms of DALYs in five out of 30 disease areas assessed: heart disease, lung and breast cancer, chronic obstructive pulmonary disease (COPD) and respiratory infections (Buck, 2014).

Symptom burden in patients with severe COPD has been compared with serious life-threatening illnesses such as lung cancer (Gore et al., 2000). The findings suggest that people with chronic lung disease experience significantly more symptoms than people with lung cancer (Gore et al., 2000). Disabling symptoms affect patients physically, psychologically and socially (Figure 56.1).

The patient's perspective

The British Lung Foundation highlighted what is important to patients is if they feel unwell, their inability to perform everyday activities and on the emotional consequences of the disease (British Lung Foundation, 2006). Over the past few decades there has been an increasing amount of qualitative research published relating to understanding patients' experiences living with particular conditions. Breathlessness is a common and distressing symptom for patients with respiratory problems. Usually, breathlessness is first noticed on climbing stairs, while carrying heavy loads or hurrying. Deterioration occurs with exacerbations of the illness and gradual progression ensues.

It is a humbling and rewarding experience listening to our patients' stories about how they are coping. The following examples give an insight into the impact of respiratory conditions such as COPD.

'If I have a bath I just sit for a bit and wait then wash myself. Even getting in and out of the bath has me puffing and panting. I sit on the end of the bath to dry myself and I'm exhausted and for the past 2 years that's the way it's been.'

'I'm alright if I'm sitting doing absolutely nothing. I can walk 5 yards then I have to stop and catch my breath for 10 minutes then go a little further.'

'I've always been active, I've been active person over the years. This is the only thing that affects me now and being inactive has been hard to get used to.'

Quality of life

For decades we have known that chronic respiratory problems such as COPD have a significant impact on patients' quality of life. The unremitting nature of respiratory illness such as COPD can have a profound effect on patients' social, family and work life (Box 56.1).

Patients often want to be 'cured' of their illness but unfortunately this is not possible. For many long-term conditions the aim of treatment is to control symptoms and improve quality of life and help patients adjust to their illness.

Coping strategies

Breathing problems affect many activities of daily living. Some patients learn to cope and adjust to the limitations inflicted upon them and take things in their stride. Others unfortunately, find it hard to cope with the impact on their lives.

When treating patients it is too easy to simply rely on assessing lung function, treating infections, encouraging patients to have the necessary vaccinations they need and checking their inhaler technique. There is no doubt that the above interventions are important but we often overlook how patients are coping with the difficulties they face on a daily basis as a result of their respiratory problem. We have been focused on lung function but measurement of lung function can adequately measure the effects of breathlessness in patients with chronic respiratory problems such as COPD.

Patients often develop positive strategies and skills to cope with the impact of their illness. Helpful strategies can be seen in Box 56.2. Here are two examples from patients that show excellent coping strategies.

'It helps if I lean over and rest on the fireplace if I cannot get my breath.'

'The doctor only sees you 5–10 minutes, they don't realise that you have them (symptoms) 24 hours a day, all the time. I have to work things out. Yesterday, I started doing the stairs. I did four stairs and I had to stop. I know it's there and I'll go back to it tomorrow and do a little more. Over a period of time I'll get it done.'

Summary

Chronic illness represents a major challenge to society and we need to identify ways of meeting the health and social needs of vulnerable patients. Nurses have a key role in helping improve patients' quality of life. By being there for patients, listening to their story and helping identify top tips to cope with the impact of chronic respiratory disease, we can all make a difference to their lives. To make a difference health and social services and the voluntary sector need to work together to identify care tailored to the patients' individual needs.

Further reading

Gore JM, Brophy CJ, Greenstone MA. (2000) How well do we care for patients with end stage chronic obstructive pulmonary disease (COPD)? A comparison of palliative care and quality of life in COPD and lung cancer. *Thorax* 55: 1000–1006.

57 Management of dyspnoea

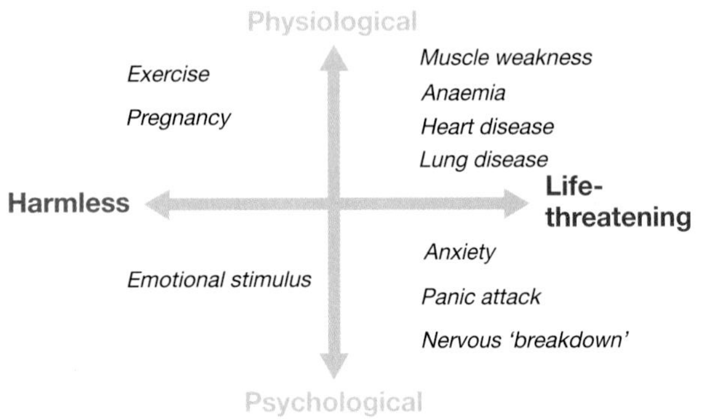
Physiological
Exercise
Pregnancy
Muscle weakness
Anaemia
Heart disease
Lung disease
Harmless
Life-threatening
Anxiety
Emotional stimulus
Panic attack
Nervous 'breakdown'
Psychological

Figure 57.1 The domains of dyspnoea

Figure 57.2 Non-pharmacological interventions for managing dyspnoea

Grouping	Intervention
Breathing	Fan therapy Breathing exercises – e.g. yoga breathing, pursed lip breathing, diaphragmatic breathing
Thinking	Counselling and support Case management Psychotherapy Cognitive behavioural therapy
Functioning	Pulmonary rehabilitation Self-management

Figure 57.3 Simple fan therapy can be effective in relieving dyspnoea

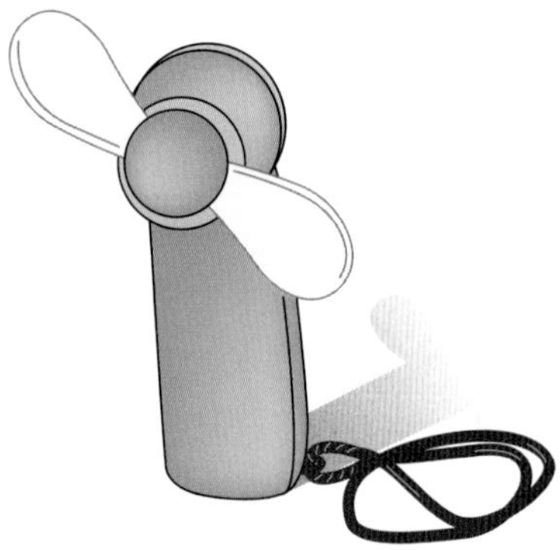

Figure 57.4 Pulmonary rehabilitation can hep strenghten muscles and reduce oxygen cost of activity

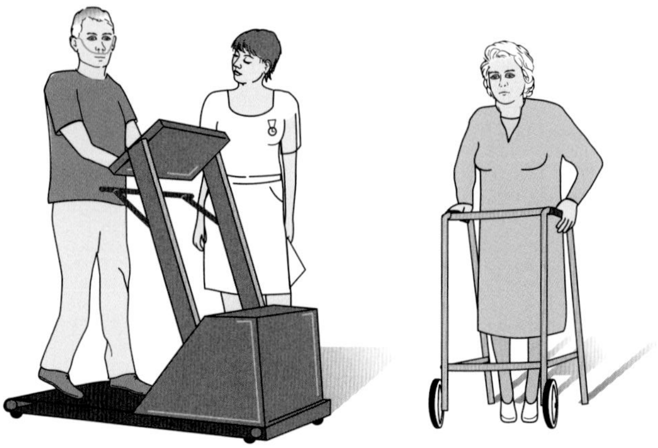

As discussed in Chapter 17, diagnosis and treatment of the initial underlying pathologic causes of dyspnoea are the recommended approach. There are many influencing factors that result in and compound dyspnoea (Figure 57.1) and managing someone with dyspnoea can present many challenges.

The therapeutic goal of symptomatic management of dyspnoea is to relieve the patient's sense of the effort of breathing. This can be achieved by pursuing one or more strategies including both pharmacological and non-pharmacological interventions.

Pharmacological management

Opioids

The use of opioids for pharmacological management of dyspnoea has the strongest evidence base. Studies have shown that acute therapy with opioids deceases exercise-induced dyspnoea and increases exercise tolerance in patients with chronic obstructive pulmonary disease (COPD). Once an effective dose has been determined, a typical opioid regimen to maintain control of chronic dyspnoea includes both sustained relief and immediate relief for opioid break-through dyspnoea. Opioids, primarily morphine, work by modulating perception of dyspnoea and there may be some decrease in respiratory drive and a decrease in anxiety. Yet, despite reassurance from limited evidence regarding the safety of using opioids, fear of overdosing and development of respiratory depression persists and limits current prescribing practices. Reassurance of both health care professionals and patients is often necessary.

Anxiolytics

Patients frequently report anxiety in association with dyspnoea. Dyspnoea can lead to anxiety and anxiety can exacerbate dyspnoea. Many patients find it difficult to distinguish between anxiety and dyspnoea. Anxiolytics (such as benzodiazepines) are frequently prescribed for patients with dyspnoea. The evidence concerning the use of benzodiazepines, which are commonly used in the management of dyspnoea, concluded that there is no evidence for a beneficial effect and this class of drugs should only be used if other first line treatment such as opioids and non-pharmacological interventions have been tried.

Oxygen

If lack of oxygen is the cause of dyspnoea then oxygen therapy may be required. However, when a patient's blood oxygen level remains normal an argument presents itself which leads to contention and confusion in practice. Evidence suggests that there is no therapeutic benefit of short burst oxygen therapy for dyspnoea and only limited evidence of reducing dyspnoea during activity with ambulatory oxygen.

However, the distressed patient may perceive that oxygen is 'doing something'. Other explanations of perceived benefit of oxygen include a cool air sensation on the face; initial studies have found that simple fan therapy has similar effects in reducing the sensation of dyspnoea. Oxygen therapy has been described as an expensive placebo but that suggests a benign therapy, yet oxygen is not without its drawbacks and side effects, including restriction of activities, impaired communication, psychological dependence and safety. Additionally, oxygen therapy poses a financial burden on health services in a time of austerity.

Inhaled therapies

If inhaled therapies are already prescribed it may be beneficial to assess inhaler technique and the appropriateness of the device. Nebulised saline 0.9% can help with expectoration. If the patient had an underlying respiratory disease then nebulised bronchodilators can also be prescribed.

Non-pharmacological management

Booth (2013) suggests three non-pharmacological intervention groupings: first, those that effect breathing, for example fan therapy, breathing exercises and neuromuscular electrical stimulation. Secondly, those that affect thinking, targeting central perception of breathlessness, for example education, relaxation techniques, cognitive behavioural therapy (CBT) and active listening. Thirdly, interventions that affect functioning, for example exercise programmes, mobility aids and pacing skills. It would seem that given the multiplexity of dyspnoea incorporation of one or several of these approaches to management is essential. For a summary of potential interventions targeting these three groupings see Figure 57.2. These interventions have varied levels of evidence. Three of the more promising approaches are outlined here.

Fan therapy

Some evidence supports the use of a hand-held fan in relieving chronic dyspnoea. Although the evidence base is still relatively limited, from a pragmatic point of view the fan is inexpensive and accessible and clinical use suggests that patients benefit. Whether this is a result of facial stimulation, placebo or an effect of self-efficacy remains unclear but justification for not utilising this on a widespread basis would be difficult (Figure 57.3).

Pulmonary rehabilitation

Pulmonary rehabilitation attempts to reverse the effects of physical deconditioning and empowers patients (and carers) to take control of their disease management (Chapter 11). Pulmonary rehabilitation efficacy on dyspnoea and health status – including fatigue, emotional function and patients' sense of control – indicates an unequivocal reduction in dyspnoea and a significant clinical improvement in health status and following pulmonary rehabilitation (Figure 57.4).

Cognitive–behavioural interventions

Dyspnoea has cognitive and emotional components in addition to the pathophysiological components and some patients will benefit from expert psychological support to help them cope with the disablement of dyspnoea (Chapter 58). Evidence has found that CBT, when used with exercise and education, can contribute to significant reductions in anxiety and depression in patients with COPD. How this transfers into the reduction and management of dyspnoea is still uncertain.

Summary

Dyspnoea is a complex phenomenon that impacts on morbidity, mortality and health care utilisation. While physiological mechanisms are important, it is also clear that psychological, social and environmental factors are also pivotal in the way that dyspnoea is experienced and controlled. Ideally, treatments need to be individually tailored to meet concerns and priorities; the inclusion of family and carers in these needs is deemed an integral part of supportive care. An 'n of 1 trial' is often necessitated with most interventions in order to assess its efficacy on an individual basis.

Further reading

Booth S. (2013) Science supporting the art of medicine: improving the management of breathlessness. *Palliat Med* 27: 483–485.

Currow DC, Higginson IJ, Johnson MJ. (2013) Breathlessness: current and emerging mechanisms, measurement and management. *Palliat Med* 27: 932–938.

58 Anxiety and depression in respiratory disease

Figure 58.1 Cycle of anxiety

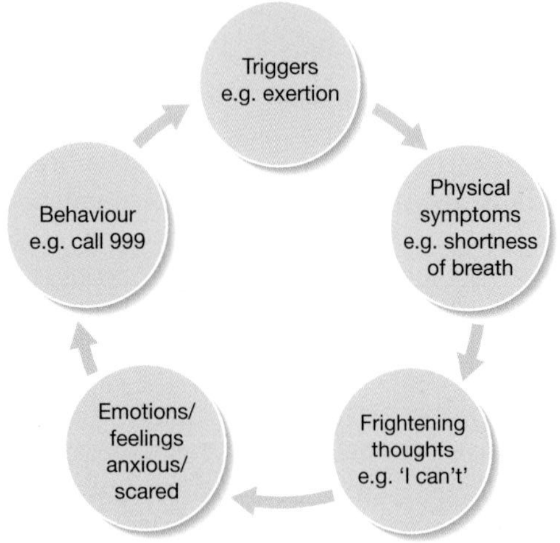
Triggers
e.g. exertion
Physical
symptoms
e.g. shortness
of breath
Frightening
thoughts
e.g. 'I can't'
Emotions/
feelings
anxious/
scared
Behaviour
e.g. call 999

Figure 58.2 Cycle of depression

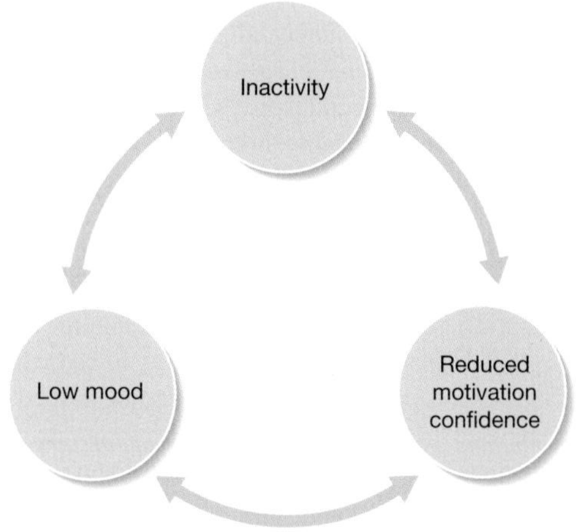
Inactivity
Reduced
motivation
confidence
Low mood

Box 58.1 Common features of panic attacks

- Triggers (e.g. exertion)
- Abrupt physical symptoms such as breathlessness and fast heart rate
- Increased self-monitoring (e.g. increased focus and awareness of breathing)
- Perceived physical, mental or behavioural catastrophe
- Apprehension and fear of future attacks
- Extensive behaviour to stay safe (e.g. avoidance of activities and exertion or seeking reassurance)
- Perceived lack of control

Box 58.2 Quick screening questions to assess mood

Over the past two weeks have you

- Been feeling down, depressed or hopeless?
- Had little interest or pleasure in doing things?
- Felt nervous, anxious or on edge?
- Been able to stop or control worrying?
- Experienced any panic attacks?

Box 58.3 Common techniques that might help reduce symptoms of anxiety and depression

- Information about respiratory problem, anxiety and depression
- Distraction
- Breathing control – slow breaths (breathe in for three and breathe out for four)
- Activity (pacing and planning activities. Doing pleasurable activities or ones that give a sense of achievement)
- Breaking tasks into small manageable realistic tasks
- Relaxation
- Mindfulness techniques
- Increasing meaningful or pleasurable activities (within physical abilities). Keep a simple list to monitor

Living with a chronic lung condition can be challenging physically, socially and psychologically. Patients have to manage unpleasant symptoms such as breathlessness and this can lead to symptoms of anxiety and depression. We have known for decades that symptoms of anxiety and depression are commonly experienced by people with lung conditions such as chronic obstructive pulmonary disease (COPD) but very little has been done about this. Psychological co-morbidities have adverse effects on the outcome of medical illnesses and have been are associated with lower levels of self-efficacy, impaired quality of life, poorer treatment outcomes and reduced survival (Ng et al., 2007). When patients are anxious they may continue to smoke to cope, decline pulmonary rehabilitation, use medication excessively and come into hospital more because they feel safe there. As a result of breathlessness it is quite understandable that symptoms of anxiety and depression develop.

Anxiety

Anxiety is an emotion experienced by us all. Anxiety is an unpleasant feeling associated with worry, fear and distressing physical symptoms. These symptoms can overlap with the symptoms of respiratory disease and be difficult to manage. Panic attacks are a severe form of anxiety and are common in patients with COPD (Figure 58.1). Patients experience episodes of extreme fear accompanied by frightening thoughts such as 'I can't get my breath, I'm going to die'. Common features of panic attacks are presented in Box 58.1. Patients become apprehensive and a vicious cycle develops. It is difficult to know the true prevalence of anxiety in patients with respiratory disease because screening is rarely undertaken. However, symptoms of anxiety has occurred in 60% of patients screened (Heslop-Marshall and De Soyza, 2014). To reduce symptoms of anxiety patients often avoid exertion which often triggers their symptoms but this leads to physical deconditioning and exacerbates the panic cycle.

Depression

Depression is a common problem for patients with long-term conditions (Figure 58.2). Depression is two to three times more common in patients with chronic physical health conditions such as COPD (NICE, 2010). Depression symptoms includes low mood, loss of interest in daily activities, loss of energy, feeling helpless, hopelessness, difficulty concentrating, no motivation and even suicidal feelings if severe. Patients with depression and long-term physical health problems have more impairment of their functional levels and higher mortality. It is therefore important to identify patients who have symptoms of anxiety and depression and treat them accordingly.

Screening

Symptoms of anxiety and depression often appear together. Screening is the first step to identify these distressing symptoms. Five simple questions can be used to screen patients (Box 58.2). If needed, psychometric questionnaires such as the Hospital Anxiety and Depression Questionnaire can be used to identify symptoms. Once symptoms of anxiety and depression have been identified the next step is effective treatment.

Treatment of anxiety and depression

Unfortunately, the treatment of anxiety and depression in respiratory patients remains poor. Guidelines recommend recommend psychological treatment, pharmacological treatment or both in combination (NICE, 2010, 2011). There are lots of ways we can help patients with symptoms of anxiety and depression.

1 Screen patients for symptoms. Using five brief screening questions can identify patients who need formal psychometric questionnaires completing to explore their symptoms further such as the Hospital Anxiety and Depression Questionnaire (Zigmond and Snaith, 1983).

2 Talk to patients. Find out what their current difficulties are. How are they managing to cope with their respiratory condition on a daily basis? Do you understand their personal story?

3 Encourage patients to exercise or go to pulmonary rehabilitation. Activity is a natural remedy for depression and benefits us all physically and psychologically. Encouraging patients to engage in enjoyable activities or activities that give them a sense of achievement within their physical capabilities can work wonders.

4 Provide self-help leaflets (e.g. Northumberland, Tyne & Wear Mental Health Trust Leaflets on panic, depression and low mood) can improve their understanding on what is happening and what they can do to help themselves.

5 Offer cognitive–behavioural therapy (CBT). CBT is one of most commonly used psychological treatments that focuses on understanding your patient's experiences, how they have developed and interpreted. CBT addresses important interactions or links between our thoughts, mood, behaviour and physical symptoms. CBT can help patients learn practical ways to cope with the impact of COPD. Research has shown that respiratory nurses can help reduce symptoms of anxiety and depression and improve quality of life in patients with respiratory problems by using CBT techniques. If your team does not offer CBT then signpost your patients to local services such as Improving Access to Psychological Therapy (IAPT) if your patient would like help with symptoms of anxiety and depression. There are a number of techniques that can be helpful for patients with breathlessness, anxiety and panic. Common techniques are shown in Box 58.3.

6 Older patients are especially vulnerable to loneliness. Encouraging your patients to engage in social activities can help with loneliness and social isolation which is often a significant problem for patients with COPD.

7 Pharmacological treatment can be required if patients have moderate to severe symptoms of depression. Raising the mood with antidepressants can help the patient to feel more able to increase their activities which can really improve how they feel. Antidepressants alone are not the answer.

8 Finding ways to support the patient cope with anxiety and depression in other ways rather than smoking can help reduce further ill health.

9 Relaxation techniques can help with symptoms of anxiety. Progressive muscle relaxation, visualisation and imagery can be used.

Summary

Symptoms of anxiety and depression are extremely common in patients with COPD and it is highly likely that other conditions have a similar effect on patients with other respiratory conditions. Screening for symptoms of anxiety and depression are recommended yet rarely undertaken. Anxiety and depression are treatable conditions and as such respiratory nurses with appropriate training are ideally placed to undertake this role and make a difference to patients' lives.

Further reading

Ng TP, Niti M, Tan WC, Cao Z, Eng P. (2007) Depressive symptoms and chronic obstructive pulmonary disease: effect on mortality, hospital readmission, symptom burden, functional status and quality of life. *Arch Intern Med* 167: 60–70.

59 Other symptom management

Figure 59.1 Cough

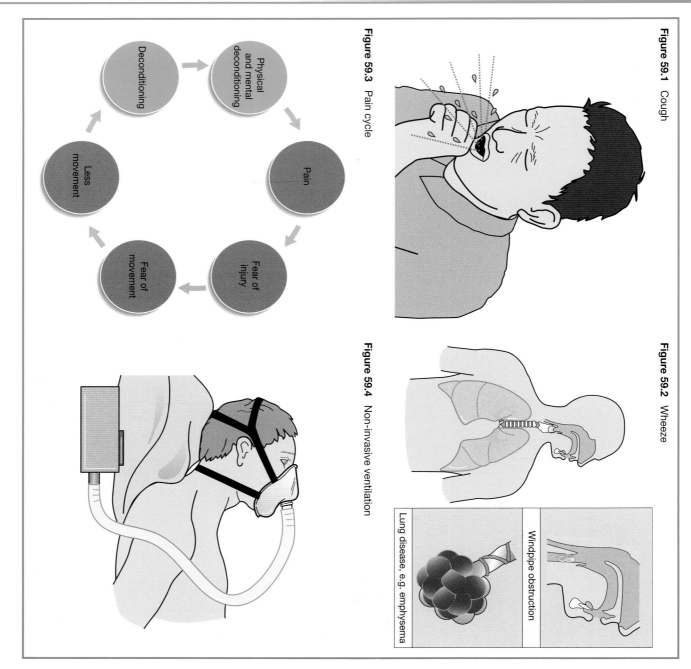

Figure 59.2 Wheeze

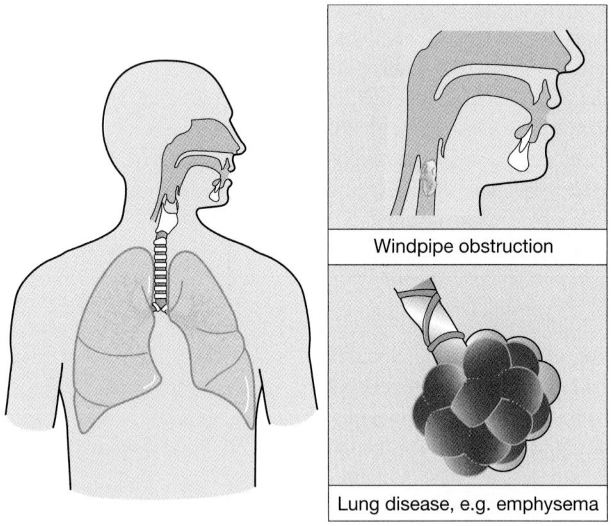
Windpipe obstruction
Lung disease, e.g. emphysema

Figure 59.3 Pain cycle

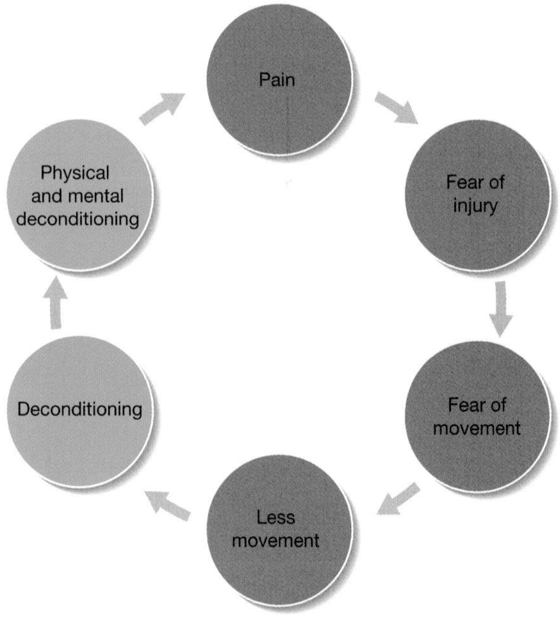
Pain
Fear of injury
Fear of movement
Less movement
Deconditioning
Physical and mental deconditioning

Figure 59.4 Non-invasive ventilation

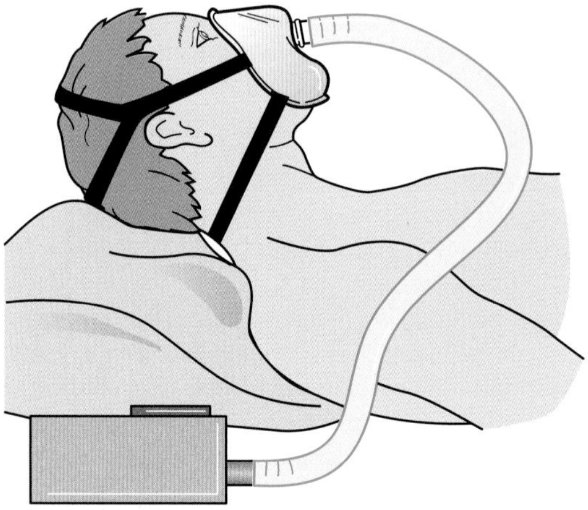

While dyspnoea, anxiety and depression are prevalent symptoms to be considered in palliative care, other symptoms can also manifest and impact significantly on patients and carers. Some of the more commonly experienced symptoms and suggested management are outlined here.

Cough

Cough is an important, usually involuntary reflex action of the respiratory tract, and acts as a defence mechanism to clear secretions and foreign bodies from the airways (Figure 59.1). Chronic cough can be evident in many respiratory conditions such as chronic obstructive pulmonary disease (COPD), asthma, eosinophilic bronchitis, post nasal drip syndrome or rhinosinusitis, bronchiectasis or pulmonary fibrosis. It can also sometimes be classed as idiopathic, where no cause is identified.

Effective control of cough is important as it can interfere with work and lifestyle and can impact upon quality of life and can exacerbate any pre-existing pain. If it persists it can lead to, or exacerbate, existing anxiety and depression or agrophobia from feelings of embarrassment and anxiety when in social environments. Effective control requires controlling the disease causing the cough and desensitising the cough pathways. This could be with an inhaler for asthma or a nasal spray for post nasal drip or oral morphine or codeine for intractable cough in a palliative patient. Each case should be assessed individually and where appropriate further investigations should be sought. This could include chest X-ray, spirometry, high-resolution computed tomography (HRCT) and bronchoscopy.

Wheeze

Wheezing is a high-pitched whistling sound heard more commonly on expiration but in severe cases can be heard on inspiration too. It is a common symptom in COPD and asthma but can also be heard with hay fever, acute bronchitis and in the presence of a swelling, growth or restriction in the airways (Figure 59.2). People with COPD experience wheeze when going out into cold air or walking into a wind but do not tend to experience wheeze at rest or at night, whereas people with asthma will experience a nocturnal wheeze and people with atopic asthma will often experience wheeze when exposed to a specific allergen. The aim when treating a wheeze is to reduce airway inflammation, usually with an inhaler but long-acting tablets can also be used. Bronchodilating inhalers relax the smooth muscles around the airways, allowing more air to enter and exit the lungs, consequently improving breathing and reducing wheeze.

Sputum

Sputum is a combination of saliva and mucous coughed up from the lower airways. It is usually white or grey but may become mucopurulent, malodorous and yellow or green with infections. Colour alone should be assessed with caution though as sputum colour can be affected by a live oak pollen drop (becoming yellowish) or by residing in a smoggy area (becoming brown). A trained professional should perform auscultation and will prescribe antibiotics and/or steroids if required.

Pain

Acute chest and/or back pain can be a common symptom when respiratory infection is present and is usually treated with antibiotics and simple analgesia but chronic pain can also be a problem in people with chronic respiratory disease and can be caused by excessive coughing or because osteoporosis, a severe thinning of the bones, is present. Osteoporosis can occur as a consequence of lung inflammation or because of steroid use, poor nutrition, inactivity and/or smoking. In severe cases, rib fracture can occur secondary to coughing. Osteoporosis should be treated first using calcium supplements and subsequent pain should initially be treated with oral analgesia. Over-the-counter remedies and prescription non-steroidal anti-inflammatory drugs (NSAIDs) should be considered for mild to moderate pain. However, in the palliative patient, where pain can be severe, opioids should be considered. Opiate medications relieve pain as well as relax breathing and should be used with caution so as not to cause excessive respiratory depression. They can be prescribed orally, intravenously or transdermally.

As opioids cause constipation and constipation can cause further pain or urinary retention, laxatives should also be considered. Patients can often develop a cycle of chronic pain that impacts on quality of life and morbidity (Figure 59.3).

Headache, blurred vision and restlessness from respiratory acidosis

As chronic respiratory disease advances and palliative input becomes more apparent some people will experience symptoms of headache, blurred vision and/or restlessness. This may be caused by a build-up of carbon dioxide (CO_2) in the blood which will in turn affect the blood pH, making it acidic. This is called respiratory acidosis or type 2 respiratory failure.

Type 1 respiratory failure is defined by a low level of oxygen and normal or low CO_2 levels. Type 2 respiratory failure is defined by a low level of oxygen with elevated CO_2 levels, also known as hypercapnia. In homeostasis the lungs take in oxygen and exhale CO_2, oxygen diffuses from the lungs into the blood and CO_2 diffuses from the blood into the lungs. Sometimes, however, the lungs cannot excrete enough CO_2 and this increase causes respiratory acidosis and symptoms of headache, blurred vision and/or restlessness.

Non-invasive ventilation (NIV) is used to improve these symptoms (Figure 59.4) and has been proven in an acute environment to reduce intubation rate and mortality in patients with COPD with decompensated respiratory acidosis (British Thoracic Guidelines, 2008). NIV can also be used in the palliative care setting as either a ceiling of treatment or a means of palliating symptoms. This can be appropriate in patients if standard medical treatment fails or the patient has chosen not to receive further treatment. In these situations it is important that any decisions made are discussed fully with the patient and family, with effective documention (Chapters 52 and 60).

Further reading

Baldwin DR, Currow D, Ahmedzai S. (2012) *Supportive Care in Respiratory Disease*, 2nd edn. Oxford University Press, Oxford.

60 NIV as a domiciliary therapy

Box 60.1 Conditions where non-invasive ventilation (NIV) is used as a domiciliary treatment

- Hyperventilation syndromes e.g. obesity, central or overlap with other conditions below
- Neuromuscular diseases e.g. motor neurone disease, Duchenne (muscular dystrophy (DMD)
- Restrictive thoracic disease e.g. kyphoscoliosis
- COPD
- Spinal cord injury

Box 60.2 Symptoms of nocturnal hypoventilation

- Morning headache (on waking)
- Fatigue
- Daytime somnolence
- Poor sleep

Table 60.1 Rational for key investigations

Investigation	Rationale
Blood gas analysis	To detect the presence of hypercapnia
Early morning blood gas	Presence of hypercapnia an indication of nocturnal hypoventilation when blood gas later in day may be normal
Overnight pulse oximetry	To detect any nocturnal hypoxaemia. May indicate cause e.g. obstructive sleep apnoea or hypoventilation
Nocturnal transcutaneous CO_2/O_2	To detect hypoventilation, hypoxaemia or hypercapnia
Sleep study – polysomnography or limited channel study	Early detection of hypoventilation e.g. during REM sleep Distinguish between causes of hypoventilation e.g. obesity or central hypoventilation, obstructive or central apnoeas
Vital capacity	Indicator of risk of developing respiratory failure in neuromuscular diseases and chest wall deformities
Maximal inspiratory or sniff nasal inspiratory pressure (MIP/SNIP)	Indicator of respiratory muscle strength, progression of condition and need for further assessment

Box 60.3 Possible benefits of domiciliary NIV

- Improved survival
- Reduction in symptoms e.g. breathlessness, daytime somnolence
- Improved sleep quality
- Resting respiratory muscles reducing fatigue
- Improved central respiratory drive
- Improved lung compliance/mechanics
- Improved cardiopulmonary and renal haemodynamics

Figure 60.1 Patient asleep with ventilator in situ

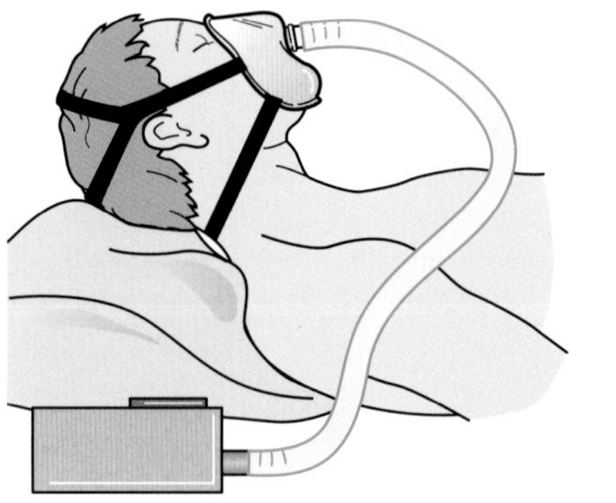

Table 60.2 Patient NIV dependency, support and equipment provision

Level	Usage	Equipment	Support
1 High dependency	>16 hrs/day, up to 24 hrs, compromised without nocturnal use	2 identical ventilators with battery back up. Inform electricity supplier	24–hr clinical and technical support
2 Low dependency	Nocturnal use only – may need for short periods in day or during acute illness	1 ventilator, battery back up not essential	9–5 working hours support, Monday to Friday

Despite domiciliary non-invasive ventilation (NIV) being used for significantly longer than acute NIV, the evidence base is less robust. Some of the most common conditions treated with NIV are outlined in Box 60.1.

Chronic obstructive pulmonary disease

Before considering NIV, patients must have a confirmed diagnosis, be on optimal treatment and clinically stable. Clinical stability can take at least a month following an acute exacerbation.

There seems to be a consensus on the indications for NIV in patients with chronic obstructive pulmonary disease (COPD):

- $p\mathrm{CO_2}$>7 kPa when clinically stable, with the following:
  - At least one episode of decompensated respiratory failure (RF) requiring acute ventilatory support
  - Daytime symptoms: morning headache, fatigue, somnolence (Box 60.2)
- Or intolerant of long-term oxygen therapy (LTOT) when clinically stable because of symptomatic hypercapnia or respiratory acidosis.

Effective treatment with NIV requires evidence of improved ventilation by a reduction in hypercapnia. This is likely to require higher inspiratory pressures which can impact on compliance.

Neuromuscular disease

NIV should be considered in those patients with daytime hypercapnia or evidence of nocturnal hypoventilation. Factors to consider when to initiate NIV include disease progression and prognosis, requirement of acute NIV and history and severity of symptoms.

These patients require regular monitoring in order to determine at which point to consider NIV. The frequency of monitoring depends on several factors:

- Likelihood of developing RF (e.g. patients with Duchenne muscular dystrophy (DMD) will inevitably develop RF but disease progression tends to be slow so may be monitored 6 monthly
- Speed of disease progression (e.g. motor neurone disease (MND) can progress rapidly so requires 2–3 monthly monitoring
- Level of symptoms (e.g. onset of orthopnoea, breathlessness or symptoms of nocturnal hypoventilation) require closer investigation and regular monitoring every 2 months
- Physiological parameters (e.g. vital capacity <50% predicted or <80% with symptoms; maximum inspiratory pressures (MIPs) <40 cmH_2O or <60 cmH_2O with symptoms; SpO_2<92% or <94% with symptoms)

Respiratory tract infections and bulbar symptoms (such as dysarthria and dysphagia) can indicate progressive respiratory muscle weakness and inability to clear secretions effectively or possible aspiration. Assessment and treatment of cough and swallow is therefore important. Severe bulbar symptoms make it more difficult to initiate and treat with NIV effectively.

Obesity hypoventilation syndrome

NIV should be considered in obese patients with daytime or nocturnal hypercapnia after other causes of hypoventilation have been excluded and obesity hypoventilation syndrome (OHS) confirmed. The presence and severity of daytime symptoms will be factors when considering initiating NIV.

OHS should be considered in obese patients (body mass index >30) with cor pulmonale or unexplained breathlessness. Up to 20% of patients with obstructive sleep apnoea syndrome (OSAS) will also have OHS. A trial of continuous positive airway pressure (CPAP) where both OSAS and OHS overlap can often be successful and NIV initiated if it fails.

Weight loss programmes should be integral in the patient's management plan, with bariatric surgery an option in patients who meet the criteria. Significant weight loss can reverse the requirement for hypoventilation and NIV.

Restrictive thoracic disease

In the UK, domiciliary NIV has been used in this group for over 30 years but despite this there is still a lack of robust evidence. However, the extensive case series data consistently demonstrate clinical benefit which may make it unethical to undertake controlled studies. In view of this there remain many unanswered clinical questions including when to initiate NIV. Patients with nocturnal hypercapnia, particularly with associated significant hypoxemia (SpO_2 <88% for >5 min) should be considered for NIV.

Where to initiate NIV

Individual centres have different approaches to setting up NIV, some admit the patient, others will initiate in an outpatient setting, in the home, or a mixture. The decision depends on resources including staff and equipment (e.g. availability of portable equipment). Other factors include the severity, complexity and clinical stability of the patient's condition and the availability of support at home.

While the patient's preference can be considered, their safety should be the priority. Ensuring effective education regarding the use of the ventilator, and ensuring the patient and/or carers are competent, must occur before the patient goes home. Written instruction must be given with appropriate contact numbers for ongoing support.

Ventilators

There are now a huge range of ventilators; some deliver a fixed pressure and others average tidal volumes with pressure adjusted to deliver the set volume. Both are effective. A back-up respiratory rate is important for patients who have difficulty triggering breaths or long periods without breathing (e.g. patients with neuromuscular disease, OHS or OSAS).

Some patients with progressive diseases can become dependent on NIV initially during sleep, but then also during the day in order to avoid significant symptoms and clinical deterioration (Figure 60.1).

Compliance and monitoring

Four hours seems to be the minimum required length of time required to provide positive clinical outcomes but patients should be encouraged to use NIV all night. Modern ventilators can provide accurate compliance data including useful information on mask leak, hypopnoeas, apnoeas and incorporate oxygen saturation to match up these events. The newer ventilators automatically transfer data securely via a wireless network to a desktop or even telephone. The frequency of monitoring will vary depending on the patient's clinical stability and likelihood of clinical change.

Oxygen

Oxygen can be entrained into the ventilator circuit but only when there is evidence of improved ventilation on NIV (significantly reduced hypercapnia), where a further increase in settings will not improve the hypoxaemia or the patient cannot tolerate further increases. Patients who continue meet the criteria for LTOT despite nocturnal NIV can be assessed and given oxygen in the day to make up >15 hours required for clinical benefit.

Further reading

Simonds AK (ed.) (2007) *Non-Invasive Respiratory Support: A Practical Handbook*, 3rd edn. Hodder Arnold, London.

61 End-of-life care

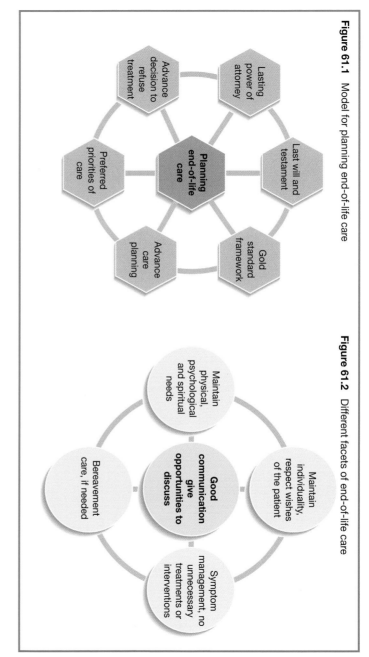

Figure 61.1 Model for planning end-of-life care

Planning end-of-life care
Last will and testament
Gold standard framework
Advance care planning
Preferred priorities of care
Advance decision to refuse treatment
Lasting power of attorney

Figure 61.2 Different facets of end-of-life care

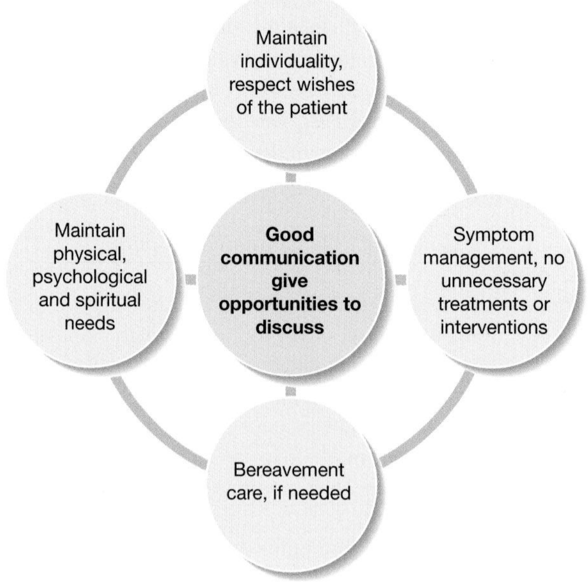
Good communication give opportunities to discuss
Maintain individuality, respect wishes of the patient
Symptom management, no unnecessary treatments or interventions
Bereavement care, if needed
Maintain physical, psychological and spiritual needs

Woody Allen, film director, actor and writer, once said 'I don't want to achieve immortality through my work. I want to achieve it through not dying.' He followed up by saying 'It's not that I'm afraid to die, I just don't want to be there when it happens', illustrating a basic human fear of death and the lack of control that we assume we have over it.

When and what we die of, we have little control over, but some of the events leading up to that might affect where and how we die and can affect the experience of death profoundly. Dame Cicely Saunders, the founder of the modern hospice movement, understood this and devoted her life's work to improving end-of-life care by improving symptom control and giving people choices over this final event in their lives. Dame Cecily once remarked that 'How people die remains in the memory of those who live on', illustrating the importance for the dying person and their families to have their preferences met.

Good end-of-life care is based on the understanding that death is inevitable, and a natural part of life.

End-of-Life Care Strategy (2008)

- To reduce inappropriate and burdensome health care interventions and to offer a choice of place of care when possible.
- To maintain the comfort, choices and quality of life of a person who is recognised to be dying (in the terminal phase).
- To support their individuality, and to care for the psychosocial and spiritual needs of the patient and their families.
- To support their families, if needed, which continues after death as bereavement care.

In order to facilitate all of this, the Department of Health has developed policies that would help and guide those caring for people approaching the end of their lives. They are all encapsulated under the Gold Standard Framework.

Advance care planning

The Gold Standards Framework allows individuals to plan their treatment and care should they become incapacitated and not be able to make decisions for themselves. It usually starts with a discussion initiated by a health care practitioner (but it can be by the patient or carer), who thinks about, talks to family and friends and then decides what care they might want if they were unable to make decisions for themselves. This might include hospital admission for acute events associated with the illness or it might be about continuing care, for instance in a nursing home or hospice, or remaining at home whatever happens.

At this point patients might decide to appoint a Lasting Power of Attorney (LPA) to make decisions regarding financial or health needs on their behalf. This can be an individual or a number of people who would agree the appropriate action with the knowledge of what the dying person has expressed that they wanted in their Advance Care Plan.

They may also want to make an Advance Decision to Refuse Treatment (ADRT; www.adrt.nhs.uk) which is very specific to the illness at hand, and treatment can only be withheld specifically for what is written down. This might be about treatments, interventions or care.

Preferred priorities of care

NHS (2011) is a document whereby several questions are asked to prompt patients to think and talk about their future care and what they might want. They can talk this over with their families and there is space to write down what they might want. Unlike the ADRT and LPA, this document is not legally binding but it can be used by families and health care practitioners to influence future decisions about treatment and care. It is important that Advance Care Plans made by patients are communicated to all health care practitioners who are caring for the patient so that the patient's wishes can be carried out: GP, secondary care doctors and nurses, ambulance crew, family and main carer.

It is important to remember that once an Advance Care Plan has been made that it is not set in stone and can be changed or modified at any time. Patients often think they will want to die at home, but as their disease progresses it might be that their needs change and so they may change their minds and would prefer to be somewhere where they can have more specialised care. This is fine and carers should not feel that they have failed. Good communication skills are invaluable for dealing with sensitive issues during the management of end-of-life care and commissioners have a responsibility to ensure their staff are adequately trained.

Community palliative care teams

Provision is variable depending on location and model of community service. The skills of Macmillan nurses are beneficial to patients with end-stage respiratory disease and referral should be considered. The use of hospice care should also be considered as many find this beneficial.

Further reading

Department of Health (2008) End of Life Care Strategy: promoting high quality care for adults at the end of their life. https://www.gov.uk/government/publications/end-of-life-care-strategy-promoting-high-quality-care-for-adults-at-the-end-of-their-life (accessed 1 March 2016).

Gold Standards Framework (2016) Advance Care Planning. http://www.goldstandardsframework.org.uk/advance-care-planning (accessed 1 March 2016).

NHS (2011) Preferred Priorities for Care. http://www.nhsiq.nhs.uk/resource-search/publications/eolc-ppc.aspx (accessed 1 March 2016).

62 Families and carers

Figure 62.1 Palliative care
Source: English Journal for Palliative Care.

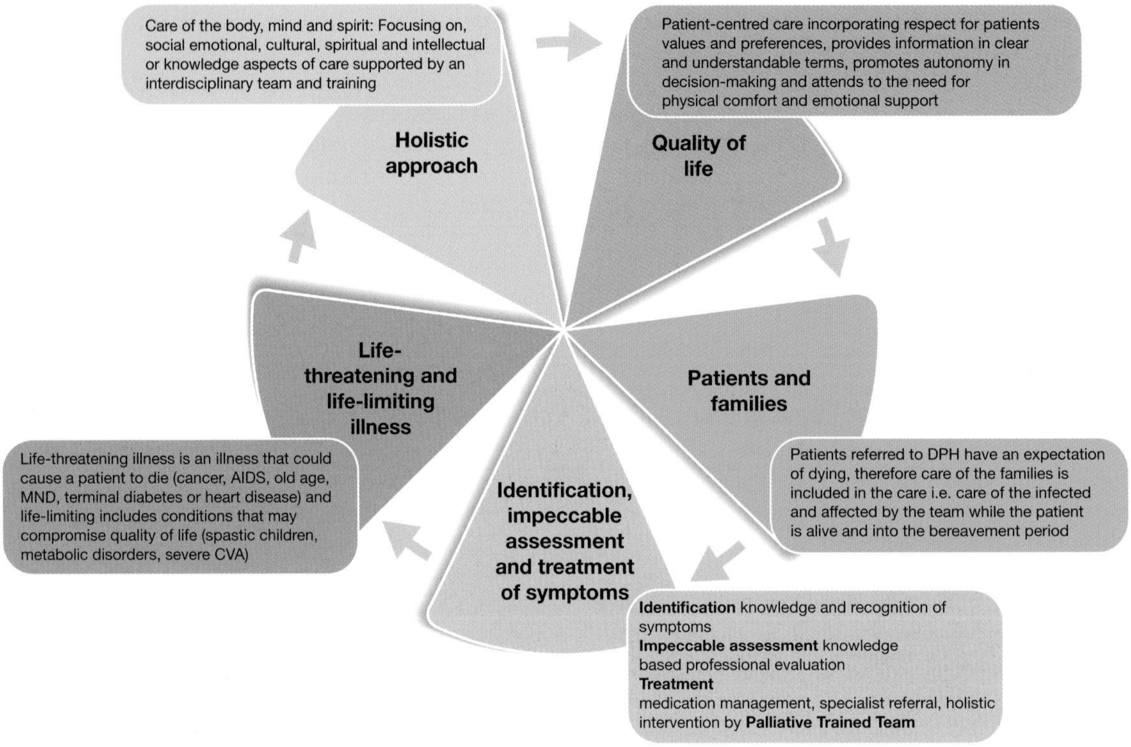
Care of the body, mind and spirit: Focusing on, social emotional, cultural, spiritual and intellectual or knowledge aspects of care supported by an interdisciplinary team and training
Holistic approach
Patient-centred care incorporating respect for patients values and preferences, provides information in clear and understandable terms, promotes autonomy in decision-making and attends to the need for physical comfort and emotional support
Quality of life
Patients and families
Patients referred to DPH have an expectation of dying, therefore care of the families is included in the care i.e. care of the infected and affected by the team while the patient is alive and into the bereavement period
Identification, impeccable assessment and treatment of symptoms
Identification knowledge and recognition of symptoms
Impeccable assessment knowledge based professional evaluation
Treatment
medication management, specialist referral, holistic intervention by Palliative Trained Team
Life-threatening and life-limiting illness
Life-threatening illness is an illness that could cause a patient to die (cancer, AIDS, old age, MND, terminal diabetes or heart disease) and life-limiting includes conditions that may compromise quality of life (spastic children, metabolic disorders, severe CVA)

Palliative care is aimed at increasing comfort and decreasing anxiety and suffering, not only for patients but for their families and carers too. Its effect on an individual and their carers can greatly influence their experience of dying.

A century ago death often occurred quite suddenly and causes tended to be infections, child birth and accidents. However, in more recent times sudden death is less common as people develop chronic progressive illness. Everyone with a chronic debilitating illness will at some point reach the stage where they require some degree of supportive care and this support can come from a palliative care team, the patient's family and friends, or both.

Many people who provide care for a loved one at a point where their loved one cannot care for themselves would not identify themselves as a 'carer', they see themselves as a mum, dad, brother, sister, son, daughter, neighbour or friend.

During the latter stages of a chronic respiratory illness many people become very breathless and lose muscle function or develop muscle pain, and gradually become unable to perform simple tasks. They rely heavily on family, friends and health care professionals to assist with simple daily tasks like washing and dressing or being able to make a sandwich or a cup of tea.

Caring is challenging, no matter how old or young the person is and feeling supported and involved is very important to a carer. When palliative input is deemed necessary the palliative and respiratory specialist teams will provide psychological and emotional support both for the patient and the carer. Anxiety and depression are not just features in the patient's life but can impact upon the carer and the family and can impact on quality of life (Chapter 58).

Breathe Easy groups

Breathe Easy groups offer support to patients and their families and can be accessed via the British Lung Foundation (BLF) who offer support and information to people with lung conditions and their families and carers. Currently, in the UK there are over 230 Breathe Easy groups. Groups typically meet once per month and members arrange health care talks and quizzes, organise social gatherings and dance or perform gentle exercises. The agenda depends on what the group's members want. Breathe Easy members are at various stages of their respiratory diseases and families and carers are encouraged to attend with their loved ones and very often experience great comfort in the realisation that they are not alone.

BLF have set up a penpal scheme so that people with a lung condition and their carers can share advice, frustrations, reassurance and encouragement. This can be particularly beneficial to patients unable to leave the house and carers who are perhaps frightened to leave their sick relative alone at home and therefore leave the house very infrequently themselves.

Family encounters when someone is dying

Death is a difficult time and can cause much distress for families before and particularly after the event. Some members of the family may be resentful while others will have a loving loyal relationship with the dying person. Some will accept the event but others will deny it. Some will be distressed by the deterioration and others will find comfort in holding their loved one's hand and talking to them. Relatives who do not live locally may feel guilt at their inability to be there while others may not want to be there because of family conflict. Carers may resent other family members for not contributing towards the daily care activities or the carer may experience their own feeling of helplessness, having depended on the dying person themselves. It is important to understand that the palliative process is distressing and emotional and requires understanding, patience and good communication on an individual basis, involving all family members.

The person reaching the end of life should be offered support to deal with the loss of their role within the family, possibly having been head of the family before and now having to accept that they need assistance. They may have been the main earner in the household and financial support and advice should be considered for the carer.

Similarly, the carer may need extra support from health care professionals in preparation for life alone. It may be that the dying person was the main carer for the current carer. Support may be required to look after the carer and can result in them requiring formal care themselves, perhaps by admission to a care organisation.

Helping the family to cope

It is essential that the family are supported and feel involved. When chronic illness disrupts the family circle it is important to try to maintain normality. Offer the patient and their family a list of helpful contacts, reassure them that you are there to help, liaise with other members of the multi-disciplinary team on their behalf and encourage family members to chat about everyday things and not to focus on the illness. Things to discuss include children, grandchildren, the family pet, work, the news, a recent shopping trip or even the weather.

Where appropriate, a period of respite should be considered in an attempt to prevent the carer from developing burnout syndrome and it should be considered that the family will grieve more easily if a good death is achieved.

Useful websites:

- www.blf.org.uk
- www.blf.org.uk/BreatheEasy
- www.blf.org.uk/Page/Penpals
- www.palliativecarenetwork.com.

Further reading

Matzo ML, Sherman DW. (2005) *Palliative Care Nursing: Quality Care to the End of Life*, 2nd edn. Springer, New York.

Nyatanga B. (2014) Avoiding burnout syndrome in palliative care. *Br J Commun Nurs* 19: 515.

References

Chapter 1: The origins of respiratory nursing

British Thoracic Society (2014) The role of the respiratory specialist in the integrated care team: a report from the British Thoracic Society. https://www.brit-thoracic.org.uk/document-library/delivery-of-respiratory-care/integrated-care/role-of-the-respiratory-specialist-in-the-integrated-care-team-june-2014/ (accessed 20 February 2016).

Castledine G. (2004) New nursing nursing roles: deciding the future for Scotland. Generalist and Specialist Nurses – complementary or conflicting roles? http://www.gov.scot/Publications/2004/04/19201/35586 (accessed 23 March 2016).

Christmann L. (1965) The influence of specialisation on the nursing profession. *Nurs Sci* December: 446–453.

Girard N. (1987) The CNS: development of the role. In Menard S. (ed.) *The Clinical Nurse Specialist: Perspectives on Practice*, John Wiley, New York; 9–33.

Giles M, Parker V, Mitchell R. (2014) Recognising the differences in the nurse consultant role across context: a study protocol. *BMC Nursing* 13: 30. doi:10.1186/1472-6955-13-30.

MacKinnon M. (2002) Diabetes nursing; a personal perspective the last 50 years. *Br J Diabetes Vasc Dis* 2: 464–467.

Oda D. (1977) Specialised role development: a three phase process. *Nurse Outlook* 25: 374–377.

Peplan H. (1965) Specialisation in professional practice. *Nurs Sci* August: 268–287.

UKCC (1992) *The Scope of Professional Practice.* UKCC, London.

UKCC (1994) *The Standards for Post-registration Education and Practice Project.* UKCC, London.

Chapter 3: Working in primary care

WHO (2015) Palliative Care Fact No. 402 http://www.who.int/mediacentre/factsheets/fs402/en/ (Accessed 13th May 2016)

Chapter 6: Respiratory public health

European Respiratory Society (ERS) (2013) Lung health in Europe: facts and figures. http://www.europeanlung.org/assets/files/publications/lung_health_in_europe_facts_and_figures_web.pdf (accessed 21 February 2016).

Royal College of Physicians (2014) National review of asthma deaths. https://www.rcplondon.ac.uk/projects/national-review-asthma-deaths (accessed 21 February 2016).

Chapter 7: The respiratory system

Peate I, Nair M. (eds.) (2011) *Fundamentals of Anatomy and Physiology for Student Nurses.* John Wiley & Sons Ltd, Oxford.

Chapter 8: Preventing respiratory disease

Department of Health (2011) *An Outcomes Strategy for Chronic Obstructive Pulmonary Disease (COPD) and Asthma.* Department of Health.

European Respiratory Society (ERS) (2013) European Lung White book: The burden of lung disease. http://www.europeanlung.org/assets/files/publications/lung_health_in_europe_facts_and_figures_web.pdf (accessed 1 March 2016).

Hazenkamp-von Arx ME, Schindler C, Ragetli MS., et al. (2011) Impacts of highway traffic exhaust in alpine valleys on the respiratory health in adults: a cross-sectional study. *Environ Health* 10: 13. doi:10.1186/1476-069X-10-13.

Marmot M. (2010) The Marmot Review. Fair Society, Healthy Lives: Strategic Review of Health Inequalities in England post 2010. www.marmotreview.org (accessed 1 March 2016).

Chapter 9: Epidemiology and contributing factors

Boulet LP, Boulay MÈ. (2011) Asthma-related comorbidities. *Expert Rev Respir Med* 5: 377–393. doi: 10.1586/ers.11.34. Review.

British Thoracic Society (BTS) (2006) A statistics report from the British Thoracic Society, 2nd edn. https://www.brit-thoracic.org.uk/document-library/delivery-of-respiratory-care/burden-of-lung-disease/burden-of-lung-disease-2006/ (accessed 22 February 2016).

Department of Health (2011) *An Outcomes Strategy for Chronic Obstructive Pulmonary Disease (COPD) and Asthma.* Department of Health.

European Respiratory Society (ERS) (2013) European Lung White Book: The burden of lung disease. http://www.europeanlung.org/assets/files/publications/lung_health_in_europe_facts_and_figures_web.pdf (accessed 22 February 2016).

Health and Safety Executive (HSE) (2014) Work related respiratory disease in Great Britain. http://www.hse.gov.uk/statistics/causdis/respiratory-diseases.pdf (accessed 22 February 2016).

McManus S, Meltzer H, Campion J. (2010) *Cigarette smoking and mental health in England. Data from the Adult Psychiatric Morbidity Survey.* National Centre for Social Research.

Netuveli G, Hurwitz B, Sheikh A. (2005) Ethnic variations in incidence of asthma episodes in England and Wales: national study of 502,482 patients in primary care. *Respir Res* 6: 120. http://dx.doi.org/10.1186/465-9921-6-120.

Office for National Statistics (ONS). (2010) Excess Winter Mortality Statistical Bulletin, November 2010. www.statistics.gov.uk/StatBase/Product.asp?vlnk=10805&Pos=1&ColRank=1&Rank=272 (accessed 22 February 2016).

Office for National Statistics (ONS). (2011) *Health.* Office for National Statistics.

Raherison C, Girodet PO. (2009) Epidemiology of COPD. *Eur Respir Rev* 18: 213–221.

World Health Organization (WHO) (2014) The top 10 causes of death. http://www.who.int/mediacentre/factsheets/fs310/en/ (accessed 22 February 2016).

Chapter 10: Smoking and smoking cessation

NICE (2008) Stop smoking services. NICE guideline PH10. https://www.nice.org.uk/guidance/ph10m (accessed 23 March 2016).

Chapter 11: Exercise and pulmonary rehabilitation

Bernard S, Ribeiro F, Malthais F, Saey D. (2014) Prescribing exercise training in pulmonary rehabilitation: a clinical experience. *Rev Port Pneumol* 20: 92–100.

British Thoracic Society (BTS) (2013) Guideline on pulmonary rehabilitation in adults: British Thoracic Society Pulmonary Rehabilitation Guideline. *Thorax* 68 (Suppl 2): 1–30.

NICE (2010) Chronic obstructive pulmonary disease in adults in over 16s: diagnosis and management. http://www.nice.org.uk/guidance/CG101 (accessed 23 March 2016).

Chapter 12: Nutrition and hydration

Steer J, Gibson GJ, Bourke SC. (2010) Predicting outcomes following hospitalisation for acute exacerbation of COPD. *Q J Med* 103: 817–829.

Chapter 13: The upper airways

Bantz SK, Zhu Z, Zheng T. (2014) The atopic march: progression from atopic dermatitis to allergic rhinitis and asthma. *J Clin Cell Immun* 5: 202.

Baser S, Ozkurt S, Topuz B, Kıter G, Karabulut H, Akdag B, Evyapan F. (2007) Peak expiratory flow monitoring to screen for asthma in patients with allergic rhinitis. *J Investig Allergol Clin Immunol* 17: 211–215.

Bergeron C, Hamid Q. (2005) Relationship between Asthma and Rhinitis: Epidemiologic, Pathophysiologic, and Therapeutic Aspects. *Allergy Asthma Clin Immunol* 1: 81–87.

British Society for Allergy and Clinical Immunology (BSACI) (2008) Rhinisinusitis and polyposis guidelines. http://www.bsaci.org/guidelines/rhinosinusitis-nasal-polyposis (accessed 1 March 2016).

Chaudhuri R, Livingston E, McMahin D, et al. (2003) Cigarette smoking impairs the therapeutic response to oral corticosteroids in chronic asthma. *Am J Respir Crit Care Med* 168: 1308–1311.

Dahl R, Nielsen L, Kips J, Foresi A, et al. (2005) Intranasal and inhaled fluticasone for pollen-induced rhinitis and asthma. *Allergy* 60: 875–881.

Chapter 15: Respiratory history taking

Bourke SJ, Burns GP. (2015) *Lecture Notes: Respiratory Medicine*, 9th edn. Wiley-Blackwell, Oxford.

Chapter 17: Measuring dyspnoea

NICE (2011) Chronic obstructive pulmonary disease quality standard [QS10]. https://www.nice.org.uk/guidance/qs10 (accessed 23 February 2016).

Parshall MB, Schwartzstein RM, Adams L, et al. (2012) An official American Thoracic Society statement: update on the mechanisms, assessment and management of dyspnoea. *Am J Respir Crit Care Med* 185: 435–432.

Chapter 18: Sputum assessment

Stockley RA, Bayley D, Hill SL, Hill AT, Crooks S, Campbell EJ. 2001. Assessment of airway neutrophils by sputum colour: correlation with airways inflammation. *Thorax* 56: 366–372.

Chapter 19: Pulse oximetry

British Thoracic Society (BTS). (2015) Guidelines for home oxygen use in adults. https://www.brit-thoracic.org.uk/document-library/clinical-information/oxygen/home-oxygen-guideline-(adults)/bts-guidelines-for-home-oxygen-use-in-adults/ (accessed 1 March 2016).

BTS/SIGN 141 (2014) Guideline on the management of asthma. https://www.brit-thoracic.org.uk/document-library/clinical-information/asthma/btssign-asthma-guideline-2014/ (accessed 1 March 2016).

Hanning CD, Alexander-Williams JM. (1995) Pulse oximetry: a practical review. *BMJ* 311: 367–370.

Kelly C. (2008) The use of pulse oximetry in primary care. *Br J Primary Care Nurs* 2: 27–29.

NICE Clinical Guideline 101 (2010) Chronic obstructive pulmonary disease: management of COPD in adults in primary and secondary care (partial update). http://www.nice.org.uk/guidance/cg101 (accessed 1 March 2016).

NICE Clinical Guideline 191 (2014) Diagnosis and management of community and hospital acquired in adults http://www.nice.org.uk/guidance/cg191 (accessed 1 March 2016).

O'Driscoll R, Howard LS, Davidson AG; British Thoracic Society (2008) Guideline for emergency oxygen use in adult patients. *Thorax* 63 (Suppl 6): 1–68.

PCRS-UK Opinion Sheet No 28 (2009) Pulse oximetry in primary care (revised 2013). https://www.pcrs-uk.org/system/files/Resources/Opinion-sheets/os28_pulse_oximetry.pdf (accessed 1 March 2016).

Chapter 20: Blood gas sampling and analysis

Leach R. (2014) *Critical Care medicine at a Glance*, 3rd edition. John Wiley & Sons, Ltd, Oxford.

Chapter 22: Assessing quality of life

Beattie M, Lauder W, Atherton I, Murphy DJ. (2014) Instruments to measure patient experience of health care quality in hospitals: a systematic review protocol. *Syst Rev* 3: 4. doi:10.1186/2046-4053-3-4.

Black N, Varaganum M, Hutchings A. (2014) Relationship between patient reported experience (PREMs) and patient reported outcomes (PROMs) in elective surgery. *BMJ Qual Saf* 23: 534–542. doi:10.1136/bmjqs-2013-002707.

Coulter A. (2002) After Bristol: putting patients at the centre. Commentary: Patient centred care: timely, but is it practical? *BMJ* 324: 648–651. doi:10.1136/bmj.324.7338.648.

Cornwell J. (2012) *Designing the future: approaches to measuring patient exprience.* Unpublished doccument: Kings Fund London.

Health Foundation (2013) *Measuring patient experience.* http://www.health.org.uk/publication/measuring-patient-experience (accessed 24 March 2016).

Hodson M, Andrew S, Roberts CM. (2013) Towards an understanding of PREMS and PROMS in COPD. *Breathe* 9: 358–364. doi:10.1183/20734735.006813.

Säilä T, Mattila E, Kaila M, Aalto P, Kaunonen M. (2008) Measuring patient assessments of the quality of outpatient care: a systematic review. *J Eval Clin Pract* 14: 148–154. doi:10.1111/j.1365-2753.2007.00824.x.

Yorke J, Moosavi SH, Shuldham C, Jones PW. (2010) Quantification of dyspnoea using descriptors: development and initial testing of the Dyspnoea-12. *Thorax* 65: 21–26. doi:10.1136/thx.2009.118521.

Chapter 23: Assessing anxiety and depression

Katon W, Lin EHB, Kroenke K, et al. (2007) The association of depression and anxiety with medical symptom burden in patients with chronic medical illness. *Gen Hosp Psychiatry* 29: 147–155. doi:10.1016/j.genhosppsych.2006.11.005.

Spitzer RL, Kroenke K, Williams JB, Löwe B. (2006) A brief measure for assessing generalized anxiety disorder: the GAD-7. *Arch Intern Med* 166: 1092–1097.

Chapter 24: Asthma

British Thoracic Society (2014) Asthma guideline. https://www.brit-thoracic.org.uk/guidelines-and-quality-standards/asthma-guideline/ (accessed 24 March 2016).

Levy M. (2014) Why asthma still kills asthma still kills. The National Review of Asthma Deaths. https://www.rcplondon.ac.uk/sites/default/files/why-asthma-still-kills-full-report.pdf (accessed 24 February 2016).

NICE (2013) Asthma: diagnosis and monitoring. https://www.nice.org.uk/guidance/indevelopment/gid-cgwave0640 (accessed 24 February 2016).

Chapter 29: Acute respiratory infections

Bourke SJ, Burns GP. (2015) *Lecture Notes: Respiratory Medicine,* 9th edn. Wiley-Blackwell, Oxford.

Chapter 30: Cystic fibrosis

Andersen DH. (1938) Cystic fibrosis of the pancreas and its relation to celiac disease: a clinical and pathological study. *Am J Dis Child* 56: 344–399. doi:10.1001/archpedi.1938.01980140114013.

Busch R. (1990) On the history of cystic fibrosis. *Acta Univ Carol Med (Praha)* 36: 13–15. PMID: 2130674.

Chapter 31: Bronchiectasis

Bilton D. (2003) Bronchiectasis. In Warrell DA, Cox TM, Firth JD, Benz EJ. (eds.) *Oxford Textbook of Medicine.* Oxford University Press, Oxford/New York.

Boyton RJ. (2008). Bronchiectasis. *Medicine* 36: 315–320.

BTS/ACPRC Guidelines (2009) Guidelines for the physiotherapy management of the adult, medical, spontaneously breathing patient. *Thorax* 64 (Suppl I): 1–51.

Ozerovitch L,Wilson R. (2011) *Independent Nurse* 22: 18–20.

Pasteur MC, Bilton D, Hill AT; British Thoracic Society Bronchiectasis (non-CF) Guideline Group (2010) Guidelines for non-CF bronchiectasis. *Thorax* 65 (Suppl I): 1–58.

Roberts HJ, Hubbard R. (2010) Trends in bronchiectasis mortality in England and Wales. *Respir Med* 104: 981–985.

Shoemark A, Ozerovitch L & Wilson R. (2007) *Respiratory Medicine* 101(6): 1163–70.

Chapter 32: Occupational and environmental lung disease

Fishwick D, Barber C, Bradshaw LM, et al. (2008) Standards of care for occupational asthma. *Thorax* 68: 240–250.

Health and Safety Executive (HSE). (2014) Work-related respiratory disease in Great Britain. http://www.hse.gov.uk/statistics/causdis/respiratory-diseases.pdf (accessed 25 February 2016).

Chapter 33: Interstitial lung disease

NICE (2013) Pirfenidone for treating idiopathic pulmonary fibrosis. NICE technology appraisal guidance TA282. https://www.nice.org.uk/guidance/ta282 (accessed 23 March 2016).

Chapter 34: Sarcoidosis

Scadding JG. (1961). Prognosis of intrathoracic sarcoidosis in England: a review of 136 cases after five years' observation. *BMJ* 2: 1165–1172.

Chapter 35: Pulmonary tuberculosis

NICE (2010) *GC117 Tuberculosis: Clinical diagnosis and management of tuberculosis, and measures for its prevention and control.* Public Health England/ NHS England (2015) Collaborative TB Strategy for England 2015–2020.

Public Health England. (2014) Tuberculosis in the UK: 2014 report. Public Health England: London.

Chapter 36: Venous thromboembolism and pulmonary embolism

Kearon C, Ginsberg JS, Douketis J, et al. (2006) An evaluation of D-dimer in the diagnosis of pulmonary embolism: a randomized trial. *Ann Intern Med* 144: 812–821.

Wells PS, Anderson DR, Rodger M, et al. (2000) Derivation of a simple clinical model to categorize patients probability of pulmonary embolism: increasing the models utility with the SimpliRED D-dimer. *Thromb Haemost* 83: 416–420.

Wells PS, Owen C, Doucette S, et al. (2006) Does this patient have deep vein thrombosis? *JAMA* 295: 199–207.

Chapter 40: Telemedicine and telehealth

Darkins AW, Carey AM. (2000) *Telemedicine and Telehealth: Principles, Policies, Performance and Pitfalls.* Springer, Ontario.

De Jongh T, Gurol-Urganci I, Vodopivec-Jamsek V, Car J, Atun R. (2012) Mobile phone messaging for facilitating self-management of long-term illnesses. *Cochrane Database Syst Rev* 12: CD007459. doi: 10.1002/14651858.CD007459.pub2.

Gellis ZD, Kenaley B, McGinty J, Bardelli E, Davitt J, Have TT. (2012) Outcomes of a telehealth intervention for homebound older adults with heart or chronic respiratory failure: a randomized controlled trial. *Gerontologist* 52: 541–552.

McLean S, Nurmatov U, Liu J, et al. (2012) Telehealthcare for chronic obstructive pulmonary disease: Cochrane Review and meta-analysis. *Br J Gen Pract* 62: e738–749.

Petrie KJ, Perry K, Broadbent E, Weinman J. (2012) A text message programme designed to modify patients' illness and treatment beliefs improves self-reported adherence to asthma preventer medication. *Br J Health Psychol* 17: 74–84.

Strandbygaard U, Thomsen SF, Backer V. (2010) A daily SMS reminder increases adherence to asthma treatment: a three-month follow-up study. *Respir Med* 104: 166–171.

Vervloet M, Linn AJ, Can Weert JCM, De Bakker DH, Bouvy ML, Van Dijk L. (2012) The effectiveness of interventions using electronic reminders to improve adherence to chronic medication: a systematic review of the literature. *J Am Med Inform Assoc* 19: 696–704.

Chapter 41: Patient education

Anderson LW, Krathwohl DR. (eds.) (2001) *A Taxonomy for Learning, Teaching, and Assessing: A Revision of Bloom's Taxonomy of Educational Objectives.* Allyn & Bacon. Boston, MA.

Chapter 43: Pharmacology and prescribing

British Thoracic Society (2014) Asthma guideline. https://www.brit-thoracic.org.uk/guidelines-and-quality-standards/asthma-guideline/ (accessed 24 March 2016).

Chapter 45: Nebuliser therapy

Bourke SJ, Burns GP. (2015) *Lecture Notes: Respiratory Medicine,* 9th edn. Wiley-Blackwell, Oxford.

Boyter AC, Carter R. (2005) How do patients use their nebuliser in the community? *Respir Med* 99: 1413–1417.

Chapter 46: Emergency oxygen therapy

Resuscitation Council (UK). (2015) Resuscitation guidelines. https://www.resus.org.uk/resuscitation-guidelines/ (accessed 23 March 2016).

Chapter 47: Domiciliary oxygen therapy

Abernethy AP, McDonald CF, Frith PA, et al. (2010) Effect of palliative oxygen versus room air in relief of breathlessness in patients with refractory dyspnoea: a double-blind, randomised controlled trial. *Lancet* 376: 784–793.

Davidson PM, Johnson MJ. (2011) Update on the role of palliative oxygen. *Curr Opin Support Palliat Care* 5: 87–91.

Eaton T, Lewis C, Young P, et al. (2004) Long term oxygen therapy improves health related quality of life. *Respir Med* 98: 285–293.

Gorecka D, Gorzelak K, Sliwinski P, et al. (1997) Effect of long term oxygen therapy on survival in patients with chronic obstructive pulmonary disease with moderate hypoxaemia. *Thorax* 52: 674–679.

Hardinge M, Annandale J, Bourne S, et al. (2015) British Thoracic Society guidelines for home oxygen use in adults. *Thorax* 70 (Suppl 1): 1–43.

Kamal AH, Maguire JM, Wheeler JL, et al. (2012) Dyspnea review for the palliative care professional: treatment goals and therapeutic options. *J Palliat Care Med* 15: 106–114.

Medical Research Council (MRC) Working Party. (1981) Long term domiciliary oxygen therapy in chronic hypoxic cor pulmonale complicating chronic bronchitis and emphysema. *Lancet* 1: 681–686.

Nocturnal Oxygen Therapy Trial (NOTT) Group. (1980) Continuous or nocturnal oxygen therapy in hypoxaemic chronic obstructive lung disease: a clinical trial. *Ann Intern Med* 93: 391.

Ringbaek TJ. (2005) Continuous oxygen therapy for hypoxic pulmonary disease. *Treat Respir Med* 4: 397–408.

Uronis HE, Ekstrom MP, Currow DC, et al. (2015) Oxygen for relief of dyspnoea in people with chronic obstructive pulmonary disease who would not qualify for home oxygen: a systematic review and meta-analysis. *Thorax* 70: 492–494.

Zielinski J. (2000) Long-term oxygen therapy in conditions other than chronic obstructive pulmonary disease. *Respir Care* 45: 172–176.

Chapter 49: Adherence and concordance

Boulet LP. (1998) Perception of the role and potential side effects of inhaled corticosteroids among asthmatic patients. *Chest* 113: 587–592.

Bucknell CE, Miller G, Lloyd SM, et al. (2012) Glasgow supported self-management trial (GSuST) for patients with moderate to severe COPD: randomised controlled trial. *BMJ* 344: e1060.

Gibson PG, Powell H. (2004) Written action plans for asthma: an evidence-based review of the key components. *Thorax* 59: 94–99.

Lavorini F, Magnan A, Dubus C, et al. (2008) Effect of incorrect use of dry powder inhalers on management of patients with asthma and COPD. *Respir Med* 102: 593–564.

Walters J, Turnock A, Walters E, et al. (2010) Action plans with limited patient education only for exacerbations of chronic obstructive pulmonary disease. *Cochrane Database Syst Rev* 5: CD005074.

Chapter 50: Respiratory failure

British Thoracic Society (BTS). (2016) Ventilatory management of acute hypercapnic respiratory failure guideline. https://www.brit-thoracic.org.uk/guidelines-and-quality-standards/ventilatory-management-of-acute-hypercapnic-respiratory-failure-guideline/ (accessed 24 March 2016).

Kaynar AM. (2015) Respiratory failure. Medscape. http://emedicine.medscape.com/article/167981-overview#showall (accessed 24 March 2016).

Tortora GJ, Anagnostakos NP, Grabowski SR. (1993) *Principles of Anatomy and Physiology*. John Wiley and Sons Inc.

Chapter 51: Pre-hospital care

Advanced Life Support Group (ALSG). (2014) Emergency Triage, 3rd edn. John Wiley & Sons Ltd, Oxford.

British Thoracic Society (2014) Asthma guideline. https://www.brit-thoracic.org.uk/guidelines-and-quality-standards/asthma-guideline/ (accessed 24 March 2016).

Jones RC, Donaldson GC, Chavannes NH, et al. (2009) Derivation and validation of a composite index of severity in chronic obstructive pulmonary disease: the DOSE Index. *Am J Respir Crit Care Med* 180: 1189–1195.

NICE (2010) Chronic obstructive pulmonary disease in over 16s: diagnosis and management. https://www.nice.org.uk/guidance/cg101/chapter/guidance (accessed 29 February 2016).

Chapter 55: Communication

Baile WF, Buckman R, Lenzi R, et al. (2000) SPIKES: a six-step protocol for delivering bad news: application to the patient with cancer. *Oncologist* 5: 302–311.

Connolly M, Perryman J, McKenna Y, et al. (2010) SAGE & THYME™: A model for training health and social care professionals in patient-focussed support. *Patient Education and Counseling* 79: 87–93.

Elkington H, White P, Addington-Hall J, et al. (2005) The healthcare needs of chronic obsructive pulmonary patients in the last year of life. *Palliat Med* 19: 485–491.

Momen N, Hadfield P, Kuhn I, Smith E, Barclay S. (2012) Discussing an uncertain future: end-of-life care conversations in chronic obstructive pulmonary disease: a systematic literature review and narrative synthesis. *Thorax* 67: 777–780.

Murray SA, Kendall M, Boyd K, Sheikh A. (2015) Illnesses trajectories and palliative care. *BMJ* 330: 1007–1011.

National End of Life Care Intelligence Network (2011) Resources. http://www.endoflifecare-intelligence.org.uk/resources/publications/ (accessed 24 March 2016).

NICE Clinical Guideline 101 (2010) Chronic obstructive pulmonary disease: management of COPD in adults in primary and secondary care (partial update). http://www.nice.org.uk/guidance/cg101 (accessed 1 March 2016).

Parker SM, Clayton JM, Hancock K, et al. (2007) A systematic review of prognostic/end-of-life communication with adults in the advanced stages of a life-limiting illness: patient/caregiver preferences for the content, style, and timing of information. *J Pain Symptom Manage* 34: 81–93.

Chapter 56: Psychosocial impact of respiratory disease

British Lung Foundation (2006) *The Burden of Lung Disease*. London.

Buck D. (2014) *How Healthy Are We? A high-level guide*. King's Fund.

Gore JM, Brophy CJ, Greenstone MA. (2000) How well do we care for patients with end stage chronic obstructive pulmonary disease (COPD)? A comparison of palliative care and quality of life in COPD and lung cancer. *Thorax* 55: 1000–1006.

World Health Organization (2008) Global Burden of Disease. http://www.who.int/healthinfo/global_burden_disease/GBD_report_2004update_full.pdf?ua=1. (accessed 29 February 2016).

Chapter 57: Management of dyspnoea

Booth S. (2013) Science supporting the art of medicine: improving the management of breathlessness. *Palliat Med* 27: 483–485.

Chapter 58: Anxiety and depression in respiratory disease

Heslop-Marshall K, De Soyza A. (2014) Are we missing anxiety in people with chronic obstructive pulmonary disease (COPD)? *Ann Depress Anxiety* 1: 1023.

Ng TP, Niti M, Tan WC, Cao Z, Eng P. (2007) Depressive symptoms and chronic obstructive pulmonary disease: effect on mortality, hospital readmission, symptom burden, functional status and quality of life. *Arch Intern Med* 167: 60–70.

NICE (2010) Depression in adults with a chronic physical health problem: recognition and management. https://www.nice.org.uk/guidance/cg91 (accessed 1 March 2016).

NICE (2011) Generalised anxiety disorder and panic in adults: management. British Psychological Society and Royal College of Psychaitrists. https://www.nice.org.uk/guidance/cg113/chapter/1-guidance (accessed 1 March 2016).

Zigmond AS, Snaith RP. (1983) The Hospital Anxiety and Depression Scale. *Acta Psychiatr Scand* 67: 361–370.

Chapter 59: Other symptom management

British Thoracic Society (BTS). (2016) Ventilatory management of acute hypercapnic respiratory failure guideline. https://www.brit-thoracic.org.uk/guidelines-and-qualitystandards/ventilatory-management-of-acute-hypercapnicrespiratory-failure-guideline/ (accessed 24 March 2016).

Index

Page numbers in *italics* denote figures, those in **bold** denote tables.